I0113227

PRAISE FOR *TURN AROUND DIABETES*

"Dr. Roshani has simplified the steps of reversing metabolic disease and covered every aspect of lifestyle change that people need. A potential life-changer."

- Dr. Jason Fung, Nephrologist, New York Times Bestselling Author of *The Obesity Code* and *The Diabetes Code*, Co-Founder of The Fasting Method

"Diabetes is rising in India, and young people are becoming more vulnerable to diabetes and similar lifestyle diseases. Dr. Roshani, through her years of experience, has suggested solutions that work for many in the Indian context. This is an interesting read for everyone, particularly the young generation."

- Dr. Anjali Tendulkar, Paediatrician, and Sachin Tendulkar, Former Indian Cricketer

"Roshani Sanghani's Turn Around Diabetes is a groundbreaking guide, brilliantly navigating the path to reversing Type 2 diabetes and managing Type 1 diabetes better through simple lifestyle changes. Combining scientific rigor with easy-to-follow language, this book stands as a beacon of hope and empowerment in those living with diabetes."

Benjamin Bikman, PhD and author of *Why We Get Sick: The Hidden Epidemic at the Root of Most Chronic Disease- and How to Fight It*

"Dr. Sanghani writes this brilliant self-care book for managing diabetes that reads like a novel and provides answers to day-to-day questions and frustrations felt by people who are trying their best to help themselves. As a diabetologist specializing in the care of older adults and also being vegetarian myself, I frequently struggle to provide a nuanced and detailed understanding of how a patient can improve their day-to-day habits. The unique perspective described in this book for people in India—a population with a variety of eating and activity habits—is useful not just for people helping themselves, but for people like me who are doctors trying to help their patients."

Medha Munshi, MD, Professor of Medicine, Harvard Medical School, Director Joslin Geriatric Diabetes Program, Geriatrician, Beth Israel Deaconess Medical Center

"I highly recommend this book if you are facing Type 1 diabetes, are trying to prevent Type 2 diabetes, or are just looking to be healthy! Dr. Sanghani has provided a comprehensive yet easy-to-understand guide-book to help you every step of the way. I'm quite confident that this book will help many people!"

> - Eric C. Westman, MD MHS, Associate Professor of Medicine, Duke University Health System, Author, *End Your Carb Confusion*

"Dr. Sanghani is a leader in lifestyle-based diabetes management. Following the very guidelines put forth in this excellent and engaging guide, I have personally achieved great gains in weight loss and diabetes management. An essential tool for anyone seeking to optimize not only their recovery from diabetes but also achieving optimal health."

> - David Jacobowitz, Senior Human Subjects Research Coordinator and Faculty Clinical Associate /University of Rochester Medical Center, Departments of Psychiatry and Geriatrics. BS, MA, CGP, CTTS, cancer survivor and recovering person with diabetes

"This book is a must-read for anyone suffering from diabetes, or caring for someone with the condition. Dr. Roshani Sanghani has provided the reader with an excellent guide on how to prevent, treat, and 'turn around' diabetes. Being a chronic health condition, education is the cornerstone to tackling this disease, and this book provides that in ample measure, in an easy to read format. She describes in great detail, various 'wheels' of care, including nutrition, sleep, exercise, and stress management. I highly recommend reading this book, and implementing the various lifestyle modification techniques described.

> - Dr. Aashish Contractor, Director - Rehabilitation and Sports Medicine Sir H.N. Reliance Foundation Hospital, Mumbai, India American College of Sports Medicine Certification Director Founding Vice-Chair, ICCPR-International Council of Cardiovascular Prevention and Rehabilitation

"Dr Roshani Sanghani is one of those rare physicians who understands and has gained expertise in a holistic approach to helping others. In her groundbreaking and eminently useful work, she manages to introduce complex concepts in an enjoyable and understandable way, making it very accessible to the reader. Her sense of humor, humility, and use of the life stories of others makes this a fascinating read, and she manages to not only delve into the "why," but provide readers practical and useful advice which can be implemented immediately. As the growing level of evidence points out, traditional approaches to treating and managing diabetes can only benefit from experts such as herself, who encourage us to step back and really think about what we do and why we do it. This book also provides excellent suggestions for those who do not have diabetes."

- Randy Brazie, M.D., Polyvagal Institute Editorial Board, Co-founder at NeuroConsulting Group, LLC, Diplomate of the American Board of Psychiatry and Neurology

"Roshani is my favorite endocrinologist—not just because she is outstanding at her work, but because she is passionate about reversing diabetes and pre-diabetes. And she puts patients' priorities before writing out a prescription—something often not taught in medical school. This book is a masterpiece in that it allows a human to change their lifestyle, and (more importantly) take their life in their hands—something that many humans leave to destiny and fate, sadly. Life is what you make of it, and Roshani guides you on how to make the most of it. If people read this book, most won't even need to consult an endocrinologist, but I don't think Roshani would be much bothered about that—that's what her passion in life has been—'take charge of your body metabolism and life, and enjoy it."

- Sujeet Rajan, MD, DETRD, DNB Director, Breath First Foundation, Consultant Respiratory Physician, Interstitial Lung Diseases/Sleep Disorders, Bombay Hospital Institute of Medical Sciences and Bhatia Hospital, Mumbai, India

"I found *Turn around Diabetes* to be thoroughly enjoyable and challenging. Equal parts practical guide and clarion call, the book challenges readers with Type 2 and Type 1 diabetes to imagine a world where deliberate behavioral changes can significantly alter results. As someone with T1D for 45 years and whose career is fairly steeped in diabetes education, I have seen my fair share of diabetes self-management instructional guides. Nevertheless, I found many ideas in the book both surprising and inspiring (e.g., the gestalt of diabetes care and the ability to reverse hypoglycemia unawareness). The idea that all of the pieces diet, (reduced carbs coupled with increased healthy proteins), sleep, stress management, and exercise matter significantly in diabetes management is effectively driven home with multiple patient narratives. Her effective use of patient narratives and vivid analogies ensures that readers can understand the concepts presented. In addition to serving as an effective learning tool, the stories and illustration of Motivational Interviewing leave the reader with the sense that Dr. Sanghani is a very caring provider who considers her patients' lived experiences when making suggestions."

- Neil Israel, President & Co-Founder, In-Range Animation, PWD (Person With Diabetes)

"I read Dr. Sanghani's book due to my husband's lifelong type 1 diabetes and my keen interest in maintaining a healthy lifestyle. This guide offers a clear path to boost insulin sensitivity and enhance overall well-being. Beyond that, it motivates me to harness my mental, physical, and spiritual resources for optimal living. Dr. Sanghani departs from traditional medical approaches, urging us to chart our own course with her insights and inspiring narratives as companions. Her candid language, humor, and personal stories empower us to test her advice and discover what works best for our individual needs. Through compassion and respect, she empowers us to freely choose our health journey, fostering greater motivation and long-lasting change."

- Suzie Israel, Chief Digital Officer & Co-Founder, In-Range Animation

"Roshani's book *Turn around Diabetes* is the most comprehensive guide I have yet to read on how to reverse diabetes relevant to both the clinician as well as a patient. Loaded with hundreds of medical references of historical significance as well as recent science and the daily practical application of all of this in real human patients, this book will make you rethink everything you have thought to be true about what we once believed to be a chronic progressive disease. It takes brave clinicians like Roshani to save the world from a completely preventable, and in most cases reversible condition, which is type two diabetes. The guide also gives great wisdom if you have type 1 diabetes which, although not reversible, can be managed in a much simpler and safer way to allow you to live a life of health. We need more clinicians around the world, teaching this and policymakers changing the food environment and maybe then we can have a healthier future."

- Mark Cucuzzella, MD, Staff Physician Martinsburg Veterans Administration Hospital, Professor West Virginia University School of Medicine, and Diplomate American Board of Obesity Medicine

"I am thoroughly impressed by Dr. Roshani Sanghani's new book *Turn around Diabetes*. As an internist, life-long educator of medical students, residents and fellows, as well as a member of the American College of Lifestyle Medicine, I applaud her four-pronged approach to better treatment of diabetes through Nutrition, Sleep, Stress Reduction and Exercise. Her experience as an endocrinologist shows through in her recognition that 'one size does not fit all' and that changes must be collaboratively identified and carefully planned. Whether you are a motivated person with diabetes looking to reduce or eliminate your medication regimen, or a provider caring for patients with diabetes, I strongly recommend you read this book."

- John M. O'Brien, MD, FACP Internist at Cook County Health, Chicago Illinois, 2004-2023, and current member of the American College of Lifestyle Medicine

Turn around Diabetes

TURN AROUND
DIABETES

The Step-by-Step Guide to Navigate Type 2 (and Type 1) Diabetes with Less Medication

Roshani Sanghani, MD
reisaanhealth.com

The material in this book is for informational and educational purposes only. It does not constitute medical advice. This does not replace or substitute for a medical consultation with your doctor for physical examination, medication management, blood test review, screening for complications, and preventive health. A healthcare professional should be consulted regarding your specific medical situation. Any product mentioned in this book does not imply endorsement of that product by the author or publisher. The author and publisher specifically disclaim any and all liability arising directly or indirectly from the use of any information contained in this book.

@Glasbergen. Cartoons reproduced with permission of Glasbergen Cartoon Service.
Cover design: Vijay Lalwani

Turn around Diabetes copyright © 2024 by Roshani Sanghani

All rights reserved. No part of this book may be used or reproduced in any manner whatsoever without written permission of the publisher, except in the case of brief quotations embodied in critical articles or reviews.

Aasaan Health LLC
651 N Broad Street Suite 201
Middletown, Delaware 19709
www.reisaanhealth.com
Send feedback to connect@reisaanhealth.com

Names: Sanghani, Roshani, author.
Title: Turn around diabetes : the step-by-step guide to navigate type 2 (and type 1) diabetes with less medication / Roshani Sanghani, MD.
Description: Middletown, DE : Aasaan Health, [2024] | Includes bibliographical references and index.
Identifiers: ISBN: 979-8-9905930-1-5 (hardcover) | 979-8-9905930-0-8 (softcover) | 979-8-9905930-2-2 (ebook) | 979-8-9905930-3-9 (audiobook)
Subjects: LCSH: Diabetes--Alternative treatment. | Diabetes--Etiology. | Diabetes--Pathophysiology. | Insulin resistance. | Metabolism--Disorders.
Classification: LCC: RC660 .S26 2024 | DDC: 616.462--dc23

Special discounts for bulk sales are available.
Please contact connect@reisaanhealth.com.

To those who would have turned around diabetes if only they knew how.
And to each of you who have decided to turn it around now.

Tell Me What You Think

Let other readers know what you thought of *Turn around Diabetes*. Please write an honest review for this book on your favorite online bookshop.

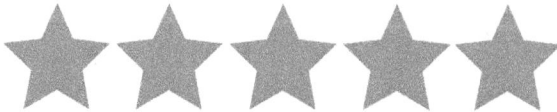

★★★★★

Disclaimer: The individuals and stories in this book are based on real events in the lives of real people. Details have been altered to protect their identity, unless specified otherwise.

Contents

PART 10: HOW TO HANDLE TYPE 1 DIABETES, TURN AROUND INSULIN RESISTANCE, AND ACHIEVE MORE STABLE GLUCOSE LEVELS WITH LESS INSULIN 397

PART 11: THE JOURNEY AHEAD. 431

Foreword by
William R. Miller, Ph.D.

I admire people who devote a career to gaining a deep understanding of their specialty, spending decades with the integration of research and practice. There is much to learn from professionals like that whose training and expertise are different from our own. Particularly valuable are those who also have a gift for writing and communicating who they know. Dr. Roshani Sanghani is that kind of gem. As an endocrinologist, she understands what is going on inside the body and its relationship to what we eat, think, and do. As a seasoned physician, she has the experience, patience, and wisdom that come from treating thousands of people with diabetes and pre-diabetes. Happily, she has taken the time to write it all down for us.

My own career has been in clinical and health psychology, in addition to which I have 18 years of lived experience as a person with Type 2 diabetes. Beyond its physical manifestations, diabetes is a disease of ambivalence. Our future health and quality of life are determined primarily by what we choose to do. When first diagnosed, I met with a diabetes educator who warned of the dire consequences of uncontrolled diabetes and listed about a dozen behavior changes that I should make in order to stay healthy. Part of me knew she was right, and another part was comfortable with living my life as I had been. That's not unique to diabetes. Dr. Roshani describes four behavioral "wheels" that can keep us rolling in the right direction. As it turns out, those four wheels are important to health whether or not you have diabetes.

In studying this book, I have appreciated both Dr. Roshani's accomplished scientific understanding of diabetes and her practical guidance for how to manage or even reverse it. Now that's a gift. The dire consequences are preventable. Solid medical information and advice are available here to take control of your diabetes and health. You also have at your fingertips (even literally) constant feedback to know how you're doing along the way. What happens from here on is up to you.

- William R. Miller, Ph.D.
Emeritus Distinguished Professor of Psychology and Psychiatry,
The University of New Mexico and Co-Founder of Motivational Interviewing

Kanika's story

It is possible to turn around diabetes and thrive again. It is possible to be happy and healthy. We bring this possibility to our clients at Reisaan Health daily–and now to you, with this book.

To help you understand the possibilities on your journey with prediabetes, type 2 diabetes or type 1 diabetes, let me tell you about Kanika. She is one of our clients, and gave me permission to narrate her experience of turning her health around. Here is her journey, in her own words.

In 2013, at the age of twenty-one, I found myself in the hospital waiting in agony for an emergency colonoscopy. The doctor was trying to diagnose the cause of my severe abdominal pain and a fever that wouldn't break. The hospital was familiar, and I expected to get only a prescription for antibiotics since this was not the first such incident. For over a decade, from as early as the year 2000 when I was 8, I had routinely experienced extreme pain in the abdomen and recurrent fevers. However, every time I had visited a doctor, it was the same old story. "You probably ate something from a restaurant, so you have a stomach infection. Take antibiotics and it will settle. Or just manage your stress better and then the pain will go away." The pain was the stressor though.

I still remember being told for years that I was imagining this pain to get attention or to escape out of difficult situations. Because of this, I spent my adolescence and much of my early adulthood downplaying my own symptoms. I didn't believe my own symptoms were real and convinced myself that my pain was imaginary. When I would go to a doctor, I would always pretend to be better than I was. Every time I went, I feared hearing again that I was only there to get more attention.

However, this time in 2013 the colonoscopy revealed that I had intestinal ulcers. I finally had a diagnosis: Crohn's Disease. This began the journey of being heavily medicated and being entirely dependent on medicines for almost another decade. Although my ulcers healed and never came back, the rest of my symptoms persisted. I would still get a fever (once a month or so) and have joint pain, abdominal pain, and severe acid reflux that needed constant antacids. My symptoms ranged from abdominal spasms to painful bloating. I was unable to stand for too long (which made going to college or socializing very difficult). This was aggravated by the fact that my menstrual cycle had become progressively irregular and painful. Eventually, I was also diagnosed with polycystic ovarian syndrome

(PCOS). To be honest, there was so much pain in my abdomen that I could hardly tell whether the pain was being caused by the PCOS, irritable bowel syndrome, or anything else.

The impact of this on my mental health was as expected: I was depressed. I did not know a single day without pain. After a while, I became immune to a certain amount of baseline suffering and would only notice once my pain exceeded a certain threshold. I repeatedly asked my doctors (and I visited many) what I could do about my symptoms. I was told to be glad that the ulcers were gone! So I accepted that chronic pain would be my way of life. I learnt to adapt by staying at home. When the pain was more than I could handle, we would go to the hospital. I would be given a shot for quick relief and be sent home. I refused to be admitted, because I had no hope of improving the quality of my daily life after being discharged. I knew that once the dose of antibiotics was complete, things would go back to usual. Some of my other symptoms included: insulin resistance, anemia, blood pressure fluctuations (low blood pressure), and lethargy. This meant that some of my doctors had started telling me it was only a matter of time before I got diabetes.

By the time I graduated and started working, pain was a part of my daily life and I did not know what life was like without it. Unfortunately, no matter how much I told myself that my symptoms were my own creation, my symptoms did not subside. I worried about my performance at work and being unable to perform my tasks without falling sick. On more than one occasion I felt faint and had to stop working or leave the office.

Before I started working with Reisaan Health, I had already tried allopathic, homeopathic, and Ayurvedic treatments to no avail. Someone I trusted suggested that I at least work with them on preventing diabetes, even if my pain could not be helped. Dr Roshani made it clear that we would focus on insulin resistance, PCOS and prediabetes. Since I did not have much to lose, I decided to give it a shot and joined the program in 2021 for six months. I cut out gluten from my diet, slowly reduced my intake of carbohydrates and eventually started fasting. I also added probiotics to my diet, reduced my sweet intake and avoided eating out for a while. I improved my nutrition and managed to consume sufficient protein all thanks to my trusty protein shake, despite being told by others that they thought I was doing drugs by taking a powder! I also worked on improving the quality of my sleep by going to bed earlier and getting my seven to eight hours. Eventually, as my health improved I felt more energetic and also started exercising. This wasn't immediate. But slowly and steadily I saw a reduction in the severity of my symptoms. While these changes were difficult to implement, I found the benefits to be more empowering than the previous status quo. For the first time, my health was in my hands and the changes I made were making a difference.

I stopped fearing food, because I started understanding what my body could and couldn't handle. I started listening to my body and still eat sweets when it makes me happy! My painful bloating, which I thought would never go away, went away. I started intermittent fasting. With every fast, I felt better. My body thanked me by giving me more energy, the ability to stand for hours and eventually run! One by one, I was able to wean off of most of my medicines under the supervision of my gastroenterologist. I was able to eat without needing an antacid. I was able to put on a pair of pants without being in pain from the elastic pressing down on my stomach. My menstrual cycle normalized, without my having to take any medicines. In short, I got my life back. I got to go out there and pursue things I was holding back on - finding love, pursuing my career and more. I got married, moved to a different city and even started lifting weights! I went from being afraid of leaving the house to starting a demanding job at a busy law firm. Things have changed from when I was a twenty-one-year old in 2021 watching life pass her by from inside her bedroom. Now, in 2024, I have experienced things which I thought were never meant for me. My PCOS sometimes flares when I get stressed out and it's a work in progress. My prediabetes is completely gone. I am grateful for every day without pain, but more than that, I am grateful that even if things go wrong now (for example, when I accidentally eat gluten or something that doesn't suit me) I know exactly how to fix it without letting it derail my life.

That is Kanika's true story.

If you, too, are ready to turn around diabetes, read on.

Introduction

As an endocrinologist committed to helping as many people take control of their diabetes as possible, I set out to make the most comprehensive guide to turning around diabetes. On one hand, as a doctor, I just want to share everything with you; all of the science, case studies, technical data, and research that I've studied over the years. On the other, as a care provider, I understand that all of that can be overwhelming, and may scare away the people that could benefit from this the most!

My solution?

I'm still going to make this the most robust, comprehensive guide that I can.

But I'm also going to give you a referential outline here so you can start with the things that apply the most to you, without being overwhelmed by all the information. My goal is that this detailed overview will help you and your loved ones find quick and detailed answers to your diabetes questions in between doctor's visits.

Here's how to get the most out of this guide.

Use this book by visualizing that you are in the driver's seat

One of the reasons people aren't able to turn around diabetes is because nobody has explained the science to them in a way that they can understand.

To simplify some of the more complex concepts in the book, I thought it best to share how this book is structured. Part 1 explains the medical science as simply as possible. As we reach Parts Two through Six, you will see the analogy I use with patients to illustrate how all of the lifestyle pieces fit together. This will keep us on the same page so that the science from Part 1 makes enough sense to power your journey without you having to go back to biology class. As you may choose to use this as a referential guide instead of consuming it first in its entirety, here is the analogy first. Use this book by visualizing that you are in the driver's seat, and your car is traveling the road toward its destination. I call this **the lifestyle car.**

The four wheels of the lifestyle car are the four major lifestyle elements: ***nutrition, sleep, stress management, and exercise, in that order.*** Once you have made sure the four wheels of your car are in good condition, you can consider going on a long drive and even putting some suitcases on top in the luggage carrier or inside the trunk. The luggage is optional and can only be safely added once your four wheels have been serviced. If you can reach your destination without the extra luggage, great! Similarly, if you can achieve your health goals with just improvements in nutrition, sleep, stress management, and exercise, then great! Much like the roof or trunk space that's available if you chose to use it, I use intermittent fasting as the fifth strategy. Fasting is an optional fifth element that can only be added safely on top of four **already aligned** lifestyle wheels. As we go into further detail, you'll understand how this analogy will be a helpful tool. I will keep coming back to this analogy to remind you of our strategies to turn your diabetes around with less medication, without restrictive dieting, without needing to change your external environment, and without buying more supplements (all under your doctor's supervision).

This interpretation will help align your mindset with the strategies that will guide you through the ups and downs of life sustainably, and in the analogy, *this* book is your GPS navigation as you maneuver bumps and detours in the road along the way. With this book guiding your journey, you will think differently about your body; learn more about how diabetes works and what you can do about it; and take charge of your life, making decisions about your lifestyle and your health. This analogy is to remind you that you can turn around the trajectory of your diabetes.

You are in the driver's seat—now here's the roadmap.

What lies ahead in this book?

This is a comprehensive take on things but made with the intention of being a guide that you can refer to in the years to come and share the information with your loved ones. For those of you using this as a reference, here's what you'll find and where:

Preface:

- Overview of how I got here.

Part 1: The Science

- The two types of diabetes, and how people with both types can turn around diabetes by addressing insulin resistance.

- The hormones that govern the body, including the master metabolic hormone: insulin. We will understand how people become insulin-resistant.

- Metabolism and nutrition—what causes difficulty losing weight, stubborn belly fat, and slowing metabolism? (Hint: It has everything to do with insulin resistance).

- Insulin resistance and accompanying conditions, including progressive diabetes.

Parts 2–6: The Lifestyle Car.

This analogy connects the four major lifestyle elements of nutrition, sleep, stress management, and exercise, and adds the optional fifth element of fasting to an already balanced and stable lifestyle. Each of the chapters focuses on the following:

Part 2: Nutrition

- End your food confusion

- Low-carbohydrate (carb), protein-centric, healthy fat focus of macronutrient distribution

- Keto, carnivore, vegan, and vegetarian diets; examples of changed eating habits without restrictive dieting; how to achieve your daily protein needs with each

- Protein malnutrition identification

- Food, hunger, and mindfulness

- How to read nutrition labels; recognize hidden ingredients, ultra-processed food; what makes junk food so addictive. (Hint: It's not your fault, and you probably don't need lifelong medication for it.)

- Whole grains versus processed grains

- Dehydration and hormone imbalances, fat storage

Part 3: Sleep

- Obstructive sleep apnea, what to do if you think you have sleep apnea

- Sleep deprivation, shift work, effect of artificial light on circadian rhythms, body clocks

- Tips to better sleep quality; We go over the impact of using food, alcohol, or screen time to fall asleep

Part 4: Stress Management

- The power of thoughts and feelings
- The power of the subconscious mind, the tendency to seek instant gratification
- Acute versus chronic stress
- Emotions versus logic, and medical conditions that are worsened by stress
- Diabetes distress, daily struggles with demands of diabetes
- Various patient solutions to feel better, change mental and emotional perspectives on life, improve their daily experiences

Part 5: Exercise

(specifically after addressing nutrition, sleep, and stress. People who aren't satisfied with their meals, are not sleeping well, and are feeling emotionally low don't benefit from being told to "just move more.")

- Why exercise is initially uncomfortable and what to do about it
- How to enjoy focusing on exercise
- Zone 2 training, increasing the health and efficiency of your metabolic powerhouse, the mitochondria; switching your metabolism to burn fat as the primary fuel
- Cardio and weight loss versus benefits of building muscle and progressive strength training

Part 6: Fasting

- How to safely fast
- How it works to burn belly fat
- Benefits of autophagy, entering deep repair mode
- How to manage common challenges during fasting
- How to adapt fasting to various life situations when choosing to use it

- Thought processes to aid success without feeling deprived when fasting

Part 7: Investigations and Prescriptions

- Common lab reports, what to look for, what to monitor
- Participating in informed decision-making regarding diabetes medication

Part 8: Doctors and Hospitals

- How to work with nutritionists, doctors, and hospitals

Part 9: Women and Children

- Women's health topics;
- Polycystic ovarian syndrome (PCOS)
- Gestational diabetes
- Postmenopausal women's health
- For parents of teenagers or adolescents with type 2 diabetes
- a family approach; changing the home environment, improving conversations around health
- Parents will understand how to begin preparing children to make healthy decisions confidently as adults

Part 10: Type 1 Diabetes

- Dedicated to people with type 1 diabetes, how to identify and work with doctors who can support your journey to more stable glucose levels with less insulin, in addition to benefiting from the lifestyle changes in other chapters

Part 11: Looking Forward

- Next steps
- Advanced skills

- How to manage diabetes in challenging situations, on vacation, under stress, or attending a work conference

This comprehensive guide is meant to help you take charge of your diabetes with your care team, and like many of the patients you'll hear from in this book—there are so many advantages to turning around diabetes. You might have felt hopeless – like there's nothing you can do about your quality of life and thestatus of your progression – but I'm here to show you how so many things can be changed for the better.

What benefits are possible when you apply the lessons in this book?*

- Remission of prediabetes
- Reduced burden of daily pills and injections
- Reduced side effects by stopping unnecessary medication
- Reduced insulin dose requirements in type 1 diabetes
- Reduced costs related to diabetes
- Increased energy
- Increased mental clarity, reversal of brain fog
- Inch loss, especially around the tummy, and breaking past weight-loss plateaus
- Reduced body fat
- Increased muscle mass and strength
- Increased agility and fitness, being able to participate more actively in life, sports, and hobbies
- A sense of empowerment and victory over what once felt like a downhill, hopeless battle
- Improvement in conditions connected to prediabetes or uncontrolled diabetes, such as the following:
    - High blood pressure
    - Fatty liver

---

* Individual results vary, and everyone needs to do this under direct medical supervision.

- Polycystic ovarian syndrome (PCOS)
- Elevated triglycerides
- Elevated uric acid
- Obesity
- Irritable bowel syndrome
- Chronic pain syndromes
- Chronic inflammation
- Seasonal allergies
- Relief from symptoms you may have thought you had to live with for the rest of your life; some may have been temporary. In the pages ahead you will learn why—and how to unlock the future you desire.

Turning things around for good

My goal is that this guide provides you with an approach that allows for the flexibility and dynamic decision-making that life demands of you. What's the point of a perfect lifestyle that won't apply when you travel or when life throws a crisis on your path? This book is meant to bridge the gap between what you know is good for your diabetes, and actually taking charge of your journey—encouraging you to make sustainable changes to give you a life of better health with less medication. Are you with me?

Let's go.

Preface: The patient who made me listen

My journey starts with a man named Dinesh.

Dinesh was fifty-eight, a tall, slim-looking man, sitting comfortably across from me in my office in one of the most respected hospitals in Mumbai in 2013. He had been sent to me by a colleague because his glucose levels were out of control despite being on four different oral medications for diabetes. All this was despite cooperating with various prescription changes over the years, which gradually went from one pill to two to four different medications.

He was on ten pills a day. He assumed the tablets had "stopped working" on his body because of years of exposure. He didn't mind new advice as long as there were no needles involved. His hemoglobin A1c (HbA1c) was 11.4 percent, indicating that his three-month average glucose was above 400 mg/dL (22.2 mmol/L).* (For reference, a normal HbA1c is below 5.7 percent, and a normal fasting glucose is below 100 mg/dL (5.5 mmol/L)). According to treatment algorithms, I was supposed to prescribe insulin to lower glucose levels immediately because of his risk of a medical emergency and complications.

But this man was not having it, flat out refusing to go on insulin. I now understood the label on the top of the referral note from his physician: "non-compliant.". I was the endocrinologist, the expert entrusted with this man's uncontrolled diabetes, and I was stuck. I didn't want to "win" just by forcing my treatment onto him. I wanted a win-win.

Before I tell you how I came to an agreement with this man, allow me to explain what helped me reach a place in my head so that I could make a difference in his life. Because many doctors, myself included, would look at his case and think:

What can a doctor do for someone with uncontrolled diabetes who doesn't want more pills or injections?

I love being an endocrinologist, but I needed more than that degree to help people like Dinesh. Endocrinology is the specialization in hormones, diabetes, and metabolism. Endocrinology held natural appeal as a career for me because of the direct relationship between habits and hormonal (endocrine) health. Although

---

* To convert mg/dL to mmol/L, divide by 18.

an endocrinologist plays the role of a specialist doctor, I went ahead and became a certified diabetes educator. My colleagues thought I was crazy, but I needed tools to help patients self-manage diabetes.

Endocrinology doesn't teach you about emotional eating, so I got certified as a mindful eating facilitator. I wanted to address the root lifestyle contributors to uncontrolled diabetes. The diabetes educator course taught me how reducing carbohydrates (carbs) could help. I started researching the science behind low-carbohydrate approaches and discovered books by Dr. Robert Lustig, Gary Taubes, and Dr. David Ludwig.

Being a doctor taught me nothing about exercise; I got certified as a personal trainer. I studied spirituality, learned stress management techniques, and read tons of self-help books.

I read the best scientific writing on sleep by authorities on the subject.

I came across the work of Dr Jason Fung and consumed whatever I could find on the science of intermittent fasting or time-restricted eating as a way to help diabetes. I got accredited in the nutritional approach to managing metabolic health.

I worked on my soft skills so that I could communicate better by listening to my patients.

Being a diabetes specialist doctor teaches you nothing about habit change; I studied behavioral economics and psychology. I was trained and certified by the Motivational Interviewing Network of Trainers (MINT) as a trainer in motivational interviewing.

Basically, I geeked out—my love for learning and self-improvement is a lifelong commitment, and it led to the discovery that people can turn around their diabetes prognosis. I realized that if it's possible, then the better question is:

Who can turn around diabetes?

Over the years, I have seen patients with diabetes achieve amazing results. I'm sharing it all with you in this book. Here are some of the types of people who have turned things around:

- A 32-year-old woman with polycystic ovarian syndrome (PCOS) and prediabetes who conceived spontaneously after years of trying unsuccessfully;

- A 59-year-old retired teacher with stabilized diabetic retinopathy and diabetic kidney damage;

- A 65-year-old man with twenty years of type 2 diabetes who got off insulin after starting strength training;

- A 26-year-old start-up founder with type 2 diabetes since the age of nineteen and a strong family history who put diabetes into remission in a year;

- A 44-year-old executive who reversed fatty liver and newly diagnosed type 2 diabetes;

- A 52-year-old chief executive officer (CEO) who always carried candy and biscuits in her purse to board meetings but broke free of her hypoglycemia and progressive weight gain;

- A 29-year-old woman with uncontrolled type 1 diabetes and wildly fluctuating glucose levels in a single day (between 40 and 400 mg/dL or 2.22 and 22.2 mmol/L) who achieved stable glucose and a normal HbA1c, requiring a fraction of the initial insulin dose;

- A 68-year-old man who had a mild heart attack and managed to reduce his glucose levels with less medication, normalized his triglycerides, and increased his high-density lipoprotein (HDL) and now goes hiking with his family;

- A 72-year-old woman who got off insulin can now wash her own clothes and has a more steady gait, with improvements in her short-term memory noted by her delighted family; and

- A 36-year-old executive whose psychiatrist was able to take him off antidepressants and sleeping pills as his prediabetes improved.

But what made all of these people choose to change their lifestyle in the first place? Well, they were clear about one thing—they wanted better glucose levels and more vitality with less medication. Regardless of whether they were dealing with prediabetes, type 1, or type 2, we worked together on their lifestyle factors so that I could safely reduce their prescription doses as their glucose levels stabilized.

How did we do this?

By addressing insulin resistance, and I'm going to walk you through how we did it—starting with Dinesh.

As we know, Dinesh was "noncompliant." He refused insulin, but he mentioned he was willing to do anything, anything at all, to avoid insulin injections. He had seen how every person in his family who had been started on insulin only got worse. The injections never stopped, and his loved ones finally died of diabetes complications. He didn't see the point of the injections and suspected they would make him sicker than he felt.

There was no further value I could add to his management as a physician.

Our common agenda was to reduce his blood glucose levels by tackling his diabetes through lifestyle changes. So, I put my role as an endocrinologist aside and put on my diabetes educator hat.

After quickly tweaking the four diabetes tablets and adding a fifth, I broached the topic of nutrition. I let him know that he had the option of reducing his carbohydrate intake to attempt to lower his glucose levels.

Dinesh was not overweight, his body mass index was normal, but his dietary carbohydrates were overflowing into his bloodstream. His daily carbohydrate intake was close to 300 grams per day, even though the Nutrient Requirements for Indians recommend 100-130 grams per day and the Dietary Guidelines for Americans recommend a daily carbohydrate intake of 130 grams per day.[1,2] If he wouldn't take insulin, but was given the option of reducing the amount of chapati (or roti, a roasted wheat flatbread) that he ate at every meal instead, would he take it?

I originally didn't believe it would work as it went against my education; I was trained to believe this was "burned-out" type 2 diabetes, where, after years of uncontrolled glucose levels, his pancreas was simply too damaged to respond to oral medication.[3] This is because we *are repeatedly told that **years** of insulin resistance will lead to the **ultimate consequence** of insulin deficiency and dependence.*

Why? Because, at some point, it does.

So in my mind, we were so close to reaching the "ultimate consequence" stage that it was theoretically unlikely for such a small reduction in carbohydrate load to make much difference. But I couldn't force him to do things my way. It was his life, his body. I had to work with this man and help him see the opportunity that reducing his roti/carbohydrate count might create.

So I scheduled him for a follow-up appointment. I made sure it wasn't further than a few days away, as the risks of not sticking to guidelines for starting insulin unnerved me. Back then, the guidelines did not mention reducing carbohydrates as a treatment option, but the diabetes educator in me knew that it might improve his glucose levels with less medication. Importantly, it gave me a way to come to an agreement with him.

I was pleasantly surprised when he coolly strode in for his next appointment. His blood sugars had dropped from the 350 mg/dL (19.4 mmol/L) range to below 200 mg/dL (11.11 mmol/L)—just by going from four to two chapatis per meal, and from ten to four chapatis per day.

Enter: A dumbstruck scientist

That day, I realized that his pancreas couldn't have been all that destroyed or burned out if just this simple change had managed to correct his glucose levels so profoundly.

This was beginning to look like he didn't have insulin deficiency or dependence at all, but it was just a case of worsening insulin resistance, which he had just "treated" by reducing his carbs.

Dinesh took this encouragement and decided to reduce his chapati and carbohydrates even more—especially if it meant I could further reduce his medications. By slowly reducing his carbohydrate intake, he was able to achieve an HbA1c of 6.6 percent with just two diabetes drugs by early 2014, and eventually, I was able to reduce his medication to just metformin. Not the results you would expect for a "noncompliant" person, right?

And yet, he had been given that unfortunate label.

What was he noncompliant with, exactly? If someone truly wanted to be non-compliant, why would they come to repeated appointments with the doctor?

Looking back, I realized I had never assessed his insulin levels. I was only staring at his high glucose levels. If I had evaluated the ability of his pancreas to make insulin (more on that in Part 1), I would have seen high insulin levels. His normal body mass index, or BMI, (calculated from height and weight) did not reveal how unhealthy his body composition was. He was thin on the outside and fat on the inside (TOFI).

It was as though this fact was glaring at me in plain sight, yet I hadn't seen it.

Why aren't we confirming whether a person's problem is high insulin + high glucose levels?

It matters because the *entire treatment approach would need to change* based on whether someone has uncontrolled glucose with high insulin or low insulin secretion.

Treating Dinesh was a major awakening for me. After that case, the way I would treat people with diabetes going forward shifted. I started actively looking for insulin resistance as a treatment opportunity. Educating patients about lifestyle changes became a mandatory part of my prescription. That same year, on World Diabetes Day 2014, I launched Mumbai's first endocrinologist-led diabetes self-management education (DSME) group classes with the support of the hospital.

Dinesh came and spoke as an invited guest.

In the decade since, I have worked with thousands of patients and witnessed people from all walks of life turning around uncontrolled diabetes. Through the rest of this book, I will share all of the steps they followed to get out of insulin resistance and turn their diabetes around.

PART 1

THE SCIENCE OF DIABETES

1.1: What is diabetes?

To take charge of your diabetes, we first have to know: What is it? Take a moment to recall how your diagnosis of diabetes was made: by high glucose readings. High glucose readings meaning,

- Fasting glucose **equal to or above 126 mg/dL** (7.0 mmol/L) on two separate occasions,

- Serum glucose level equal to or above 200 mg/dL (11.1 mmol/L) either at a random test or two hours after a 75 g oral glucose tolerance test (OGTT), and

- HbA1c (reflecting 90-day average glucose) equal to or above 6.5 percent on two separate measurements,

High blood glucose ultimately will lead to a diabetes diagnosis. Knowing what is considered high, as well as what is considered normal, will help you and your medical team to track your health accurately. That then brings up the question: **What's a normal glucose reading?**

A normal fasting glucose is **below 100 mg/dL (5.55 mmol/L)**. Most normal people cannot visualize what that even means. Let me walk you through some math.

First, 100 mg of glucose per deciliter of blood is the same as 1,000 mg of glucose in 1,000 mL—which is the same as 5,000 mg (5 g) of glucose in five liters of blood.

If the average adult is considered to have five liters of blood in their body, then we normally have around five grams of glucose in our bloodstream.

Five grams of sugar is one teaspoon. Having the equivalent of two teaspoons of sugar dissolved in your blood would translate to a glucose level of **200 mg/dL** (11.11 mmol/L). This means that going from normal blood glucose (**100 mg/dL** or 5.55 mmol/L) to the cutoff for diabetes (**126 mg/dL** or 7.0 mmol/L) translates to going from that one teaspoon, to just over one and a quarter teaspoons of sugar in the entire bloodstream.

The math shows that *the difference between normal blood glucose and un-controlled diabetes is less than one additional teaspoon of sugar dissolved in your blood*.

So, what is diabetes exactly? First, it's important to understand it is not a monolith; there are two main types of diabetes.[*] The word *diabetes* means "the fluid runs through," referring to the excessive urination and thirst of uncontrolled diabetes, and *mellitus* means "sweet urine," referring to the time when scientists noticed the urine of people with diabetes tasted sweet.

These names were assigned centuries ago when physicians did not have the luxury of laboratory testing. They were trying to make sense of a condition that has now, sadly, become a household name.

Here is an oversimplified table of major differences illustrated between the two types of diabetes:

	Type 1	Type 2
Cause	Destruction of pancreatic beta cells due to genetic, autoimmune, inflammatory damage, surgical removal of the pancreas, or unknown causes Not caused by lifestyle	Familial and lifestyle causes
Treatment	Insulin-dependent from diagnosis Urgently need insulin to survive	Non–insulin dependent at diagnosis Treatment starts with pills and can progress to injectable medication and insulin

---

[*] For a historical timeline of our understanding of diabetes over the centuries and the naming of the condition as diabetes and then the later addition of the word mellitus, see Marianna Karamanou, Athanase Protogerou, Gregory Tsoucalas, George Androutsos, and Effie Poulakou-Rebelakou, "Milestones in the History of Diabetes Mellitus: The Main Contributors," World Journal of Diabetes 7, no. 1 (2016): 1–7, https://www.ncbi.nlm.nih.gov/pmc/articles/PMC4707300/; and Kenneth S. Polonsky, "The Past 200 Years in Diabetes," New England Journal of Medicine 367 (2012): 1332–1340, https://www.nejm.org/doi/10.1056/NEJMra1110560.

	Type 1	Type 2
Reversibility	As of today's writing, there is no widely available cure, although research is ongoing. For the time being, we still need insulin therapy to treat type 1 diabetes, and lifestyle changes help keep the dose to the minimum	Can be put into "remission" through aggressive lifestyle change when the C-peptide level shows sufficient insulin production by the body
Symptoms at diagnosis	Excessive urination, thirst, weight loss, and hunger	In modern times, often no symptoms Often discovered on routine testing or screening Can also have symptoms of high glucose: excess urination, thirst, weight loss, and hunger
Weight trend before diagnosis	Weight loss	Gradual weight gain If very high glucose, can cause weight loss
Main defect	Insulin deficiency	Insulin resistance
Made worse by	High insulin doses and insulin resistance	Weight gain around the belly
Glucose transport	Glucose not entering cells in absence of insulin	Defective glucose transport
Predominance	This was the noticeable form of diabetes centuries ago because of severe and rapidly progressive symptoms before lab testing of blood was possible.	The dominant type of diabetes in modern times Earlier diagnosis occurs by routine blood tests, often before symptoms start
Serum glucose	High	High
Serum C-peptide	Low to undetectable C-peptide and insulin levels at diagnosis[1]	High levels of C-peptide and insulin at diagnosis Late-stage type 2 can have low C-peptide levels as a result of pancreatic beta-cell failure and "burnout"

	Type 1	Type 2
Ketoacidosis	A possible life-threatening complication due to lack of insulin or extreme stress/ illness. Can be triggered by SGLT-2 medication	Rare in type 2 diabetes, can be triggered by SGLT-2 medication[*]

This is why it's important to look at glucose and C-peptide levels.[**]

Author Note: Going forward, when I use the term *diabetes medication*, I mean tablets and/or insulin.

Diabetes is more than just a glucose problem—it's also an insulin problem!

Insulin resistance is present when a patient has **both** high glucose levels and **high** insulin levels (or doses), and it's what makes diabetes progressively more difficult to treat. But can you get unstuck?

From all of my patients and case studies, it seems you can. But before you can make a plan, we have to know—what is insulin resistance?

---

* Severe type 2 diabetes can rarely present with some overlapping symptoms of Type 1. That's outside the scope of this book.

** J. Roth, I. Whitford, R. Dankner, and L. Szulc, "How the Immunoassay Transformed C-Peptide from a Duckling into a Swan," Diabetologia 55 (2012): 865–869, https://doi.org/10.1007/s00125-011-2421-0.

1.2: What's insulin resistance, and why you're stuck

If you have high glucose levels despite having high insulin levels (or doses), you are looking at full-blown insulin resistance.

Insulin resistance is what makes type 2 and type 1 diabetes **progressively difficult to manage;** addressing insulin resistance helps you turn around diabetes. This means better glucose levels with less medication and less insulin for both type 1 and type 2 diabetes.* If that's your goal, like it is for my patients, then let's solve the first mystery: **what's keeping you stuck in insulin resistance?**

We can inherit a tendency for insulin resistance from our parents. Some of that tendency is coded in our DNA, and some of the tendency is coded in the habits we learn while growing up.

In essence, DNA loads the gun, and lifestyle pulls the trigger.

Modern lifestyles are keeping us stuck. It takes just one flat tire for your other tires to be overworked and in trouble, and then it's just a matter of time before your lifestyle car slows and breaks down in the middle of the road. Any one area of your lifestyle could be a major contributor to burdening the remaining areas, resulting in misalignment and tension.

Different lifestyle choices within nutrition, sleep habits, stress management, and exercise can keep people confined in a vicious cycle of insulin resistance. As insulin resistance is an integral driver of increasing prescriptions for diabetes, let's understand what factors could contribute to this hormone imbalance. Before we go deeper, here's an overview of how certain decisions can keep you stuck.

Nutrition

A diet high in carbohydrates will *keep you hungry* all day, especially **addictive or highly-processed carbohydrates and sugar**, which can then *perpetuate crav-*

---

* Type 1 diabetes cannot be cured as of this writing. Most cases of type 2 diabetes can go into remission, as long as the pancreas is still making enough insulin. I explain this in part 1.3.

ings and energy crashes that keep your brain wanting more all day long. It can lead to **constant snacking**, which ultimately, *requires insulin exposure all day*. A diet that causes **high insulin**, however, *perpetuates weight gain*, which worsens insulin resistance, creating a vicious cycle. Once **insulin resistance** is reached, it causes *leptin resistance*, which makes the brain feel like it's hungry, starving, and craving food all day. Combined with the fact that **protein-deficient meals** cause *cravings and a lack of satiety* all day and that certain foods **disrupt gut health—** *you have an altered gut microbiome and gut-brain axis*. In addition, **carb heavy meals** create *lethargy and low energy*, which, if **you need food to fall asleep**, isn't helped by the fact that it can *cause acid reflux* if you eat right before bed—**affecting your quality and amount of sleep**.

Sleep

Not only is it possible to be kept awake from acid reflux, but **staying up late** triggers *food cravings*, and **late-night meals** *disrupt the body clock and create an unhealthy gut*. **Sleep deprivation** directly *increases insulin resistance and glucose levels*. **Late-night screen time** can *reduce sleep quality*—and **poor sleep quality** triggers *food cravings and increased hunger* the next day. A **poorly rested brain** is less able to learn and use creativity to *find new solutions and solve old problems*, so **waking up with a tired brain** makes *you reach for food* all day. What's worse is that sleep deprivation makes it *harder to choose healthy foods* and resist temptation. In addition, **undiagnosed or untreated sleep apnea** *worsens insulin resistance*, but regardless—poor sleep *makes you irritable, hungry and stressed*.

Stress

We all know that **chronic stress** *prevents restful sleep*. Stress often *increases food cravings, emotional eating*, and worsens **acidity** (acid reflux) that *makes you want to keep eating*. Additionally, chronic stress **reduces natural endorphins and serotonin** (your natural feel-good chemicals). The stress hormone, **cortisol, stays at high levels**, *worsening insulin resistance, energy levels and mood*. Low energy and mood *reduce the willingness to exercise*—and that's assuming you wanted to in the first place!

Exercise

We've already acknowledged that a **high-carb, protein-deficient diet; poor sleep; and high stress** can lead to *low energy*. We also know that **low energy levels** *reduce your ability to move*. A **lack of exercise** *deprives you of natural endorphins* (your natural feel-good anti-depressant chemicals) and a **protein-de-**

ficient diet causes a *lack of muscle gain* despite any attempts to get fit. The **lack of results** despite dragging yourself to exercise makes it *demotivating to be consistent*, which furthers the cycle.

These four major lifestyle areas can come together to keep the person stuck. Insulin resistance progresses, and we are left with a "chronic progressive" pattern of diabetes.

When I come across a complex pattern like this, I try to reframe the problem with a solution-oriented, first-principles approach. If this is a vicious cycle, how can I unravel it with what I already know? The good news is that by focusing on each of the lifestyle elements we'll walk through step by step, you can start chipping away at the vicious cycle and reduce insulin resistance. Throughout the book, I'll show you how real people made lifestyle changes, one baby step at a time, to improve their health. Because I've seen thousands of people do it for themselves, I want you to have access to all I've learned from working with them. I'm going to show you how you can do this, too.

1.3 Remission versus reversal of diabetes and metabolic syndrome

While I believe that most people with diabetes can benefit from this guide, I want to be clear about an emerging shift in diabetes terminology. Instead of saying *diabetes reversal*, we might prefer the term t*ype 2 diabetes remission* because it is still a chronic condition that can "relapse" if you go back to the lifestyle that caused the condition.[2] Because type 1 diabetes cannot be reversed as of this writing, I will focus on showing you ways to turn diabetes around so that you are not on a chronically progressive and worsening downhill path. By sharing how people have changed their lives, I am offering you an alternate path for type 2 and type 1 diabetes. The purpose is to help you develop clarity to decide *why* you want to change, what to change, and how to do that so you can get unstuck (and stay unstuck). That way, you can navigate more easily toward your unique goals.

Metabolic syndrome

When it comes to turning your diabetes prognosis around, you may have heard the term **metabolic syndrome**, or "syndrome X." **Metabolic syndrome** is another term that refers to insulin resistance syndrome. It correlated with a higher risk of heart disease, diabetes, stroke, and all-cause mortality.[3]

The official definition of metabolic syndrome from the NIH is characterized as a person who has a combination of any three of the following:

1. **Visceral/android obesity:** waist circumference at *the largest point* being larger than 40 inches (101 cm) in a man, or thirty-five inches (89 cm) in a woman;

1. **High blood pressure:** above 130/85 mm Hg or being treated for high BP;

1. **High fasting glucose:** above 100 mg/dL (5.5 mmol/L);

1. **High triglycerides:** above 150 mg/dL;

1. **Low high-density lipoprotein HDL:** below 50 mg/dL in a woman or below 40 mg/dL in a man; and did you notice?

We don't find low-density lipoprotein (LDL) or total cholesterol on this list of symptoms at all! The good news is that you can turn around diabetes and reverse metabolic syndrome (even improve HDL cholesterol, which is supposed to be genetically determined) through lifestyle change.[4]

Metabolic psychiatry and metabolic neurology

Metabolic psychiatry and metabolic neurology are exciting fields that look at the relationship between metabolic health and brain health. World-class institutions like Stanford and Harvard now have entire departments devoted to looking at a metabolic and nutritional approach to mental health. Dr. Chris Palmer's book *Brain Energy* and Dr Georgia Ede's new book *Change your Diet Change your Mind* revolutionizes the way we should be looking at mental health by taking a metabolic and lifestyle approach to the brain and nervous system.

Insulin resistance in the brain seems to be linked with multiple neurodegenerative conditions like Alzheimer's and Parkinson's through "brain glucose hypometabolism". This is a situation in which the brain is running low on fuel. It is unable to use glucose for fuel despite high insulin and glucose levels, and also unable to use ketones for fuel because of those same high insulin levels. The good news is that the approaches outlined in this book for diabetes have a direct positive impact on the metabolic approach to mental health, too.

It's clear that there's a common link, and you know you are getting closer to the truth when one answer holds true in multiple scenarios. By understanding insulin resistance in terms of its contributing factors, and how it affects the body, we can begin to search for answers on how to turn our diabetes around.

1.4: Hormones and homeostasis

Homeostasis is the body's self-regulating system that keeps the internal environment stable in terms of blood pressure, body temperature, electrolytes, glucose level, and so much more. Healthy hormone systems are what create and maintain homeostasis, and any shift in these hormone systems can cause a variety of symptoms.

You'll notice how I keep calling them "systems," instead of just "hormones." Much like the shift to say "remission" over "reversal," it helps to use words that establish a baseline expectation. In this case, it's not just hormones—*it's a system of highly adaptive and dynamic intelligence by which the sensory organs receive inputs*. These systems get the bulk of their stimulation from two places:

1. The external environment: Inputs from sight, sound, taste, touch, and smell get converted to information that is then given meaning—finally being converted into instructions that tell target organs what to do. For example:

- **Smell food** → meal is available → prepare saliva and digestive juice. Activate gut motility.

- **See a predator** → danger → secrete cortisol and switch to fight-fright-flight mode.

2. Or, the internal environment: These inputs are better seen as "status updates"

- **You drink a lot of water** → water absorbed from the gut enters the bloodstream → increased blood volume → **stretch of heart muscle** → **informs the kidney** → urinates a precise amount of excess water out to maintain sodium and water balance.

- You eat a carb-rich meal → **glucose surge** → **insulin release** → move glucose into storage → store excess as fat.

The phrase *insulin resistance* gets thrown around a lot so I don't want to assume that you know exactly what insulin is.

Or what a hormone is. Or what metabolism is.

So, let's clear up a few points so that the rest of the book makes sense when we talk about how to address insulin resistance at the root. Because let's face it, right? The only way to achieve better health with less medication is to learn everything about our obstacles. That's how we gain an advantage and turn things around. Knowledge becomes my medicine for you.

So let's start here: *insulin is not the enemy.*

Insulin is the master metabolic hormone.

Hormones as long-distance biochemical messengers

As I explained before, endocrinologists think of hormones in terms of systems. They help align the various agendas of all the different organs into focusing on the agenda that matters most: the survival, health, and balance of the individual.

Hormones enable different organs and tissues to coordinate and talk to each other. They are biochemical messengers secreted by endocrine glands directly into the bloodstream to send instructions and signals to distant parts of the body.* When these instructions reach the target cell, the cells respond by activating or suppressing various parts of the DNA. When a specific part of DNA is activated, a specific protein molecule is manufactured to carry out the required response. This then sends a feedback message to the gland as confirmation to complete the message loop so that the body maintains the balance it loves.

What is special about hormones is they can carry messages far away from their original gland, making sure all systems are on the same page. In this way, each specialized organ performs its own specific task while hormones coordinate the body as a whole.

Let's be clear: Not all secretions are hormones.

Let's say you watch a movie that has a very happy ending. Your brain interprets the movie and generates a feeling of joy, sending "feel-good," happy hormones all across the entire body, generating a warm, fuzzy, happy response. Your facial expression softens, your shoulders relax, and you enter a slightly euphoric state. If you are the happy-tears type, your brain signal may tell the tear glands to secrete some tears, which are only released locally in your eyes. You don't cry from your shoulders.

---

* Endocrinology in the study of hormones and metabolism. Insulin being one of the master hormones that regulate metabolism, the study of insulin comes under endocrinology, too. When we graduate from the endocrinology fellowship, we are certified in the speciality of hormones, diabetes and metabolism. Endocrinologists are the medical doctors that have received the highest level of specialized training when it comes to prescribing medications for diabetes, including insulin.

The feel-good chemicals from the brain that influence the entire body are the hormones. Your tears are secretions, but they are not hormones.

Picture the endocrine system as an office –

Imagine a large, healthy company with various buildings across a large campus. By sending interdepartmental mail and messages the coworkers can cooperate, each smoothly doing their job while updating the entire staff in other buildings to ensure overall alignment with the headquarters' goals.

Our healthcare system has a different specialist for each organ system, such as a **cardiologist** for your *heart and circulatory system*, and a **nephrologist** for your *kidneys and excretory system*. An **endocrinologist** specializes in *hormones, diabetes, metabolism, and the endocrine system.*

Imagine what it would be like for your specialist doctors for each organ to speak to each other daily, in real-time, about your health! Whether the doctors keep in touch or not, you can be sure that your heart, kidney, muscle, liver, and pancreas are talking to each other all day, every day, with the specialized message delivery service of hormones; it's why I love endocrinology. Hormones unite the systems into one major balancing masterpiece, and some of the more well-known hormones and the top messages they send through the bloodstream can be found in this incomplete list:

Endocrine gland	Major hormones	Major messages/actions
Tail of pancreas	Insulin Glucagon	Glucose and fat metabolism, growth, appetite, energy balance, weight management
Thyroid gland	Thyroid hormone	Metabolic rate in all tissues, brain function
Adipose (fat) tissue: 1. White fat/white adipose tissue (WAT) 2. Brown fat/brown adipose tissue (BAT)	Leptin and adipokines like adiponectin Resistin*	Regulate satiety Nutrient and energy metabolism Insulin resistance/sensitivity White fat wants to store energy, and brown fat wants to burn it.
Muscle	Myokines like irisin	Regulate fat metabolism, converting white fat to beige fat by making more brown fat

---

* Resistin is an inflammatory marker of atherosclerosis in humans.

Endocrine gland	Major hormones	Major messages/actions
Fat, muscle, pancreas, and liver	Fibroblast growth factor 21 (FGF-21)	Glucose and fat metabolism
Stomach	Ghrelin	Stimulate hunger, influence fat storage*
Gut (small intestine)	Incretins, glucagon-like peptide-1(GLP-1), and gastric inhibitory polypeptide (GIP)	Glucose metabolism, hunger, satiety, appetite, regulate stomach emptying
Hypothalamus	Orexins[5,6] Gonadotropin-releasing hormone (GnRH), thyrotropin-releasing hormone (TRH), corticotropin-releasing hormone (CRH)	Sleep, vigilance, feeding, energy balance balance Regulates appetite via leptin Regulate the pituitary gland
Adrenal gland	Cortisol Aldosterone Sex steroid hormones	Stress response, blood pressure Sodium and potassium regulation Sexual characteristics
Pineal	Melatonin	Sleep-wake circadian cycle
Testes	Testosterone	Male sexual characteristics
Ovaries	Estrogen, progesterone	Female sexual characteristics
Pituitary gland	Growth hormone, thyroid-stimulating hormone (TSH), adrenocorticotropic hormone (ACTH), luteinizing hormone (LH), follicle-stimulating hormone (FSH), prolactin, vasopressin	Puberty, growth, stress response, lactation and more Water balance
Parathyroid gland	Parathyroid hormone	Calcium, vitamin D, magnesium, and bone metabolism
Bone	Osteocalcin	Glucose metabolism, regulates testosterone secretion, and muscle mass

---

* Ghrelin, a gastrointestinal hormone regulates energy balance and lipid metabolism.

Endocrine gland	Major hormones	Major messages/actions
Kidney	Renin Erythropoietin	Blood pressure, sodium, and potassium regulation Red blood cell production
Heart muscle	Atrial natriuretic peptide (ANP) Brain natriuretic peptide (BNP)	Regulate blood volume Salt and water balance

So, what's the connection between hormones, weight, and metabolism? As noted earlier, insulin is the master metabolic hormone because it's one of the hormones *we all need to survive*. As it's associated with energy abundance, it's common to be told that you are struggling to lose weight because of your hormones, or even to blame it all on a slow metabolism. The thing is—your hormones are *in charge* of metabolism.

1.5: Understanding metabolism and the master metabolic hormone

Metabolism is the sum of the biochemical processes carried out by all living things to use energy from the environment to support the functions inside living cells. It's the sum of building new tissues (anabolism); and the breakdown, recycling, and excretion of old tissues (catabolism). When it comes to metabolism, you'll find physics, chemistry, and biology all alive and in action in one place.

The easiest way to illustrate insulin action is to use the analogy of **"The three musketeers of glucose metabolism:"**[7]

1. **Skeletal muscle**, or the *glucose taker*—especially after meals, taking up around 80 percent of postmeal glucose; the

1. **Liver**, or the *glucose provider*, maintains stable glucose levels even when fasting; and the

1. **Pancreas**, or the *glucose regulator*, coordinates insulin responses to keep glucose levels normal by promoting the skeletal muscle to take up the postmeal glucose, and by controlling the overnight fasting glucose provided by the liver.

As you prepare to eat a meal, the body realizes that a fuel supply is coming. Insulin, the master metabolic hormone, is secreted by beta cells in the tail of the pancreas. The regulator guides energy uptake and storage throughout the body.

Insulin, the master metabolic hormone

Without insulin, there are no three musketeers, and the food you digest doesn't enter the cells of your body.* That's why a person who has been recently diagnosed with type 1 diabetes will report weight loss before they identify the high glucose levels that make the diagnosis. Without enough insulin to get their nutrients inside the cells, they are storing less energy and losing weight—why would they ever suspect high blood sugar?

Food is what triggers the pancreas to begin sending metabolic messages via insulin to the main insulin response organs: liver, muscle, and fat. Your digestive system breaks down carbohydrates into glucose, which is then stored as glycogen in the liver and muscle, and if there is still extra energy, it is stored as fat in the fat cells.** Dietary carbohydrates create the most glucose and therefore require the highest amount of insulin. Less insulin is required for protein, and dietary fat requires the least amount of insulin.***

A high-insulin environment after meals is one where you put the energy from food into storage, but you can't access it until insulin levels drop again.

A high-insulin environment is like depositing cash in the bank with no way to withdraw it for spending. Insulin's job is to store carbohydrates and fat—basically, *store energy* for a rainy day. As long as energy is flowing in, high insulin levels will keep directing incoming fuel into storage and accumulate savings. In this way, insulin works as an anabolic (growth-promoting) hormone. Under healthy conditions, insulin tells the body to STORE fuel in the following ways:

- Store more glucose as glycogen in the liver.

- Reduce glucose production in the liver.

- Package fat as triglyceride (very low-density lipoprotein [VLDL]) in the liver.

- Take up glucose into the muscle.

---

* I learned more about the practical role of insulin in storing nutrients and the pathophysiology of obesity from reading the following than I did during my fellowship: Gary Taubes, Why We Get Fat (New York: Anchor, 2011); Robert Lustig, Fat Chance (New York: PLUME, 2012); Jason Fung, The Obesity Code (Vancouver: Greystone Books, 2015); David Ludwig, Always Hungry (New York: Grand Central Life & Style, 2016); Jason Fung, The Complete Guide to Fasting (Las Vegas: Victory Belt Publishing, 2016); and Jason Fung, The Diabetes Code (Vancouver: Greystone Books, 2018).

** Glycogen is just a long chain of many glucose molecules.

*** This is why a keto or very low-carb diet reduces the insulin requirement in type 1 diabetes and the medication requirement in type 2 diabetes.

- Store more glycogen in muscle.

- Promote fat storage as triglycerides in fat cells, especially white fat (white adipose tissue [WAT]).

- Block breakdown and utilization of fat.

Seeing this list of packaging and storing energy as fat in a healthy body, it becomes clear that body fat can be a good thing.

Especially when it's brown.

1.6: How fat and insulin are trying to help us

You're probably wondering what that even *means*. Here's the background. If insulin helps you store digested food as energy to be used inside the cells—so that you can go about living life—then extra fuel gets stored as fat. This energy management system worked very well for our ancestors who lived thousands of years ago, before the agricultural revolution, when it was common for hunter-gatherer humans to experience periodic food shortages. During food shortages, insulin levels dropped, making the stored fat available as a source of energy to fuel hunting and gathering.* Now here's where it gets interesting.

Our body mostly tends to have **white adipose tissue** (WAT) or white fat, which wants to store fuel, but it's the *brown* **adipose tissue** (BAT), commonly known as brown fat, that is insulin sensitive and wants to burn stored fuel to generate heat (thermogenesis) and energy.

BAT is rich in mitochondria, which not only gives brown fat its color but also the thermogenic property of burning fuel instead of storing it. How? Mitochondria are brown in color from being iron-rich and are considered the energy powerhouse of the cell.[8] They are where all the efficient energy generation in the body happens. They will be featured throughout the book because whether you are eating or fasting, your mitochondria are always making **adenosine triphosphate** (ATP), the energy currency of every living cell in the body.

Body fat helped hunter-gatherer humans survive spells of food shortage and kept them warm in extreme winter months.

Fat was good. Insulin was good because it helped us hold on to fat. We were insulin-sensitive. That meant normal amounts of insulin could store the right amount of fuel to get the job done.

It turns out that there are beneficial metabolic effects that come from activating brown fat through cold exposure—maybe that's the reason you see so many

---

* Starvation is still a real problem in many parts of the world affected by famine, poverty, and war. That is outside the scope of this book.

influencers embracing cold therapy, including cold-water plunges and immersion. [9]According to Dr Ben Bikman, a leading expert on insulin resistance, brown fat is activated and starts burning glucose around 18°C (64°F). Perhaps that was also the logic behind the 1980s blockbuster Bollywood Hindi song urging people to have a cold-water bath.

Research suggests that something as simple as increased room temperatures can impair the metabolic benefits of brown fat and reverse the switch. Sleeping at 24°C (75°F) reduced benefits previously achieved from sleeping at 19°C (66°F).[10] While bedroom temperatures have gradually increased from 19°C to 21.5°C (66°F to 71°F) over the last three decades in the United States, millions of people in India, Southeast Asia, and equatorial regions sleep without air-conditioning and are exposed to warmer temperatures—likely blunting the activation of brown fat. Since brown fat keeps you warm, it's unlikely to be activated when it's too hot.[11] Research suggests that South Asians may also have genetic differences that prevent BAT activation when exposed to cold, possibly due to higher endocannabinoid (EC) activity.[12] The EC system is your brain's natural version of marijuana—a higher endocannabinoid level is responsible for the "munchies": increased food intake, increased fuel storage, and lower energy spending.[13] These are still loose hypotheses at this point, and we need more research in these areas to better understand how hormones interact with the environment to drive weight gain and obesity.

Even though we have just gone over how body fat, (especially brown fat) is a good thing, too much white fat or dysfunctional fat can be a bad thing.

Too much white fat can become an unwanted fourth musketeer that contributes to insulin resistance (from the three musketeers earlier in this chapter).

We need insulin to survive. And yet, too much insulin can become a bad thing, known as *insulin resistance*. That is what happens to everyone with type 2 diabetes and can also happen if someone with type 1 diabetes is on very high doses of insulin. Let's now tackle how insulin resistance causes difficulty losing weight, stubborn belly fat, slowing metabolism, and diabetes that starts going the wrong way.

1.7: The root of chronic progressive disease: Insulin resistance

A broken thermostat: When homeostasis breaks down

We just discussed how insulin works in the body, and homeostasis is how the body uses sophisticated automatic feedback loops to keep things in balance. Now let's see what it's like when insulin resistance sets in: insulin doesn't *work*, even though it's present (either your own insulin or taken through shots). *Insulin resistance is when the body doesn't respond correctly to the messages that insulin is trying to deliver.*

We know that all systems communicate with each other through checks and balances; internal body mechanisms maintain a constant rhythm for the organism to stay alive. *Broken homeostatic mechanisms are the onset of disease.* It's difficult to visualize insulin resistance because you can't see it or feel it. Here is a more tangible example. In terms of our body temperature, let's understand what could happen if the homeostasis thermostat were to break down.

When we are in a very hot environment, the body begins to increase blood flow to the skin to release body heat, which is why we look flushed. We begin sweating to cool off, we try to get out of direct sunlight and we activate the thirst system and the search for water. Too much heat without access to enough water can overwhelm our thermostat causing a heat stroke, or even death.

On the other hand, when we feel cold and we start to shiver, it means our muscles are contracting to generate heat. We look for warmer places to take shelter and maybe put on an extra layer of clothes to stop losing body heat. Too much freezing weather without sufficient heating, and we can die of cold.

Homeostasis regulates all of those systems and signals—and yet that's only a fraction of its workload. Our bodies balance multiple survival needs by being flexible.

Metabolic flexibility or metabolic resilience

In the case of metabolism, *the mechanism to detect energy shifts, counter-regulate, set things right, autocorrect,* and *self-repair* is called **metabolic flexibility**.

A healthy person eating one large, rich meal at a wedding or holiday will not get type 2 diabetes overnight thanks to their metabolic flexibility. Their satiety signals tell them, "I'm done," and they will go into hibernation, or what we call a food coma, causing them to want to sleep it off—possibly skipping the next meal. This allows the internal systems to recalibrate, and they will come back to balance.

All natural systems have a threshold, beyond which they can get overwhelmed and dysfunctional. That's when disease can set in. The more rigid a system, the easier it is to break. The more flexible and responsive a system is, the more adaptive and resilient it remains.

The root mechanism of insulin resistance

Insulin is necessary for life, dynamically increasing or decreasing multiple times a day, depending on the situation. It is only when there is unrelenting, excessive pressure on our metabolism that things break down. In the case of modern sedentary, overfed lifestyles, a vicious cycle sets up insulin resistance. Every time you eat something, even if it's the healthiest food on the planet, it creates an insulin spike. Five meals means five insulin spikes.

Too much insulin being secreted (or injected) for too long without any restorative breaks from high insulin levels is called *chronic hyperinsulinemia* and is a hallmark of insulin resistance.

In prediabetes and type 2 diabetes, this means insulin is being secreted but is not able to do its job effectively. Conversely, in type 1 diabetes, chronic hyperinsulinemia means exposure to higher and higher insulin doses without sufficient periods of low insulin levels.*

Insulin resistance can be the starting point of many chronic diseases, including type 2 diabetes, obesity, hypertension, fatty liver, high triglycerides, polycystic ovaries, cardiovascular disease, Alzheimer's disease, inflammatory conditions, and even cancer. During the COVID pandemic, insulin resistance was linked with worse outcomes in people admitted to the hospital.[14]

Research is still underway to try to figure out what exactly flips the switch into the deranged fuel metabolism of insulin resistance. This is probably a multifactorial multi-switch event. We probably won't reach a universal agreement on a single trigger that sets the problem off (and therefore no single cure). While the researchers debate and try to figure it out, this book will help you focus on the lifestyle changes that we know can turn things around. The syndrome of insulin resistance creates unhealthy changes among the three musketeers; the muscles, liver, and pancreas. This causes unwanted involvement of the fourth musketeer, the fat cells. The following key patterns have been linked to diabetes, and look something like this:[15]

- **Muscle** (the glucose *taker*) displays deranged glucose uptake and metabolism inside the muscle cells, deranged glycogen metabolism, and accumulation of toxic fat inside muscle cells (fatty muscle/intramuscular fat/intramyocellular lipid/myosteatosis), and ultimately a reduced ability to use fat as fuel with excess glucose being diverted to the liver.

- **Liver** (the glucose *provider*) displays deranged glucose uptake by the liver cells and increased glucose production (gluconeogenesis). While there is reduced storage of glucose as glycogen by the liver, there is also an increased breakdown of glycogen (glycogenolysis) resulting in higher net glucose output. This, plus the liver creating triglycerides from excess sugar can lead to toxic triglyceride accumulation inside the cells, resulting in a fatty liver (hepatosteatosis) which is also called nonalcoholic (NAFLD) or metabolic associated fatty liver disease (MAFLD).

- The **pancreas** (the glucose *regulator*) can initially increase the secretion of insulin to keep pushing glucose levels to normal, but along with accumulation of toxic pancreatic fat (fatty pancreas) ultimately,

---

* If you have type 1 diabetes, you probably have insulin resistance if you keep needing more insulin (over one unit per kg body weight per day). Although type 1 diabetes does not have a cure at this point in time, if you have type 1 diabetes, you will learn about lifestyle changes that reduce insulin resistance and bring insulin requirements down. Do this under medical supervision so that your doctor can reduce your insulin dose to avoid serious hypoglycemia.

the pancreatic beta-cells will burn out and fail to secrete insulin. That would be the "burned-out" state of type 2 diabetes I thought Dinesh had reached.

- **Excessive fat cells** go from being good fat to being the fourth unwelcome musketeer when there is an excess of triglyceride in white fat (adipose) cells. Toxic, inflammatory cytokines are released from these unhealthy fat cells, worsening insulin resistance. The body ends up dumping triglycerides into circulation that increase cardiac risk.

- **Blood** is where we diagnose diabetes when we find raised glucose levels and hemoglobin A1c (HbA1c) levels. The blood also carries the increased load of inflammatory substances that make insulin resistance worse: toxic fat particles, raised triglyceride or very low-density lipoprotein (VLDL), and raised uric acid levels. Chronically elevated insulin levels make insulin resistance worse.

Your muscles, liver, pancreas, and fat tissue try very hard for years to prevent rising blood glucose levels, prediabetes, type 2 diabetes and inflammation. Once the capacity of these systems is exceeded and they begin dumping waste into the bloodstream, you see a rapid rise in glucose levels, despite the presence of high amounts of insulin. That's the telltale sign that something is broken and backward. Insulin is supposed to bring glucose levels *down*.

Over the years, as the three, and eventually four, musketeers lose their battle to maintain balance, the buildup of waste changes the blood composition, and this creates changes in the blood vessels. High glucose levels cause chronic oxidative stress from toxic reactive oxygen species (ROS) and nitrogen species (RONS) that overwhelm the natural antioxidant systems causing damage throughout the body. High blood glucose levels interact with blood molecules, forming advanced glycation end products (AGE) which *accelerate* aging, inflammation, and diabetes.

This kicks off a chain of events where the aging vessels allow unhealthy fats to enter the vessel wall lining (endothelium), which triggers inflammation, ultimately damaging both small vessels (microvascular damage) and large blood vessels (macrovascular damage). The immune system sends protective white blood cells which, attempting to repair the damage by swallowing the unhealthy fats, become inflamed foam cells. There is still fat to be consumed, so those foam cells send distress signals for help and when more white blood cells arrive, it causes a pileup of reactive junk—eventually forming an atherosclerotic plaque, the hallmark of cardiovascular disease.

Bad things keep bad company

After discussing the capability of the fourth musketeer to cause cardiovascular disease, I think it's becoming clear that it's not just chronic progressive *diabetes* we are talking about now. I wonder if you could guess what other chronic conditions are associated with insulin resistance.

Give yourself a moment to think about what else you think is influenced by insulin resistance (I even shared some in this chapter if you can remember!) and see how many are on this list:

- Prediabetes and type 2 diabetes
- Obesity, especially around the belly (tummy or visceral fat)
- High blood pressure
- Cardiovascular disease
- Cancer
- Fatty liver
- Worse COVID outcomes
- Alzheimer's dementia and Parkinson's
- High triglycerides
- High uric acid and gout
- Polycystic ovarian syndrome (PCOS) and gestational diabetes
- Chronic inflammation, chronic pain, and fibromyalgia
- Irritable bowel syndrome (BS), Small intestinal bacterial overgrowth (SIBO), leaky gut, and poor gut health.[16,17,18]

That's a lot of unwanted health issues, and when a patient finds the three musketeers at their maximum capacity, they need a helping hand. In this case, we have a vehicle that can help them return to homeostasis, heal, rest and recover, but here's the thing: we are going to have to service the vehicle first.

It's time to service the lifestyle car, starting with one of the most powerful wheels—nutrition.

Part 1 summary

- Insulin resistance is at the core of progressive uncontrolled diabetes and multiple chronic medical conditions.

- The four wheels of the lifestyle car with the fifth optional element of fasting show you how to turn around insulin resistance and uncontrolled diabetes.

- You are in the driver's seat. This book is your navigation guide after consulting your physician.

- There are 2 main types of diabetes: Type 1 diabetes, a condition of too little insulin secretion in the body and Type 2 diabetes, a condition of too much insulin secretion in the body.

- There are three "musketeers" that normally manage glucose metabolism: muscle (the taker), liver (the provider) and pancreas (the regulator).

- A high insulin environment means fuel is being stored, to be used for energy when insulin levels go low again.

- You know you have insulin resistance if you have high glucose levels in spite of high circulating insulin levels (or high insulin doses in type 1 diabetes).

- Insulin resistance is the loss of metabolic flexibility, where the body is predominantly running on carbohydrates from food and unable to use stored fat.

- When systems break down, the three musketeers become dysfunctional with toxic inflammatory involvement of body fat and the entire bloodstream.

For Bonus Materials, Visit the Website Here:

PART 2

THE FIRST WHEEL OF THE LIFESTYLE CAR: NUTRITION

2.1: The end of food confusion and addiction

This book doesn't have a single magic diet, because there isn't one. If there was one ideal diet in the world, we would all know exactly which one it is, and the global epidemics of type 2 diabetes and obesity would be cured. Each dieting philosophy insists it's the best; still, everyone hasn't embraced one way of eating. That means there is a lot of variation in what works for different people, what they find sustainable, what foods are available to them, and what they are able or willing to do in the context of their reality. Unfortunately, that hasn't been made clear—hopefully not on purpose.

As a result of not knowing how to customize their approach to nutrition, people end up wondering why the right answer for "everyone else" never works for them. People end up becoming consumers of various diets because they haven't found **the one**, *the* diet that *actually* works. People keep searching for answers because the previous attempt didn't work.

This steady need fuels innovation and commerce, and *that's* why new diets keep popping up.

While the marketplace keeps creating and selling cookie-cutter answers, this chapter and the ones that follow will teach you how to think about nutrition. Knowing how to think about food and eating will empower you with enough knowledge and body experience to design a custom approach to nutrition that works for you. Despite all the noise and confusion, there are many ways to succeed.

CAUTION: *Changing your food is a very powerful way to change your blood glucose levels. Do not do this without medical supervision. Your doctor needs to adjust your current medication to make sure you don't develop dangerously low blood glucose (hypoglycemia) as the levels come down with the changes you make.*

Food addiction

Rahul confessed to me that he had a weakness for junk food. He admitted that whenever he saw junk food, he wanted it. Once he started eating it, he could never stop at one bite. He always wanted more. Before he knew it, he would have finished a whole bag of chips without really deciding to.

I told him he was not weak but that he was, in fact, normal.

It's normal to feel addicted to addictive foods.

Just like it's normal to scrape your knee if you fall off your bicycle, because getting injured from that is not your personal failing, right?

Why don't you blame your scraped knee on a personal weakness, some moral or mental failure? Because no industry benefits from making you doubt your cycling ability. Nobody has invested *millions* of dollars into brainwashing you that you are flawed as a cyclist.

Food addiction is normal because millions of dollars of proprietary research have gone into actually making each fast-food product or snack addictive. Big Food companies collaborated with experts from the tobacco industry to make recipes addictive by increasing their salience (noticeability) and effect on the dopamine (reward) pathways in the brain. Tobacco marketing teams took over food marketing to influence buyers.[1]

You assume guilt and shame, thinking it's your weakness when you overeat junk, when in fact, the formula specifically creates insatiable cravings. The junk "food" has been designed to be hyper-palatable and to bypass "sensory-specific satiety (SSS)."

To understand the term SSS, think of a healthy vegetable or protein source. Let's assume it's spinach, dal, or meat. After you eat a certain amount of plain spinach, you will know you are done. Most people don't feel addicted to the point of overeating spinach. That's because the brain recognizes whole spinach and its sensory-specific satiety (SSS) level.

You are not mentally weak, and we know this because your **brain** recognizes natural food.

Social conditioning and marketing messages have convinced and brainwashed consumers that overconsumption happens purely as a result of individual weakness. Meanwhile food giants continue innovating new addictive recipes that have fats and carbohydrates combined in unnatural ratios that don't exist in real food.[2]

In comparison to spinach, I want you to think about french fries. Or popcorn. Every culture seems to have some variation of these "finger-licking-good" snacks and comfort foods, and most people don't stop at one. What are they made of? Carbs, salt, and fat.

If you were to eat those ingredients separately – the potato or corn by itself, the salt by itself, or the fat by itself– you would not find any of the ingredients addictive individually. Because your **brain** recognizes them when they are experienced one by one. It's the human-made *combinations* that are addictive because everything from the combination of flavors to the sound of opening the bag has been planned. The color, smell, and texture of each morsel are part of a **multisensory** experience—purposely created to override the "specificity" of **sensory-specific satiety**. Now, they have you hypnotized before you even take the first bite!

Scientists are paid by the food industry to run experiments and calculate the perfect formula to put inside a package. People are put in magnetic resonance imaging (MRI) machines to observe what part of the brain lights up when exposed to various artificial combinations of texture and flavor. Researchers are looking to hit the "bliss point" so precisely that they know you will love it, won't seem to get enough, will keep craving more, and will think it's all your fault. The formula is built so that there is no satiety from it, and you are willing to go for "all you can eat."

So the popular Hindi ad saying *"dil maange more,"* (which translates to "the heart wants more") should really say "we keep your brain wanting more."[*]

The "No one can eat just one," ad campaign was actually honest.[**] You were warned about getting hooked.

The latest research confirms that sugar and fat, when combined, create an additive hedonic (pleasurable) effect on the dopamine pathway. The sense of reward from a dopamine hit increases overeating compared to fat or sugar alone.[3] It makes it clear that the goals of fast-food corporations are directly at odds with the goals of preventive health care. And this is not a localized issue—countries around the world sell addictive foods, and we have the global diabetes epidemic to show for it.

Dr. Robert Lustig, a pediatric endocrinologist with special expertise in obesity, specifically obtained a master's degree in law so that he could impact the food industry through policy change.[4]

As Rahul thought about this, he said aloud, "And the more I stay addicted to food, the more I need medication. I just realized that even when visiting the pharmacy to pick up my diabetes medication, addictive foods are available for purchase at the checkout register! It seems like someone benefits twice from my suffering—when I buy junk and when I buy drugs! Is the fox guarding the henhouse?"

---

[*] Pepsi ad campaign in the late 90s showing Bollywood movie stars and Indian cricket players all wanting "more."

[**] Lay's Chips campaign in India featuring "Bet you can't eat just one"; see https://www.youtube.com/watch?v=dTVIrhnt5x4.

And while he wasn't wrong, just promising to cut out those addictive foods simply isn't enough to fix nutrition.

2.2: Why calorie-restricted diets fail

Recall from Part 1.5 how a high-insulin environment acts like an energy trap, where not only is your fuel being stored in the cells in a way that it can't be used, but it's also getting stored in toxic ways that are making you sick.

Enter: Mona.

Mona was a 55-year-old financial advisor who had lived with diabetes for over twenty years. Her food was always home-cooked. She believed in eating light meals, with fruit as the between-meals snack, so that she stayed below 1,200 calories per day. She suspected she wasn't getting enough calories, but she was afraid of gaining weight. She always carried chocolate and biscuits in her purse just in case her glucose level dropped in a work meeting. It had happened once, and the episode was so scary that she made sure to always eat some low-fat multigrain crackers or puffed rice snacks before stepping into long meetings. Not only did she dread weighing herself, but the fear of low-glucose reactions at work was making her anxiety even worse, and she felt trapped without a way to get off so many medications. Despite being a numbers woman, she couldn't get a grip on the numbers displayed on her glucometer or weighing scale.

Enter: Vicky.

Vicky was very concerned about his diabetes. He lost both of his parents to diabetes in their sixties, before they could even see his kids. He didn't want to suffer the way they did; he wanted a healthy life after retirement. He followed all of the advice of his doctors, who kept telling him to lose weight through diet and exercise. He did his research, read a lot about low-fat diets on the internet and was walking a few times a week. Despite the walks and eating small, frequent, low-calorie meals, he was still gaining weight, and his pants were getting tight around the waist. Still looking for answers, he decided to see me, because no matter what he tried, things seemed to be getting worse.

While we know that all weight loss eventually comes down to a calorie deficit, it's important to be clear about what a calorie is. Calories, more precisely, *kilocalories*, are human-made measurements of the heat that is generated when scientists take a particular food and burn it completely inside a sealed container. The method is called *bomb calorimetry*. Nowadays, food manufacturers don't literally burn food to see what heat it generates; they derive calorie estimates from the known macronutrients (carbs, proteins, and fat). A gram of carbohydrate and protein will generate four calories each and a gram of fat generates nine. This is taught in biology class.

But the thing biology class doesn't make clear about calorie deficits is that the body doesn't communicate internally via calories. *There are no calorie receptors in the body.*

The body has evolved to sense, interpret, and signal nutrient availability for millennia before both the bomb calorimeter and processed food were invented.

How?

Through hormones, especially insulin.

Every time you eat, your body sees fuel coming and releases insulin. The higher the carbs in the meal, the higher the insulin response. This keeps you hungry and wanting to eat something throughout the day.

Why?

Because carbohydrates turn directly into glucose after they are digested, giving you a short rise, then a crash in energy; and because low-calorie often means low-fat (since per gram, fat has the most calories), you *lose the satiety benefits of natural healthy fat.* When a diet is low-calorie, not only is it low in fat, but is often also low in protein, the other macronutrient that offers satiety.

This means that eating small, frequent, low-calorie, carbohydrate-predominant meals causes repeated insulin responses that keep telling the body to "store fuel and store fat." *The stored fuel can only be used when insulin levels go down again, but the small frequent meals keep insulin levels up.* The combination of receiving insufficient calories plus the inability to access stored calories (due to the insulin lock), *forces the metabolic rate to slow down*; the body also loses lean muscle—especially on a low-calorie diet without resistance training or adequate protein.

Not only are you *storing fat and losing muscle,* but when the diet ends, you regain the weight back in the form of fat—and then some. The number on the scale doesn't tell you about this bad transaction and leaves you with a worsening body composition. If that wasn't medically bad enough, the entire experience of a low-calorie diet is usually miserable because you are feeling hungry and tired all the time.

Like I said, bad deal.

So really, it's no wonder that calorie-restricted diets haven't solved the world's obesity and diabetes epidemics. They don't address the carbohydrate-insulin hormone imbalance, the metabolic impact or the psychological experience.

Even though the debate still rages on between the energy balance model (EBM; calories in, calories out [CICO]) versus the carbohydrate-insulin model (CIM), we can thank the CIM for explaining why low-carbohydrate (under 130 grams of carbs/day) and keto (under 20–50 g of carbs per day) diets have worked so well at improving diabetes.[5,6]

This research has informed the methods that I have shared with my patients. My practice is centered on discussing the differences between calorie-restricted diets and fasting (more on that in Part 6). We then customize everything to patients' personal preferences, lifestyle needs, and how their body responds. I have seen people succeed on less than 100-130 grams of carbs per day.

So with that in mind: What were Mona and Vicky to do?

Both Mona and Vicky had tried the low-calorie approach and their diabetes had only gotten worse over time. They were gaining fat around the belly even though they were eating less food, pointing to slowing metabolic rates and worsening insulin resistance.

With repeated weight-loss attempts, they remained overweight but undermuscled; this unhealthy body composition is called *sarcopenic obesity* (SO).[7]

They were surprised when I told them how, despite being overweight, they were malnourished in terms of the primary macronutrient—protein.

I had them stop weighing themselves every day. Instead of counting calories, I had them count protein. When we found that they weren't getting enough protein, I told them they needed more of it. If you start by telling a person who is hungry all day to eat less of the carbs they have been surviving on, they will probably not like you and will probably not last very long following that advice!

The word *protein* originates from the Greek word *proteios*, which means "first place" or "primary." The Greek physicians knew how essential protein was to build everything that we are made of, and by getting enough protein on your plate at each meal *first*, you will be able to reduce your carbs naturally without feeling deprived or hungry.

As many people suffer from protein deficiency, the rest of this chapter is focused on the importance of counting protein and how to integrate the practice into whatever eating pattern you prefer, making it more effortless and therefore sustainable to reduce carbs.

Unfortunately, many patients protest when I tell them they need more protein, or that they may be deficient. A 2023 review of the Indian protein deficiency epidemic confirms that more than 80 percent of Indians fail to reach sixty grams of protein per day, and yet these patients assume their diet is fine for one or more of the following reasons:[8]

- **They have been eating home-cooked meals.**

Sorry, but eating traditional light, low-fat home-cooked meals does not rule out a carbohydrate-predominant, protein-deficient diet.

- **Their plate is "balanced" by following the plate method.**

I actually used to recommend the plate method around 12 years ago! It was a better tool than nothing at all, and I even had a laminated printout of a portioned plate on display at my hospital desk to generate awareness about portion control. Now that I have been counting people's macros for over a decade, I know that simply eyeballing a plate will often result in protein deficiency. I teach patients how to explicitly count the grams until they know how to eyeball enough protein. The plate method is also risky as it tends to keep carbohydrates as the majority macronutrient, suggesting that they are essential even though they are not.

- **Their blood tests show normal albumin and globulin levels in the blood.**

By the time a blood test shows low albumin levels indicating malnutrition, they are already extremely ill from it. Most people walking around with protein deficiencies are not starving for calories, but their cells are very starved, or malnourished, in terms of protein. Remember, a gram of carb and a gram of protein both give four calories each, but protein is essential while carbs are not.

None of these are reason enough to assume you are getting enough protein, especially because, I typically find out my patients are malnourished by going through their food logs and counting everything they eat. They say health is wealth. I say you should know your daily protein balance as well as you know your bank balance. You probably want both health and wealth for a comfortable retirement.

If you have never consciously ensured that you are getting enough protein, then **before telling yourself protein counting is not for you** and moving on to the next segment, **check if you have any of the symptoms described in the next section.**

2.3: Symptoms of protein deficiency and adult protein malnutrition syndrome

Most people don't know how to count their protein intake on the tips of their fingers (although they should). Most doctors don't know how to count them either (and I have interviewed many nutritionists who are not adept at counting macros from a patient's food log). The good news is that it's a skill that can be learned even if you aren't a health professional. Most of us are creatures of habit, and we end up eating similar things across a span of a few weeks. Once you get familiar with counting the top foods that give you sufficient protein, you will know more about nutrition than most doctors around you and can alleviate any of the symptoms of protein deficiency you may be suffering from. The following symptoms can be caused or worsened by protein malnutrition:

- Chronic fatigue and lethargy
- Feeling hungry, having low energy, and feeling weak all day
- Poor muscle gains despite exercise
- Delayed recovery from workouts
- Muscle loss, skinny arms and legs, "looking weak"
- Low immunity, repeated infections
- Delayed healing from injury
- Chronic body pain, joint pain, and muscle aches
- Digestive complaints, chronic diarrhea, bloating, and gas
- Hair falling out, hair thinning, poor hair quality

- Reduced skin quality
- High uric acid (due to a carbohydrate-predominant diet)
- Poor sleep, low mood
- Fat-loss plateau, especially stubborn fat around the waist
- Swelling and puffiness under the skin from water retention (edema)
- Slowing metabolism
- Chronic inflammation

If you see your symptoms listed here, you could be from among the group who fail to reach sixty grams of protein per day, and any of these symptoms might have taken you to different medical specialist doctors. They run tests, say nothing much is wrong on the reports, and send you off with various pills based on the predominant symptoms. This makes it entirely possible for most adults with protein malnutrition and insulin resistance to not receive an actual diagnosis.

Based on the most major symptoms, they may get an unsatisfying label of chronic fatigue syndrome, fibromyalgia, fat inclusion myositis, unexplained myopathy, mixed connective tissue disease, adrenal fatigue syndrome, or irritable bowel syndrome. None of these have a clear cause or cure, but they affect daily living and quality of life, and tend to get better with "lifestyle changes." This one problem of protein malnutrition can result in you seeing many doctors and gathering multiple, often disjointed opinions. Sometimes it seems like lifestyle change is the "last resort" when there isn't a miracle drug to prescribe. Often, these "alternative medicine", lifestyle medicine or functional medicine approaches are explored by frustrated patients seeking answers when they are no longer feeling helped by "mainstream" medicine.

Essentially, there are various medical specialists and alternative healers out there who are busy treating symptoms of protein malnutrition—whether they know it or not. This is particularly true in a vegetarian-predominant country like India. The fact that it's so prevalent makes you wonder why there aren't more diagnoses of protein malnutrition.

Adult Protein Malnutrition Syndrome is a term I created to explain what I was seeing in patients going about their daily lives with protein deficiency and insulin resistance.

Yes—I made it up. The reason we don't see more diagnoses of protein malnutrition is because this isn't a condition doctors are taught to routinely look for in walking and talking people in the outpatient setting. The only time doctors come across protein deficiencies in medical training tends to be during extreme situations.

In my final year of medical school, for example, I was on a pediatrics rotation and we had **one** chapter on severe protein malnutrition. We studied pictures of little kids from rural India and Africa with skinny arms and legs but bloated tummies.* Their skin was like paper, and their hair was thin. They were swollen from water retention, barely surviving on low-quality carbohydrates, and their weak muscles were wasting away from insufficient protein. The treatment?

Careful and measured *refeeding*, so that their digestive tracts could learn to process richer nutrient loads.

When it comes to adults, protein needs were only considered in intensive care units (ICUs) when patients hadn't eaten in days as they were fighting deadly ailments. Some of the sickest patients struggled to retain protein in the right body compartments, rapidly losing muscle mass *despite* us attempting to refeed them via tubes into the stomach or directly into their veins. In both extremes, whether caring for babies in famines or adults in ICUs, nutrition had to be monitored carefully.

But since I didn't specialize in pediatrics, nor did I work in ICUs, I didn't think about protein much for years.

As I started focusing on lifestyle and nutrition in my endocrine practice, I began noticing how patients' bodies responded after I insisted they got enough protein to proceed with their diabetes management. Some of them were able to increase protein intake without any hiccups. Some (especially those with a plant-based or vegetarian diet) often took much longer to adapt to sufficient protein in terms of satiety and gut symptoms. The folks adding pure animal protein seemed to have fewer digestive complaints as they ramped up protein.

What was consistent, whether they took the plant or the animal approach, was that many of the seventeen symptoms in the previous list started disappearing as their protein intake started approaching target levels.

But I wasn't aiming to treat those symptoms!

I was just correcting obvious malnutrition and aiming for better glucose levels with less medication. The body did the rest and didn't stop at reversing just insulin resistance. It seemed to be using the protein to fix other "vague" problems, too.

My entire outlook on diabetes began to shift as I looked around and saw an entire population of protein-malnourished adults walking about in society, with waistlines increased by harmful fat. I realized how many of them were merely in between two extremes: not sick enough to be in the hospital, and not well enough to thrive.

But how did they all get there?

---

* India still has one of the worst rates of childhood malnutrition in the world, ranking 94th among 107 countries in the Global Hunger index 2020, with approximately one in three malnourished children globally being Indian. See: Mohan, Viswanathan, Vasudevan Sudha, Shanmugam Shobana, Rajagopal Gayathri, and Kamala Krishnaswamy. "Are Unhealthy Diets Contributing to the Rapid Rise of Type 2 Diabetes in India?" Translational Nutrition, 2023. https://doi.org/10.1016/j.tjnut.2023.02.028.

While seeing patients and making recommendations, I've noticed that I get this question at least fifty times a month: "How long will I have to keep this high-protein diet? Won't it be harmful long term to eat so much protein?"

After a thousand times, I realized that there was a major **behavioral** component to the phenomena.

Besides the other lifestyle factors that everyone faces globally, the replacement of quality protein with cheaper processed powdered carbohydrates is pushing India ahead of most of the world in the diabetes epidemic. This swap is influencing India's metabolic crisis, but word on the street seems to justify misplaced fear, exaggerating false rumors surrounding protein. Being unscientific, inaccurate or partial truths twisted out of context doesn't stop alarming claims from becoming headlines on social media and news outlets. These repeated impressions eventually influence people to **behave** in a way where they actively avoid protein, completely missing two key things. First, that protein is a vital building block and second, that they might just be protein malnourished.

2.4: How is protein a building block?

We have all heard that DNA carries our genetic code. Do you accept that you were originally made from just one strand of DNA from each of your biological parents?

How did that DNA become *you*?

DNA stands for **deoxyribonucleic acid**, where an exact sequence of nucleotides makes a gene, and each gene contributes to the blueprint of your body through specific codes for specific amino acids. If you string amino acids together in a particular sequence, you'll get a specific protein.*

That's it. *DNA codes for protein and protein alone.*

For example, when your body was being made, the DNA strands you got from your biological parents at conception had to decide if the nose would be like your mother, your father, or someone else from the family. Based on that outcome, the protein instructions determining nose shape (different amounts of cartilage in different proportions with different types of skin folds and skin color) would be laid down with precise design instructions, and you would be born displaying your unique version of the family nose.

But DNA doesn't just determine what you look like. Your body is constantly observing the internal and external environment. It decides what response is needed. That information dynamically guides the intelligent DNA blueprint to open and close relevant sections of code to manufacture the necessary proteins (like deciding which files from your laptop to select for printing and how many copies to make). Everything your living body does is via DNA-protein signaling. Everything.

Too sunny outside? Let's open the DNA segment for melanin (the natural skin pigment protein that makes skin dark). The DNA prints some extra melanin copies to make your skin darker (a suntan) so that we prevent sunburn.

Chronically dehydrated? Your hydration-sensing system will detect the imbalance and send signals to the DNA segments to manufacture sophisticated hormone responses for thirst and water recycling.

---

* Fun fact: Insulin was the first protein to be sequenced and this led to the Nobel Prize being awarded to Sanger in 1958 for their work on protein sequencing.

Knowing how vital proteins are, it becomes apparent that if you don't get enough protein in your diet, your DNA might struggle to continue making healthy proteins.

To understand how protein deficiency can completely mess up whatever your entire being is trying to do via your DNA, let's imagine you are trying to print a file that's on your laptop. Perhaps you want to print two color copies of a specific image. You open the folder, select the file and send the instructions to the printer.

Imagine the printer is running out of ink.

You might end up with a printout that's unacceptable. Maybe you can't see the image clearly, or the color is distorted. Or you run out of the correct paper quality so you feed in a cheap substitute, which misfeeds into the machine, gets partially chewed up, and gets thrown out all crumpled and damaged.

That's what it's like if your DNA is trying to convert genetic blueprints into healthy protein copies but doesn't have enough high-quality raw material to make the final product correctly. You end up with damaged, dysfunctional proteins. The body is then built with unhealthy structural and functional molecules, and we begin to see how those seventeen symptoms can be explained by a protein-deficient diet.

Would you want to keep taking prescription drugs for chronic symptoms, or would you want to treat a major root cause by fixing malnutrition?

If protein is necessary for so many life functions, then it's time we dispel the myth that you only need a lot of protein if you're trying to build muscle. The truth is that **you need these building blocks even if you're not a "bodybuilder."** So for those of us who are *not* bodybuilders and *also* are not getting enough protein—what's the healthy medium?

2.5: How much protein is enough, and why replace carbs with protein?

Most nutrition guidelines mention we need 0.8 grams of protein per kilogram of body weight (g/kg BW) per day based on the US Recommended Dietary Allowance (RDA). At levels below 0.8 g/kg BW (below 0.4 gram protein per pound BW per day), you would be considered officially malnourished.*

Using the RDA as my guide, I prescribed the target of 0.8 g/kg BW for my patients for many years. Over time, I noticed my patients weren't gaining enough muscle mass despite hitting their protein goal and putting effort into their strength training—particularly the vegetarians.

Because the RDA was calculated by factoring in nitrogen balance (not amino acid metabolism) and these calculations were based on the data from young, healthy males in their twenties, experts claim that the RDA doesn't reflect the needs of the average person above the age of forty. Research now strongly suggests that the current **guideline of 0.8 g/kg BW is is insufficient** for optimal organ function.[9] Based on this, I have updated my recommendation for protein intake, and now state that it should be at least 1.2 grams of protein per kilogram of body weight (g/kg BW) per day divided across the major meals.

We know now that the efficiency of protein use goes down with aging. In one study, researchers observed elderly people in their seventies over three years. They compared those who ate 0.8 g/kg BW per day to those who consumed 1.2 g/kg BW of protein per day and found that the group with the higher protein intake lost less muscle mass over those three years. This reinforces the importance of higher protein intake to prevent the muscle loss (sarcopenia) associated with aging.[10]

A higher protein intake of 1.6 g/kg BW has been found to be safe and effective at preserving muscle while allowing fat loss. Research has proven that high-

---

* To convert body weight in pounds to kilograms, divide by 2.2

er protein combined with exercise provided more total weight loss, specifically more fat loss and less muscle loss in the group that supported exercise with 1.6 g/kg BW versus 0.8 g/kg BW.[11]

The protein intake of 1.6 g/kg BW recommended by experts, is for an average, healthy adult. For those who have diabetic kidney disease, the minimum recommended protein intake is 0.8 g/kg BW per day, not less than that.[12] Sometimes people hear you have kidney disease and just knee-jerk tell you to "reduce protein" without confirming whether you are even at the 0.8 g/kg BW! Without actually counting your intake, you will not be having an intelligent discussion.

Most people I work with are actually getting way below 0.8g/kg BW and need to increase their intake to fulfill their minimum needs, but if someone is on dialysis, they need 1–1.2 g/kg BW per day, which is higher than the 0.8 recommended to patients with stage three or higher diabetic chronic kidney disease (CKD). This is because patients on dialysis see increased protein wasting, according to the *Standards of Care in Diabetes*—2024 guidelines published by the American Diabetes Association.[13]

My recommendations are for those of you who are not on dialysis or suffering from kidney damage. Before I give my thoughts, it may be helpful to note that people have safely consumed high-protein diets of 1.6 to 2 g/kg BW per day without any kidney damage.[14] If you have any anxieties surrounding the change, you can do this under the supervision of a well-informed professional to ensure your nutrition is balanced.

With that in mind, I recommend that you **start the day with around thirty grams of protein in the first meal.** By breaking your overnight fast, you activate the **mechanistic target of rapamycin** (mTOR), which is an important protein that senses nutrient availability and promotes cell growth, division, and survival by blocking protein breakdown. Healthy muscle growth happens when there are *alternating periods of high and low mechanistic target of rapamycin complex 1* (mTORC1) activity, which is naturally the case with healthy feeding and fasting cycles respectively.[15]

I tell my patients to aim **for approximately twenty to thirty-five grams of protein per meal (depending on their weight), over approximately three to four meals per day**, providing 2.2–3 grams of the essential branched-chain amino acid leucine, per meal, to stimulate mTORC1 and build muscle protein.16

Having a protein-focused breakfast might take some effort, especially because the food industry has us thinking of mostly carbohydrate options for our mornings, but working on it helps my patients reach their goals. Previous research has indicated that there isn't any added benefit of consuming more than forty-five grams of protein in a single meal,, so the idea is to spread your protein target evenly throughout the day while getting enough at the main meals without feeling too hungry or too stuffed.[17,18] This is particularly true for people eating plant-based protein.

Fresh research, however, has just challenged the existence of this protein ceiling, asserting that there might not even be an upper limit to the body's anabolic response to protein intake and that perhaps higher amounts of slow-release protein can still be used without being "wasted."[19] This all goes to show how our understanding keeps evolving, and scientific research is the only way to continue to study and learn how our metabolism can be optimized. While more research is being done on that, it's been shown that reducing carbs by sixty grams per day and increasing protein by the same sixty grams per day can reverse prediabetes.

We can see this in the results of a six-month trial of men and women with obesity.[20] This study focused on people with obesity, minimal physical activity, and prediabetes. The experiment showed that shifting the diet from approximately 60 grams of protein to 120 grams of protein per day while reducing carbs from approximately 220 grams to 160 grams per day caused positive health changes that, if you're reading this, you are most certainly interested in! They found that with these dietary changes, the study participants showed:

- 100 percent remission of prediabetes
- Increased lean muscle percentage
- Reduced fat mass percentage
- Weight loss
- Improved insulin sensitivity
- Improved cardiovascular risk factors
- Reduced markers of inflammation (cytokines)
- Reduced oxidative stress

Isn't that impressive? When you realize that one gram of protein has the same calories as one gram of carbs (four calories each), and they were eating the same caloric amounts, just in different protein and carb densities, it seems so simple!

But realistically, most people don't know what sixty grams of carbs or protein looks like. This is confirmed by most of my Indian patients with insulin resistance; most of them don't know they are getting less than sixty grams of protein per day when we first meet. That realization led us to design an app for our patients to help them understand the grams of carbs and protein in their food—**but, how can you do this for yourself?** Most people assume there's a perfect diet, so they ask:

2.6 So is the keto, carnivore, or vegan diet the best?

That's nutrition politics.

Polarized protein positions.

Extreme ideologies on social media, with influencers canceling other dietary approaches that don't match their own.

Rigid elimination rules.

None of these helped my patients design a sustainable lifestyle or food plan that worked for them. They all told me, "I tried. It worked briefly but I couldn't sustain it. My fault."

Despite trying their best, these people were left blaming themselves for the lack of results, believing perhaps that one of the extreme positions was the "right" answer, even if they couldn't follow it.

To make things worse, the system often doubts them by saying, "They must be cheating or not trying hard enough."

Fanatic supporters of one particular eating type will demonize a person who didn't get results, insisting that their own form of dietary "ism" is the only proper way to eat. People don't know whether to listen to the clinical MDs or the PhDs because everyone is saying something different.

It may have been the same for you, and perhaps that's why you are reading this book.

*The right diet for you is one you can sustain because **diabetes is a long game.*** I see no point in asking you to align with a dietary pattern that doesn't resonate with or work for you.

If you reach the top of Mount Everest, it won't matter whether you got there by taking the northern or the southern approach. What matters is what transpired between you and the mountain. Once you achieve metabolic health (normal blood work; inch loss from the waist; increasing energy, stamina, and strength; increased muscle mass; and feeling more alive and healthy with the lowest possible medication dose), it won't matter how you got there. Success commands respect by speaking for itself.

So, here's my position. And *please*, whether you choose to follow a keto, vegan, whole-food, or carnivore diet or any other approach—treat other people's food preferences with kindness and respect. Nobody is trying to melt our planet. Nobody wants to make the next generation sick. Nobody is trying to commit suicide through their food choices. Nobody is purposely trying to suffer. If you feel inspired to share your perspective and perhaps "educate" someone about your views, they will be more likely to listen to you if you speak to them with compassion. Assuming others have bad intentions is not a helpful strategy. Guilting or shaming others isn't a durable way of advancing your agenda—if you truly have one.

Regardless of whichever protein philosophy you chose, **start with baby steps** towards getting enough protein. **Visualize yourself eating that food** for the rest of your life. How does the visual make you feel? If you decide you want to eat more eggs, visualize doing that for the rest of your life. Do you like the idea of eating more eggs? If you hate the idea of eating eggs, you are unlikely to keep eating them and they probably won't be of much help to you, so there is no point forcing yourself to eat them even for a day. If you enjoy your new protein option, then you are more likely to eat it again, because you enjoyed the process. That's how getting enough protein can become a habit, and from there, a new lifestyle. It's not really sustainable to keep doing things you don't enjoy. Aim to get more **whole, high-quality, unprocessed, naturally-sourced** sources to increase your protein intake. That's one truth all of these -isms agree on—get enough high-quality protein at each meal.

As you increase protein, you will feel more satiated. Hunger levels will drop, and your ability to eat previously "normal" portions of food will reduce rapidly. This is how your satiety hormones naturally regulate portion control, and **animal protein is one of the easiest and fastest ways to achieve your daily protein goals.** I see the least digestive trouble and the most rapid improvements in metabolic health when people go this route. It's also much easier to stay low-carb and feel satiated when using animal protein versus plant protein. So, if animal protein works with your religious or cultural beliefs, your body will respond rapidly with positive results.

Keto means less than twenty to fifty grams of carbs per day, which is easier to maintain on an animal-based protein diet, and my patients who can achieve it feel great very quickly. They usually enjoy it so much they prefer to stay on it as much as possible.

When it comes to vegetarians or vegans, they will need to put more effort and thought into meeting their protein target due to a few unique challenges. With vegetarianism being a prevalent and deeply-rooted concept in Indian culture, as well as being a vegetarian myself, I have to work creatively within these patient preferences. They have come up with interesting ways to sneak more protein into their traditional recipes. Personally, I have found my own low-carb balance to get enough protein while building muscle and maintaining metabolic health as a vegetarian.

All this leads me to believe, besides the other lifestyle and genetic causes, that the predominantly vegetarian diet is pushing more Indians toward diabetes. **The vegetarian diet, as a default, is lacking balance between protein and carbs, and it's harder for people to reduce carbohydrate intake on a plant-based diet.**

That means **nutrition changes alone are usually not enough for a vegetarian to completely turn around insulin resistance** or uncontrolled diabetes. Keto-vegetarian or very low-carb vegetarian will bring glucose levels down, but this can be a difficult lifestyle to sustain and may also compromise nutrition if you are not careful. That's why **you should work with a professional to make sure you are getting enough nutrients**, especially because many plant-based sources lack some essential amino acids and are therefore considered incomplete protein sources. There are a few exceptions, including unprocessed soybeans, quinoa, and a few others that provide all the amino acids, and are therefore complete proteins.

Researchers are still learning about the bioavailability of amino acids and differences in quality among various plant-based protein sources.

Through research, we have learned that there are certain antinutrients in plant-based sources, and further study has taught us that the antinutrient effects can be reduced through soaking, and other cooking methods.[21] On the other hand, for example, we know that processing a grain or legume can reduce the bioavailability of protein, but we aren't sure by how much.

No matter how much we have learned, or how many questions we have, we still need to make food decisions every day until more research is presented. But until then, I like to tell my patients that our hunter-gatherer ancestors were probably flexitarian omnivores. They didn't have the protective comfort of technology, transportation, or electricity, and probably ate when the opportunity arose, so it's likely that our return to health in modern times will take more than choosing one diet of eating ancient grains or meats alone.

Ultimately, nutrition happens to be one of the most powerful initial lifestyle changes to start with, and while we will build on this in later chapters, there are a few things I want you to take away from this. I want you to remember to **take baby steps,** and **do what feels right for you** because if you enjoy it today, *you might repeat it tomorrow*. Understanding that there is *no single right* way to turn around your diabetes is the first step to making the best decision for you.

2.7: The different diet preferences: From theory to reality

L ife happens.

How you **choose** to show up in life is your **lifestyle**.

Daily **choices** form **habits**.

Small **tweaks** in daily choices form **new habits**.

Sustainable tweaks build a **sustainable lifestyle**.

This is what I am sharing.

I don't want the knowledge gained from this book to become one more diet in your life, because I am not here to blame anyone for their situation. I want to empower you to try changes that you could see yourself living with every day. This is why it is so important that we start from individuals' current reality and not from some perfect hypothetical rulebook. It's much more powerful to begin change from within the messy reality of a person's actual day-to-day choices.

With that in mind, I would like to discuss how different types of diets have helped different kinds of patients turn around their diabetes.

The Flexitarian–Raghu

Raghu was a sixty-one-year-old man who had been struggling with obesity for over twenty years. He had tried every calorie-restricted diet, seen every top dietitian in the city, and had developed diabetes five years before I met him. By the time we met, he was tired of following diets and taking the increasing list of medications.

In Raghu, I saw a man who had faithfully followed all the advice he was given. Years of dieting had conditioned him to choose low-fat, low-calorie options, leaving him tired and hungry all day long, and yet, he hadn't given up. Trying ten different diets isn't something a person does if they are not interested in losing weight! He had decided, once again, to work with us to find a solution. Talk about determination to get better!

After my team and I explained our protein guidelines to him, he was struggling to visualize how to incorporate these ideas into his day.

Being vegetarian on most days of the week, he realized through using our app that he was not even reaching half of his protein target, and his food was adding more carbohydrates than protein. We suggested some tweaks in his options, giving us a plan that looked similar to this:

Original food combo	Protein	Carbs	Modified food quantity	Protein	Carbs
Breakfast: Oats + 2 fresh fruits + half cup milk	15	45	Breakfast: Half the oats + half the fruit + more milk + 1 scoop whey protein supplement	35	25
Lunch or dinner: 2 slices of bread/roti + 3 cubes paneer + half cup daal + half cup french beans + half cup homemade yogurt + half serving of soybeans	26	47	Lunch or dinner: 1 slice bread/roti + 6 cubes paneer + half cup daal + 1 cup french beans + half cup homemade yogurt + 1 full serving of soybeans	47	37

Originally, his carb intake at breakfast was forty-five grams from fruit and oats, with no dedicated protein source besides the quarter-cup of milk in the oats. We suggested reducing this carb intake (fruit and oats) by half and adding a high-quality protein source of his choice to the breakfast, perhaps a few eggs or a protein shake as a last resort if he didn't have enough whole-food options to complete the protein requirements.*

At lunch or dinner, he was having either two slices of bread or two roti with half a cup each of whole soybeans, dal, yogurt, and paneer (fresh Indian cheese). We suggested doubling the quantity of low-carb protein sources, such as soybeans and paneer, while simultaneously reducing the bread or roti intake to half.

---

* I always encourage whole unprocessed food first. If someone chooses to be vegetarian or vegan for personal reasons, they still need to get their daily protein, and they need to be much more deliberate about their choices at each meal. In a world of trade-offs, this usually means needing a protein supplement to complete the protein deficit. We will discuss how to select a supplement in a few pages. Find a way to get protein to target that works for your beliefs and values! That's the only way for it to become a habit.

As a flexitarian, there were days of the week that he was having animal protein, such as meat, fish, or poultry and he used those as low-carb ways to replace the daal and yogurt to get more protein.

If he was traveling for work on a vegetarian day, he ordered paneer paratha and asked the chef to give him one extra paneer stuffing ball to be served *without* the outer dough covering. The staff were initially confused, but as long as he was paying for two parathas, the restaurant didn't mind. This way, he doubled his paneer and kept the carb intake the same while enjoying one yummy hot paneer paratha!

This simple switch in his existing menu caused a frictionless but powerful improvement in his daily protein totals, while easily reducing the carbohydrate load. He also found it easier to achieve his protein targets on days when he included more nonvegetarian food in his menu.[*]

The Vegan–Maitri

Maitri brought me an additional challenge of wanting to pursue a vegan lifestyle in addition to the desire to reverse her insulin resistance. She also had a traveling lifestyle and realized that the mainstream food and travel industries were not helping her health goals, and she didn't want to be at their mercy anymore; so she needed an approach that would work both at home and also in a hotel room.

We really had to get creative here.

In my experience, it's almost *impossible* to stay low-carb and get protein to 1.2 g/kg BW per day over the long term without a supplement. She did some trial and error to find a plant-based protein supplement that she liked enough to consume consistently and carry along in her luggage. For her, it was important to find one that had a combination of protein isolates from quinoa, pea, and brown rice, so that the entire amino acid profile was complete.

Once Maitri made some switches to her meals to get her protein intake to the target level, this is what her meals looked like:

---

[*] Unique terminology for Indian eating preferences: Pure vegetarian means plant based and dairy are OK but eggs and gelatin are not OK. Eggetarian means plant based plus eggs and dairy are OK. Nonvegetarian means plant based is OK; poultry, seafood, shellfish, red meat, eggs, and dairy are OK

Original food combo	Protein	Carbs	Modified food quantity	Protein	Carbs
Breakfast: 1 cup poha (cooked rice flakes) or cornflakes with oat milk and 1 cheela (savory lentil crepe)	6	45	Breakfast: 2 cheelas with pea protein supplement in the batter + olive oil	30	50
Lunch or dinner: 1 cup rice + half cup kidney beans + half cup green salad	8	60	Lunch or dinner: sprinkle rice on top of 1 cup kidney beans + half cup green salad + nuts, seeds, and nut butter + avocado + 1 scoop plant-based protein supplement	43	40

This helped her protein intake reach closer to the target while the carbohydrate totals also stayed similar. She was able to lower her carb intake on days that she replaced the legumes with lower-carb protein from soybean, tofu, or tempeh. At home, Maitri started increasing the size of the tofu in her homemade stuffed tofu paratha (stuffed wheat flatbread) so that the dough ball was smaller than the tofu stuffing ball.

The Animal-based diet–Layla

Layla had spent years avoiding animal products at each meal because she had been conditioned to avoid red meat, shrimp, and pan-fried fish daily. She loved these foods, but thought they were bad for her heart. Once we discussed how we don't have (and probably won't have in the near future) any clean, randomized, long-term dietary trials on any diet being ideal, and that it makes sense to eat as naturally as possible, her decision became a lot easier.

Here is how Layla changed her diet:

Original food combo	Protein	Carbs	Modified food quantity	Protien	Carbs
Breakfast: 1 chapati or 1 slice bread + 1 egg white + 1 fruit	4	35	Breakfast: 1 almond flour roti + chicken mince patties with whole eggs	48	0
Lunch or dinner: 1 cheela + 1 cup chickpeas or legumes + green salad + grilled fish/chicken twice a week	22 (vegetarian days), 47 (animal protein days)	60	Lunch or dinner: red meat curry or grilled fish/chicken + green vegetables + 1 fruit	40	15

She decided to choose naturally-raised, fresh meat that wasn't overcooked along with poultry and wild caught fatty fish. She made her roti with almond flour instead of wheat because she wanted to keep a roti in her daily diet, and she kept one fruit at lunch as her carb of choice. She would occasionally eat dessert when out with friends, but it started tasting too sweet after a few weeks, even with the keto options. Her glucose numbers came down very rapidly just by making these changes in her foods.

Eventually, she didn't want the roti and moved to a mostly animal protein–based diet. Her need for dessert disappeared rapidly. She reached a point where she was eating less than fifty grams of carbs per day and felt better than she had in years. I had to rapidly adjust her medication accordingly to make sure she didn't experience severe low glucose levels (hypoglycemia), which was made possible by closely tracking her numbers as she made her dietary changes.

Layla, like all of my current patients, was using our app to track her food choices.

Before my own app was launched, my patients and I relied on available food-tracking apps to log food. On one hand, these apps helped patients learn how their meals were mostly carbs with very little protein or healthy fat. This explained why they were hungry all the time.

On the other hand, most people got distracted by the calorie count or weight-loss targets, and tried keeping their calories under some arbitrary number suggested by the app even though I wasn't asking them to. These apps also did not establish a person's emotional and social relationships with their food. Many apps came with minimal or low-quality coaching support that was disconnected from the medical care team, and therefore, was not safe for a person on diabetes medication.

Some of the top apps even had accuracy issues, with nutrition data being crowdsourced from users, and therefore, you could search for a slice of bread, a roti, or a bowl of rice, and get fifteen different macro counts. I was looking at noisy data and could not be sure whether my patients were selecting what they really ate.

My team and I finally decided to make our own app to help our patients log their food more accurately and focus on the things that helped them build deeper awareness about how their choices were affecting their daily changes in mood and hunger. Using the app data to guide coaching calls with our healthcare team gives people the incentive to log their food diligently because they know a trusted human being on the other side is studying the data. The app has been a success over the last three years and user generated feedback is helping us improve its features so users can track their progress, and learn how their different lifestyle choices are impacting their health.

Through this data and the constant analysis of our patients' symptoms, decisions and outcomes, we have been able to identify some common causes of all-day hunger, and also have the data to support the solutions.

2.8: Common causes and solutions for all-day hunger or cravings

A s patients came to us, we would track their entire journey. When we compared their original diet and symptoms to their modified results, we realized that while they were all coming to us for the same reason (feeling hungry all day)—their hunger was being triggered in different ways. Without the data and the volume and diversity of patients, we may not have realized how many causes of hunger we were solving.

If you are trying to turn diabetes around but find yourself losing the battle due to hunger and cravings, this list of common causes and their solutions may be a helpful place to start:

- **Cause of hunger:** High carb intake, 100+ grams/day

Treat the root cause by reducing your carb intake *after* confirming with your doctor that your medication profile is safe to treat your diabetes with nutrition therapy and therapeutic carbohydrate restriction (TCR).

- **Cause of hunger:** High glucose levels (hyperglycemia)

Treat the root cause *by reducing your carb intake after* confirming with your doctor that it's safe to treat your diabetes with nutrition therapy.

- **Cause of hunger:** Crashing glucose levels, from an uncontrolled high back toward normal

Treat the root cause by *seeing your doctor to reduce the medication* that causes low glucose. The rapid fall of glucose can trigger cravings even before you hit a true low blood glucose.

- **Cause of hunger:** High insulin dose causing insulin resistance making stored fuel inaccessible

Treat the root cause by *seeing your doctor to adjust insulin and reduce* *carb intake* under medical supervision.

- **Cause of hunger:** Low glucose levels (hypoglycemia = below 70 mg/dL or 3.8 mmol/L)

Treat the root cause by discussing with your doctor immediately to *adjust medication/insulin before reducing carb intake*, as **hypoglycemia is a medical emergency** that needs to be treated with simple, easy-to-absorb carbs at that moment.

- **Cause of hunger:** Poor sleep quality and quantity

Treat the root cause by *improving sleep hygiene* and seeing your doctor to *decide if you need testing for sleep apnea* (see Part 3).

- **Cause of hunger:** Insufficient healthy fat/calorie/energy intake

Treat the root cause by increasing natural healthy fat intake to the point of satiety (see list coming in a few sections).

- **Cause of hunger:** Insufficient protein intake (possibly insufficient intake of the essential amino acid tryptophan)

Treat the root cause by achieving at least 1.2 grams of protein per kg BW per day (0.8 if kidney disease) of good quality complete protein.

- **Cause of hunger:** Sodium losses after reducing carbs

Treat the root cause by monitoring salt intake and blood pressure (BP) so that your doctor can adjust BP medication.[22] High insulin levels cause sodium retention. Many people experience a lower BP after going low-carb because the lower insulin requirements cause the body to throw out excess sodium in the urine. *Salt losses can trigger cravings* that feel like hunger. Only change salt intake under medical supervision, as not everyone's BP goes up when increasing salt.[23,*]

- **Cause of hunger:** High intake of processed foods that bypass sensory-specific satiety (SSS) and cannot trigger natural satiety

Treat the root cause by replacing whole, unprocessed, natural food that looks similar to how it exists in nature. If it has added ingredients, it's processed.

- **Cause of hunger:** Dehydration that can be mistaken for hunger

Treat the root cause by ensuring three to four liters of water a day, especially in warm climates, as thirst can be mistaken for food cravings and

---

* Do not increase salt intake without consulting your doctor if you are on blood pressure medications.

fatigue. Urine should be pale and odorless if you are well hydrated.*

This is by no means an exhaustive list, but it's definitely a high-impact place to start your journey if you are battling endless food cravings. I often find patients are incredibly surprised that *thirst can mimic hunger*.

---

* Discuss your fluid targets with your doctor if you are a heart failure patient with fluid restrictions.

2.9: Thirst, hunger, and hydration

If protein is the basic building block of the body, water is the basic conductor of all information throughout the body. Water is the main component of your body, comprising around 60 percent of you!

Just like we need protein on a daily basis, we need water, too. Water helps with every function the body performs every day: digestion, making blood, maintaining body temperature, repairing tissue, transfer of information between organs, making lymph, bathing the nervous system in nourishing cerebrospinal fluid, directing immune responses, excreting waste, and so much more.

Did you know that being dehydrated can trigger hormone responses that tell your body to hold on to more fat?[24]

It's true—when the body gets dehydrated, your water-balancing system puts you into "camel mode," where it holds on to fat because fat can become a source of water. Eating very salty junk food not only leaves you feeling dehydrated and thirsty, but also triggers fructose production that gets converted to fat as a way to generate water.[25] Dietary fructose and sugar can make this worse.

High glucose levels can worsen dehydration. As the kidneys filter and clean the blood, they try to clear the toxic glucose levels. Excess glucose gets thrown out of the body through the urine—but the rowdy glucose doesn't leave the party alone. It osmotically drags water out of the system, too, causing net water losses, more concentrated blood, and higher glucose levels, unless you actively replace the water.

Staying hydrated can help prevent high glucose levels from spiraling further upward. The weather in your area may also determine how much water you feel like drinking, as many of us drink less water when it feels cold outside. It's possible that if you have become used to chronic dehydration, you may not even remember what normal thirst feels like.

You may need to **consciously** drink enough water and stay well hydrated in order to restore your normal thirst signals. Some people carry around large water bottles with markings; some set up water challenges in the office. Some use a water-drinking app that makes a splashing sound every hour as a reminder to drink a glass of water. Find what it takes for you to stay hydrated and work with your healthcare provider to safely hydrate yourself.

All of my patients report better skin quality, increased energy, and better glucose levels when they drink enough water. This also helps their kidneys flush out the toxic glucose levels.

Many ask, what's the best fluid to drink for basic hydration?

Plain water.

You don't need electrolyte water, alkaline water, artificially flavored water, amino acid water, mineral water, distilled water, protein water, charged water, or reverse osmosis–filtered water. You definitely don't need sports drinks or energy drinks that have glucose. Just normal drinking water.

2.10: Counting protein in common sources

What I want you to notice is that many plant-based foods are praised for their protein content without realizing that they are barely different from the food they are replacing.*

Plant-based	Protein	Carbs
Half cup** *cooked*** whole legumes/lentils/pulses: green gram/ Bengal gram/chickpeas/kidney beans/black-eyed beans	8	22
Half cup *cooked* whole soybeans	16	9
Half cup tofu	20	5
Half cup tempeh	16	7
Half cup wheat flour****	7	48
Half cup cooked whole millet	3	20
Half cup cooked whole quinoa	4	21
Half cup cooked whole rice	2	22
Half cup cooked whole wheat	3.5	25
2 tablespoons mixed nuts	4	4
2 tablespoons mixed seeds	4	4
2 tablespoons hemp hearts	6	2

* References for nutrition data: nutritionvalue.org, fatsecret.com, fatsecret.co.za, verywellfit.com, carbmanager.com, nutritionix.com/usda. Whole eggs, whey protein, meat, poultry and seafood are complete proteins.

** Cup size will vary based on how tightly you fill food into the cup. If you chop certain foods more finely, you will pack more food into the same cup. So use this table as a general guide, not a replacement to working with a nutrition professional. Also, don't obsess over single-digit gram differences. Get a general sense of your top choices and move ahead.

*** Cooked versus raw and dry versus soaked makes a difference in nutrition counts because of changes in water content.

**** Read further to understand glycemic index of whole wheat flour versus whole wheat grain.

Plant-based	Protein	Carbs
2 tablespoons nutritional yeast	8	5
2 tablespoons unsweetened nut butter	7	6
½ cup *cooked* spinach	3	3
½ cup *cooked* broccoli	2	3
½ cup *cooked* mushrooms	2	4
1 serving scoop of plant-based protein powder (pea/brown rice)	25	1

Dairy	Protein	Carbs
½ cup homemade yogurt/curd	4	6
½ cup Greek yogurt/hung curd	12	4
½ cup skyr yogurt	15	4
2 tablespoons hard fresh cheese	5	1
2 tablespoons soft fresh cheese	2	1
½ cup crumbled paneer	14	1
1 serving scoop of whey protein powder	25	1
1 serving scoop casein powder	25	1

Egg	Protein	Carbs
Egg white	3.5	0
Whole egg	6	0

Meat/Poultry/Seafood*	Protein	Carbs
100 grams of *raw* chicken mince	19	0
½ cup *cooked* chicken mince	17	0
100 grams of raw fish	19	0
100 grams of *cooked* fish	23	0
100 grams of raw red meat	17	0
100 grams of *cooked* red meat	25	0

* I have grouped the major animal proteins here because it is so much easier to achieve protein targets from these categories without feeling deprived or stuffed while also staying low carb. There can be around a 5-gram difference between certain types of fish or meat, but in the grand scheme of things, people attempting to reach at least 1.2 grams per kilogram of body weight per day will easily cross this threshold when using these foods. It's the plant-based folks who need to search for every extra five grams they can add. The predominantly vegetarian population I work with on a daily basis is protein deficient and needs to count more carefully.

For example, switching from wheat to millet doesn't change your protein/carbohydrate profile by much, and neither does using quinoa instead of rice. I am not talking about gluten here. I am talking about proteins and carbohydrates, the main macronutrients we are focusing on in this chapter.

Maybe someone somewhere noticed a two gram difference between quinoa and rice and made a particular item famous for protein. My suggestion is to choose what you love, aim for variety, and aim for unprocessed actual whole food that gets protein to target.

2.11: How vegetarians and vegans can get enough protein

When it comes to a plant-based diet, there are often a few more challenges when it comes to getting enough high-quality protein. I know this, I acknowledge this, and I want to help you with this. If you are struggling with any of the following issues, I am offering the solutions I have found through my practice as a doctor—and also as a vegetarian myself.

The first issue we run into is that **many plant-based protein sources often come with 2.5 grams of carbs per gram of protein**—which makes following any low carb guidelines even more difficult. *My solution to this is to consider that eating beans, legumes, quinoa, and millet to get forty grams of protein* automatically comes with about 100 grams of complex carbs. So be sure to add in lower carb protein sources to get the rest of your protein while managing glucose levels.

While plant-based proteins are available in different forms, we run the risk of missing out on some amino acids. **Many plant-based proteins are considered "incomplete,"** or lacking the combination of all essential amino acids. You absolutely need variety to get enough essential amino acids like lysine, but the good news is, there are complete proteins that are vegan-friendly. By *including unprocessed soy, chia seeds, spirulina, and nutritional yeast*, you can increase your intake of the essential amino acids found in their complete proteins. Just remember to count, because some of these sources offer less than fifteen grams of protein per serving and you won't end up eating bucketfuls of them.

While those complete proteins can help you balance your diet, one of the unique struggles with plant-based options is that **the bioavailability of essential amino acids may be less than expected because of differences in protein quality,** so the protein target may need to be **higher** than calculated if relying exclusively on vegetarian sources. I recommend that you go beyond the label claims of food manufacturers and develop a deeper understanding of vegan-friendly, quality protein options that don't need intense processing.[26] Anecdotally, on my last trip to the United States to visit friends and family, I ended up trying many versions of mock meats and vegan ready-to-eat protein. Most of them were frozen, and claimed fifteen to twenty grams of protein per serving. The ingredient lists were extremely long, more than I was comfortable with, but I made the trade-off because we were on holiday. I was surprised at how hungry and unsatiated I felt after eating most of them. I already knew what it felt like when I ate whole food to get my day's protein. **Processed food doesn't even come close to triggering satiety.**

As plants are heavy in fiber, so too, are whole food plant based protein sources. If you find that **the protein is so rich in fiber that you find your meals bordering on stuffing yourself to finish**, my professional advice is to *start your meal with protein and vegetable sources*, and then see how hungry you are for carbohydrates. As we will cover in Part 2.16, carbs are not essential in the diet.

Whether or not fiber turns out to be the reason that **you can only make small strides toward your protein goals at meals before finding yourself satiated**, have hope. It's a simple remedy! If you find yourself full before you can get enough protein, it can be as simple as *taking a dedicated protein supplement after you eat your fill of whole foods*, as the one trade-off.

Many patients upon making these adjustments make comments that they **"can't digest" it, or that it's resulting in gastric upset.** *First, assess your habits:* are you eating slowly and mindfully, or are you more likely to chug a protein shake while multitasking? If it's the latter, you may not have given the stomach and brain enough time to prepare for protein with the cephalic phase of stomach acid secretion, which kick starts protein digestion before the meal reaches the small intestine.*

For those who didn't quite suffer from gastric upset, I've heard complaints that **adding new protein triggers uncomfortable gas and bloating**. This can be caused by the natural sugars in plant-based protein sources, also referred to as fermentable oligosaccharides, disaccharides, monosaccharides, and polyols—or FODMAP. Since a low-FODMAP diet limits important vegetarian protein sources, one way is to *try to introduce one new item at a time and allow two weeks for the gut microbiome and digestive capacity to settle*.

Finally, for those who find the adjustment easy, aside from **the diet feeling "heavy,"** *you may need some time*. If you've been on a protein-malnourished, low-fat, high-carb diet for most of your life, this new quantity of protein may signal satiety in a way that you have never experienced. Since protein provides more satiety than carbs do, it's possible that your body just doesn't know what getting enough protein feels like. We know *feeling full is the opposite of feeling hungry*—which one would you prefer?

---

* The brain phase of digestion, which starts the secretion of digestive juices when the mind anticipates a meal is coming soon.

It's important to get enough protein, but add it in slowly if you have any sensitivities, or if you have been on one particular diet for a length of time. Eat your protein before anything else, and most importantly, go at your own pace.

2.12: How to read labels for protein

When it comes to nutrition labels, I always think of my patient Ruhana. After hearing that getting more protein would reduce hunger, reduce cravings, and help her build muscle, Ruhana was very motivated. She visited the nearest health food store and stocked up on protein bars to round out her stash of leftover dietitian-recommended protein biscuits from when her mom was discharged from the hospital. Being pressed for time, Ruhana didn't study the fine print or tiny nutrition numbers on the back; she simply noticed the words "protein" and "diabetes-friendly" in bright, colorful font on the front of the package and decided this was an ideal protein source. She's a busy person, and it was too much to think about whether the food was a complete protein by providing the essential amino acids.

You're probably a busy person, too.

Busy. Cognitively overloaded. Burdened with too many decisions every day.

There's what to wear, when to complete tasks, what needs to be done for the home, what series to watch on TV, or what Instagram reel to open. On top of all of that, you are reading this book and considering which new decisions you want to make when it comes to food. Our overloaded minds don't like spending too much energy on deliberation. Our minds want to move on easily, quickly, and effortlessly, even if that risks some inaccurate decisions.[27]

Unfortunately, being busy can cost us our health if we end up buying foods without really understanding their nutritional content. Learning something new demands mental bandwidth and conscious attention, a mental resource busy people are often depleted of, and that's why the food industry tries to make it easier for you to decide what to buy with creative messaging on the front of food packages. Even if you've never slowed down to turn the package around to make sense of the nutritional information or ingredient list, it's okay, because you are reading this page right now.

I am here to make it easier for you to learn to navigate the back of packages and identify **ultra-processed foods**. To be clear: these are *"food substances never or rarely used in kitchens, or classes of additives whose function is to make the final product palatable or more appealing;"* and further, the "processes and ingredients used to manufacture ultra-processed foods are designed to create highly profitable products (low-cost ingredients, long shelf life, emphatic branding), convenient (ready-to-consume) hyper-palatable products liable to displace freshly prepared dishes and meals made from all other NOVA food groups."[28]

The NOVA system classifies foods according to the amount of processing used to produce them; and Nina Teicholz, a science journalist with a PhD in nutrition, has an interesting take on the NOVA system. Dr. Teicholz recently explained how renaming junk food as "ultra-processed food" can be dangerous, depending on what criteria are used to define "processing" and what biases might exist within organizations that do the classification.[29] She makes a point to mention that sticking to calling it junk food will probably reduce confusion and misinterpretation by food companies that want to take advantage of loopholes in the NOVA naming system—which we know is quite likely based on all of their other branding and marketing tactics.

How to read the nutrition label and ingredient list

When it comes to processed food, there is always a nutrition label and an ingredient list. In regards to the nutrition label, look for a balance between carbs and protein; look for how much sugar it has. Remember, we are looking at increasing protein for improving diabetes with less medication. How is the added sugar helping that goal? I don't see the point of a protein bar or protein cookie loaded with more sugar than protein for anyone, but especially not not for someone with diabetes.

You can find the *amount* of sugar found on the nutrition panel, but it's the ingredient list that tells you what *kind* it is. Every few years there is a new ingredient (think: MSG, oils, sugars, trans fats, etc.) that you "should be avoiding," ultimately, there is no *one* thing you should be watching out for. If you want to be more aware of what is going into your body and their effects, some of the things you may want to start looking for include **emulsifiers, refined oils, hydrogenated fats, chemical preservatives**, and processed carbohydrates. This is by no means an exhaustive list, but it's a good place to start.

Emulsifiers, to begin with, are added to protein supplements for mouth feel. There'll often be hidden **sugars, gums,** and **starches** added to food because the protein concentrate itself does not have great texture or moisture. Examples like *soy lecithin* and *sunflower lecithin* are often *highly* processed and may cause gut inflammation, similar to **refined oils**. These are usually something like **sunflower oil** or **rice bran oil**.[30] These oils are rich in the potentially inflammatory polyunsaturated fatty acids (PUFAs), or omega-6, which can be *especially* harmful when the ratio of omega-6 to omega-3 in our urbanized diet is already too high.

While the "chemical" in **"chemical preservatives"** may seem straightforward, the ingredients list may not be. The chemical additives extend shelf life by making a food indigestible to bacteria, pests, and fungus, but *is often an unrecognizable name followed by "(for freshness)."* Personally, I've always been fascinated by how many preservatives we use to preserve packaged food compared to the generations before us who preserved natural staples with only salt!

Much like how the word "chemical" is never found in a list of ingredients, neither are **"processed carbohydrates."** Instead, you'll see them listed as the final product, like *beetroot powder, apple fiber, starch powder, rice flour, millet flakes, lotus (foxnut) seeds, grain flakes, or rice puffs*. These sound like healthy things on their own, but the reality is that these are starches that have been broken down through manufacturing into a product that is super convenient and portable. This is done because these processed versions can be eaten with minimal chewing and without any cooking, and as a result, they also have a much higher impact on glucose levels than their actual whole-fruit, whole-vegetable and whole-grain counterparts.

How to translate important marketing points to the ingredient list

When it comes to what's in your food, there are quite a few things to take in. There's obviously the nutrition panel and the ingredients, but it also helps to understand and recognize where the marketing and legal teams have a spot on the wrappers—you should be looking at the front, too! I say this because a lot of companies want to get your attention—but they must do so legally.

For example, the **whole grain lies:** a *whole grain should look whole when you see it, cook it, touch it and chew it.* A powder, a puff, or a flake cannot be a whole grain. Maybe it was a whole grain – a long time ago in a field far away – and while that *legally* may make it a grain, biologically, it isn't quite the same.

While the whole grain lies are pretty straightforward, it's different when you find foods that advertise things like "*sugar-free.*" If they say that there's "**no refined sugar,**" or "no added sugar:" look for hidden sugar. The front of the label is *allowed* to be vague and misleading, so much so that from 2013 to 2023, Dr. Robert Lustig's hidden sugar list grew from fifty-six items to 262 items.[31] It seems wrong, but really: Shouldn't something that claims to be healthy have more protein than carbs *easily*? When it comes down to it, *jaggery* is sugar. *Brown sugar* is sugar. The only way you'll know if it's actually "no sugar" or simply *no white sugar listed,* is by reading to identify the actual sugars and carb content listed. When in doubt, ask yourself this: Is the food industry trying to help you?

And even if there are no sugars listed—be suspicious if it tastes sweet and promises to be healthy! **Sugar substitutes** and **non-caloric non-nutritive sweeteners (NNS)** are used because they don't have calories nor do they spike the glucose level, but how long do you feel satiated, and how soon do you crave sweets, after having foods with sugar substitutes?

These questions have been the mark of an official and valid concern since 2015 in terms of sugar substitutes' effect on the gut microbiome, insulin resistance, metabolic syndrome, conditioned metabolic responses, glucose management, and effect on our sense of taste.[32] As of now, many are still legal and unregulated, regardless of the concerns, questions, and research. They only get away with it because we don't have long-term clinical trial data on their effects on health.

Other legal and marketing partnerships have their wrapper workarounds, especially when it comes to artificial flavors and colors.

Regardless of what's legal, we know that whole, unprocessed food doesn't have any **artificial flavors**. If we have to make a trade-off and use a supplement to get to our protein target, why are we okay with so many artificial additives being added to our health journey? We can question whether any natural protein tastes like cookies or berries, but we should also be asking: Does "**nature identical**" mean "natural" or "artificial?"

Just like there are natural flavors, some of the **permitted colors** come from natural sources, such as the carmine pigment derived from crushed red insects. Other shades of food color are artificial and can be made from petroleum (**red 40**). These have been linked to food allergies, altered gut microbiomes, and a correlation with mental health conditions like autism and attention deficit–hyperactivity disorder (ADHD).[33,34,35] Correlation does not prove that artificial colors cause behavior problems, but a correlation has paradoxical implications for parents of children on the spectrum who might give their children brightly (artificially) colored junk foods as treats or rewards for good behavior. Amidst all this uncertainty, governments don't have consensus—it's important to note that there are only six synthetic colors that are approved by *both* the United States and the European Union, even though both regions have over thirty approved color additives each.[36]

When it's time to eat

While you may do all of the shopping and control all of the food in the house, there are still a couple of things to watch for even after you've done all that work.

First, be sure to pay attention to the **serving size** listed. You have gotten the perfect snack, only to finish the package without realizing you ate twice as much as what you read on the label. It's not your fault! Often the manufacturers will do this so they can list more servings on the box, delivered in a few packages, containing two to three servings each—*but the back panel still lists the nutrition information per single serving.* Other times it's misleading because the serving size may be a single bar, but the information is mentioned in grams, and most of us are too busy to actually do the math to convert the units and figure out how much we are getting.

Then, if you're aware of the serving size, enjoy! And watch out for the **addictive mouth feel**—something you'll only find by eating it. Some foods are designed to create a pleasurable sensation in your mouth that keeps you wanting more oral gratification. Besides all the time spent reading labels, it takes effort to know what you're eating. Sometimes, they're going to trick you even if the label is perfect.

2.13: Deciding about protein supplements

I get asked a lot about my recommendation for protein supplements. These "supplements" are not medications and don't undergo the rigorous testing that medications do, so there isn't as much robust scientific data around supplements. Even so, people need guidance on how to choose, so they ask their doctor or lifestyle coach because that's often the most trusted person they can ask.

So what's best? Bars? Shakes?

When it comes to **protein bars**, the inclusion of unnecessary additives makes them unacceptable to me. This is because, frankly, I haven't found any protein bar worth recommending owing to the ingredient lists that include emulsifiers, sweeteners, and other binding agents that overshadow the supplement's intended role of trying to provide protein.

As far as **protein powder** goes, people are often afraid of powder because it's processed. Sure, plant-based protein powders are definitely processed because the carbohydrate has been separated from the protein and the natural structure has been completely changed. But much like reading the labels, we are just trying to make the best decision, and I ask my patients to always attempt to reach protein through natural, unprocessed, whole food first. If we are struggling to hit our goals and would like to remove the pressure a bit, *then* we can add in a protein powder. However, when I suggest this, I often get asked, "Is it dangerous to take a powder?" I have three replies to this question:

First, I point out to them: They *are already eating processed powdered carbohydrates:* any flour or food that contains flour, any ready-to-eat food that has powdered grains (that used to be whole once upon a time) that now melt in your mouth, or homemade food that has powdered the grain and processed it until it's unrecognizable from its original form. Sourdough bread, for example, used to be a wheat grain. After harvest, the wheat was ground to a powder. Then the dough was allowed to ferment. Then it was baked. Three levels of processing. The humble Indian idli that everyone considers to be "light" because it's fat-free has been processed even more. Idli rice is usually parboiled after harvesting. That means soaking, steaming, and drying. That's three steps of processing. Then, when you want to eat idli, you soak the parboiled rice overnight: then you grind the grain into a batter; you let that batter ferment next. And then, you steam it. That's seven steps of processing in total. Processed carbs are harming human metabolic health more than protein powder—but you decide. If you want to eat whole and unprocessed everything, that's great, just get your protein to target.

Second, for those who already have insulin resistance, I ask them to *check what role carbohydrate powders have played* in their metabolic and hormonal imbalance. Is this fear of protein powder based on any facts? I tell them to do the math to see if they are even close to sufficient protein intake because I have not yet met a person who ruined their health by increasing their protein intake. I meet sick people every day, who have faithfully been taking carbohydrate powders and medications to chase them, without achieving better health. Check your facts.

And finally, if nothing else can combat their hesitance, I'm always sure to make it clear: *protein malnutrition is dangerous*. If you can achieve your protein targets without a powdered supplement, great. Just don't be malnourished.

Dairy-based protein powders

Whey protein concentrate is the least processed of protein supplements, and I advise my patients to select one that has just that single ingredient: whey protein. That's it.

Whey protein is what you get by simply dehydrating the liquid whey that separates from curdled milk, cheese, or yogurt. It has a high bioavailability and is rapidly digested and easily absorbed. Casein, on the other hand, is derived from the solid (precipitated) component of milk and takes longer to digest than whey. Both of these are complete proteins, but if you have significant lactose intolerance, see if a whey protein isolate works better. Remember, protein doesn't need to taste sweet or be flavored like chocolate or strawberries.

Plant-based protein powders

Plant-based protein supplements qualify as ultra-processed foods because you need a factory to split the protein and carbs apart, most commonly from a rice grain, quinoa grain or a pea—a process which isn't natural at all. The least processed, low-carb option would be soy milk powder, which comes from dehydrating soy milk. Soy milk has been made in Asian homes for centuries, so it does not have to involve heavy, factory-level processing depending on the brand, but you can decide what trade-offs you can live with.

As a vegetarian, I have found a solution in searching for a single-ingredient protein supplement, shaking it with water and gulping it, telling myself that it's giving me the number of grams my body needs. Although it's true that my hunter-gatherer ancestors certainly did not consume powdered protein that had the carbohydrate component stripped away, I am not living anything close to an ancestral life in 2024. I have already made a series of trade-offs by choosing urbanized, industrialized city life with a desk job. So instead of making myself miserable chasing perfection, I chose something that worked, and I moved on. As long as my metabolic health and strength are where I want them, I am satisfied; find what works for you.

Making a powder-based protein supplement more palatable

Because the only animal protein I eat consistently is free-range whole eggs, I always need a plant-based supplement to cover the gaps. While I am getting my protein to target for my health, I'm always looking for ways to minimize the additives I consume. The food and sports supplement industry has been trying to solve this problem while prioritizing convenience, palatability, and taste—and that's where this becomes a personal choice to decide if adding all those extras is worth it. I recommend that you read the NOVA classification for a better understanding of the levels of processing food can undergo, but once you make your choice, it's all about making it work for you.[37]

One of my patients decided she needed her supplement to taste good if she was going to stick with it long-term. She understood how to read labels and found a single-ingredient whey protein she liked.

She then started innovating with homemade recipes, such as adding crushed ice cubes, coffee or cacao powder and vanilla extract to create a milkshake experience.

Another patient added powdered spices like cumin (jeera), carom or caraway (ajwain), turmeric (haldi), and rock salt to her pea, brown rice, and quinoa protein blend.

One time, I was trying to find tasty ways to consume pea protein powder and came up with a masala smoothie recipe similar to the sattu drink found in Kolkata, but with fewer carbs. I blended the scoop of pea protein, a pinch of salt, half a fresh green chili, a dash of red chili powder, a pinch of chaat masala, a teaspoon of extra-virgin olive oil (for a smooth mouthfeel), and a glass of water together, garnished with a few cilantro leaves. A spicy, savory protein kick.

Whether you enjoy five whole eggs a day, a vegan single-ingredient shake, or a steak to cover a thirty gram protein deficit, just do whatever it takes to get to your protein goals.

2.14: For lower glucose levels with less medication, how do you know what you can eat?

After all this, you might still be wondering what you can actually eat. After learning how to get enough protein in the day based on body weight, how to spread protein across the day's three to four meals, and how to read the information on labels, patients still wonder:

- But can I eat sweet fruits like bananas, mangoes, and grapes?
- Can I eat dessert?
- How often can I eat out to maintain my social life?

These are common questions, questions that I get **often** because we *struggle to visualize that a different relationship with carbs is possible.*

The Mayo Clinic says people should get 225-325 grams of carbs per day, and the typical American diet says Americans take in 250 grams of carbohydrates a day.[38,39] In my practice, people of Indian origin with uncontrolled diabetes consume from 200 to over 300 grams of carbs per day before they start working with us, which is consistent with data published from across five sites in India.[40]

Those ranges are well within the limits set by the Mayo Clinic, and yet, people eating that way became my patients. There is increasing evidence that we need to offer people the option to reduce carb intake to achieve better diabetes with less medication.[41] As per the 2024 Standards of Care in Diabetes, published by the American Diabetes Association, the studies looking at the optimal amount of carbohydrates for people with diabetes *have been inconclusive about the "optimal amount"* but say that *monitoring carbohydrate intake is a key strategy* in managing glucose levels in type 1 and type 2 diabetes.

As I have said before, I want to help you build a solution that works for the rest of your life. Not just for a month; not just as a drastic fad. Frankly, I don't even know how your individual body is going to process your food choices at the time of reading this book.

When it comes to my patients asking me whether or not they can eat *this* from the menu, or have *that* fruit that's really sweet, I will tell you exactly what I tell them.

But first: using continuous glucose monitoring

If you want to know what to eat, it helps to know how your food affects your glucose levels, and a continuous glucose monitoring (CGM) device can play a role here. The painless convenience of having a wearable device on your upper arm that gives you nearly instant feedback becomes a powerful self-monitoring tool. We set up dashboards with our clients' CGM data and use the data to coach them on what seems to be working and what further lifestyle adjustments can help. It's always advisable to work with your healthcare professional to interpret your CGM data when you are on diabetes medication.

CGM is not as accurate as a finger prick using a glucometer because it's not testing your blood, but it gives you a general sense of glucose trends after various meals or activities. During times of rapid glucose fluctuation, severe highs, or severe lows, the CGM can be quite inaccurate and lags beyond the true readings, so always use your glucometer when you want to know your exact glucose level. As always, it's your health, and your decision, but as we discuss how to make the most accurate decisions for you, it may involve a few more finger-pricks.

Figuring it out: What can I eat?

Let's say you want to know if you can eat a banana or not because you love bananas.

First, I want you to **confirm with your doctor** that it's safe to change your diet.

If you are planning to combine the banana with a meal to reduce the number of between-meals insulin spikes (remember Part 1.7), you can check the glucose level before and after that meal, and see what happens if you **get thirty grams of protein** before the banana. Note the numbers down somewhere (For example, my patients log these meals and glucose readings in our app).

If you are eating it as a snack, **check your glucose** level on your glucometer, **eat the banana**, and **check the reading in two hours.** Note it down.

Then, *in a few days*, **eat that same meal again, without the banana. Check the difference.**

Let's say you notice that the glucose is 180 mg/dL (10 mmol/L) after eating the meal with the banana, and 160 mg/dL (8.8 mmol/L) without the banana. That's not surprising, considering that the banana has natural sugar—this is where you get to decide what to do.

See, if you came to a doctor's office with a postmeal glucose level above 140 mg/dL (7.7 mmol/L), the doctor might want to push that glucose down with a heavier prescription. But you, my friend, have a choice. If you want to keep your glucose down with less medication *and* keep the banana, you get to review the whole meal and see what *other carbs* were present along with the banana, and potentially reduce them instead.

Common carb sources you can reduce

When you see your postmeal glucose crossing 140 mg/dL (7.7 mmol/L), there are some common high-carbohydrate foods you can reduce by 50 percent that will make a huge impact. The reason I advise cutting a carb by 50 percent is because this way, your menu stays the same; only the proportions change. I always coach my patients to **get enough protein in the meal before thinking about reducing carbs**. They are more satiated that way. It feels less drastic (and therefore more sustainable) than trying to stop a beloved food completely when you are still hungry! Always review diabetes prescriptions with your doctor before reducing the carbs, and see what swaps you can make.

Fruit is on the list. Sure, it's natural. Keep it if you want it for the fiber and *micronutrients*, but consider reducing it for its *macronutrient* (carb) that is raising your blood glucose. To keep the **fruit** or even the **dessert**, you can play with the balance of things grains. From **wheat, rice, barley, buckwheat,** and **oats** to **millet** and **quinoa**, grains in all their forms can be eaten less of. You could swap out or reduce **bread** and **pasta** in all forms (even if legally advertised brown or multigrain, it is completely processed), and check if you want to reduce **packaged junk food and snacks** (potato chips, crackers, cookies, and biscuits) and sugar-sweetened beverages, soda/cola/pop, or fruit juice, which deliver large loads of sugar at high speed into your gut and place a large metabolic load on the liver.

You can gain some wiggle room by reducing **starchy vegetables: potatoes, sweet potatoes, beets, carrots, corn**, and really any **underground roots**.

For vegetarians, you may end up keeping the beans/legumes/pulses as a protein source. It's important to remember from the protein table in Part 2.10 that most of these come with close to 2.5 times the grams of carbs, *per* gram of protein. For example, a serving of cooked chickpeas will have 8 grams of protein and twenty-four grams of carbs, essentially driving your carb count toward 80–100 g/day without really getting the protein to target. Working with a professional can help here as this is where we coach our patients on how to customize something that works for them.

"But what about glycemic index and glycemic load when choosing carbs or fruit?"

I get this question a lot when people come to me for a more custom approach. Although websites and nutrition experts profess these highly technical terms to persuade you to eat more of this and less of that, I take a more practical self-directed approach. The concept I want you to know here is how a particular carbohydrate affects *your* glucose levels and insulin needs at a *particular stage in your journey.*

A juiced fruit has a higher glycemic index than a whole fruit.

A flour can deliver a higher glycemic load than the whole seed, kernel or grain.

When you turn something into powder or liquid, you destroy its natural layers. The outer covering was meant to resist pests, germinate in the soil, and provide instant underground nutrition as starch to the growing baby plant. Flour or juice makes the simple carbohydrates immediately available to your body, whereas your digestive system would have had to slowly work its way through the outer protective covering if the food had been eaten whole. The best way to know the glycemic load or index of your meal is by running the same experiment that we discussed earlier with the banana; eat the food in question, and check your glucose levels before and two hours after the meal to see the effect. If the glucose level goes high, you know how that carbohydrate load affects you. You can then decide what carb you want to keep or reduce. While we will later discuss in Part 5 how having more muscle mass can reduce the glycemic impact of food, for now, we are focused solely on what we can change regarding food.

Now, let's set up that hypothetical banana situation as an experiment, where eating your normal meal **and** a banana is the starting point we will compare our data to—also called the control. In this scenario, **the control meal** might look something like this:

- two servings of bread/roti
- Banana
- Vegetables
- ½ cup yogurt
- ½ cup kidney beans (rajma)
- ¼ cup rice
- Two spoons of dessert

Let's say that the pre-meal blood glucose (BG) was 110 mg/dL (6.1mmol/L); and two hours postmeal, BG was at 160 mg/dL (8.8 mmol/L).

Now what?

If you ask me if you can keep the bananas, rice, or dessert, I will say, "It's up to you!" My opinion doesn't matter. Let's not fool ourselves that you will stop eating bananas, even if you love them, just because I said so. You ate the banana because you probably wanted to, and that's fine by me.

Instead, let's look at the fact that *your body* has an opinion already. Your body is already telling us that it's unable to handle that particular carbohydrate load.

Your protein in this particular meal has not reached close to thirty grams, so maybe you could increase the quantity of yogurt. On the other hand, if you increase the kidney beans to get more protein, you'll also get more carbs with the protein (remember the protein source chart a few pages ago?). You could think of some low-carb protein options to add to this meal, such as nuts, seeds, or animal protein if that's part of your options. You will feel more full with that increased protein of thirty grams in the meal.

If your goal is to get that 160 mg/dL (8.8 mmol/L) down with fewer meds and still eat the banana, you then have the option of reducing your carbohydrate load from that meal in many different ways. You can experiment with your changes and compare your numbers to your control meal, and then assess which changes make you happiest. Your experimentation with different options and swaps may look like this:

- **Experiment 1:** You could skip either the roti/bread or the rice, but keep the banana.

- **Experiment 2:** You could keep both roti and rice, but reduce their proportion by 50 percent each, and keep the whole banana.

- **Experiment 3:** You could reduce the banana and dessert portion by 50 percent, keeping the same bread and rice.

- **Experiment 4:** You could try all kinds of combinations here to see what method works best for you by adding or removing different carbs to the mix.

And guess what? By reducing the overall carb total of the meal by 50 percent, I have seen many patients make rapid progress in turning around their diabetes. What's even better is that this motivates them to focus on getting enough protein while further lowering their carbohydrate intake, alongside investing in *other areas of their lifestyle*. By taking charge of practices such as improving sleep, stress management, strength training exercise, and even intermittent fasting on top of informed food decisions, a year later, we find that the body's ability to handle the occasional fruit, rice, restaurant food, pasta, bread, or dessert has actually improved! Patients even find that their glucose does not spike as high as it used to with the same foods, so if you have ever "quit" your favorite food or dessert—check what needs to change. You can improve your metabolic flexibility. I have seen people turn things around.

Too often I have seen people who "let go" of their favorite foods, like bananas or mangoes, for years. What was the point of all that sacrifice if their diabetes still never went away? Well, it's not the one serving of fruit or one dessert that makes or breaks this—their diabetes didn't turn around because they likely weren't advised on reversing the root problem of insulin resistance. So, instead of feeling like a child who has to ask a parent's permission to stay out late at night and feeling guilty if you "break the rules," how about flipping the script so that you are in charge of your food choices? It's more fun (and more sustainable) when you decide and let your body tell you what to do.

Listening to your body: Mental or physical hunger?

I should take a minute to differentiate between physical hunger–your stomach growling in the upper left or mid-central region of your abdomen, near the bottom of your left rib cage (not your entire paunch, all over your belly, or circling your bellybutton)–and mental hunger (cravings, ideas, and thoughts urging you to eat). Insulin resistance develops over years of habits and exposure to different stimuli, and the chosen response to those stimuli. Some of the habits can ultimately have consequences beyond just insulin resistance. The creation of eating habits based on mental hunger might have the unintended consequence of losing contact with what genuine physical hunger feels like. If you have found yourself eating because:

- it's time to eat or just more convenient to eat now;
- you're in a good mood or bad mood;
- you're low on energy or high on energy post-exercise;
- of social pressure or loneliness;
- you shouldn't waste;
- you didn't hydrate;
- you're trying to fall asleep or stay awake;
- you're overwhelmed or bored;
- or because of any other reason outside of your stomach quietly rumbling; you may have a stronger association with mental hunger rather than physical hunger.

Pro tip: If you're not sure whether your hunger is physical or mental, ask yourself this: would you be sure if you needed to sneeze? Do you have to think or wonder about it? Needing to sneeze is a physical bodily feeling, starting in the nose. You don't rationalize with yourself about how sneezing later would be inconvenient; that would be a mental idea about sneezing. True hunger is unmistakable once you recognise it. It's a feeling that starts in the empty stomach.

> *Disclaimer: If you've struggled with any kind of eating disorder, the tracking of glucose logs, counting of macros, or working on listening to your body may cause anxiety or feel like a trigger, so please work with your healthcare professional to decide how to best use this advice.*

We want to understand how to reduce carbs in a way that suits you, but we can't do it well unless we are in tune and *comfortable* with what your body is sharing. With the understanding that we are always talking about *physical* hunger, let's discuss what I recommend when it comes to reducing carbs.

2.15: Carbohydrate-reduction guidelines

Before anything else: **get your medication and insulin safely adjusted**. Work with your healthcare professional to prevent hypoglycemia *before* reducing carbs, as you will need regular follow-up and supervision if you are on medications for blood pressure, triglycerides, diabetes, and uric acid.

After making sure you're cleared and ready if choosing carbs to keep, **choose whole, unprocessed foods that keep you full for longer.** Carbs aren't inherently bad, but **processed carbs make overeating easy.** They go down without chewing or satiety signaling, requiring high insulin. This increases hunger and blocks leptin signals of satiety. How? High insulin levels cause insulin resistance and signal the body to store fat. Leptin resistance keeps your brain thinking you are hungry all day. This is what we call the **carbohydrate-insulin model** (CIM) of weight gain and obesity.

Look for whole and unprocessed carbohydrates because as we learned from how labels use marketing to trick you: **Light doesn't automatically mean healthy.** Low-fat processed carbs are often perceived as healthy, even though the grain has been completely processed and delivers a high-carb load.

Common Indian snacks like *rice puffs* (kurmura), *millet* (jowar, bajra, ragi) *snacks of all shapes and sizes, savory rice or corn flakes* (chivda), *instant rice flakes* (poha), *instant wheat* (upma), *tapioca starch* (sabudana), *millet crackers* (khakhra), *lotus seed puffs* (makhana or fox nuts), *instant oats, various porridges* and anything made of *flour* will surprise you if you monitor your glucose levels before and after, so why take an influencer's or food company's word for it?

While it may be easy to decide which carbs you want to keep eating, it's hard to know *how much*. Some diabetes nutrition recommendations talk about "reducing" their carb intake from 65–75 percent of total daily calories to 50–55 percent, but this might take the average person from 300 grams to 220 grams of carbs per day.[42] The agreement is that **a low-carb lifestyle is between 80–100 grams of carbs per day.**

Most people don't really know what any of that looks like in daily life. If we take an average combination of vegetarian foods like:

two slices of bread or two rotis of six-inch diameter (30 g carbs)

- + ⅓ cup of cooked rice (15 g carbs)

- + ½ cup of legumes/pulses (15 g carbs)

- + one cup of yogurt (12 g carbs)

- + one cup of cauliflower (5 g carbs),

we get close to eighty grams of carbs, and as you can see, this combination quickly reaches the low-carb threshold but is still very far from the daily protein target for the average adult.

This is where we work with our patients through our app and coaching to help them start making tweaks to their meals to keep carbs low while getting enough protein because **the sequence matters.** *Starting the meal with protein and vegetables and keeping the carbs for last has been shown to reduce the impact on blood glucose levels.*[43] So, you can try changing the sequence and see how that affects your levels. **Once you get enough protein, you can decide which carbs to keep and in what quantity, based on your physical hunger.** This also keeps you in the driver's seat of the lifestyle car, getting to choose the carbs you want to keep so that you don't feel deprived or restricted.

Depending on what your favorite kind of carbs are, there is a chance that you can reduce the impact of your chosen foods on glucose by leveraging *resistant starch*, an indigestible form of complex carbohydrates that may provide fiber and gut health benefits while causing lower glucose spikes. One way to **increase the resistant starch in your favorite carbs is to cook them, cool them in the fridge at four degrees Celsius for a day, and then eat them reheated the next day.** Don't just take someone else's word for it—what matters is how your body responds.

Try it out and measure your glucose levels two hours after eating freshly cooked carbohydrates versus cooled and reheated ones to see if there is a favorable impact on your glucose response.

If you like meat and animal protein more than starches, there's something else you can try—the keto diet. The **keto diet focuses on less than 20–50 grams of carbs per day to help you stay in nutritional ketosis**. I have seen it work. It's been shown to be safe and has many benefits for those who have made it a way of life. They have reported better health with less medication. So if it works as a lifestyle and you feel great about it, more power to you.

Creating your own diet and choosing how you view food also helps you plan around life events like weddings, parties, and outings. You can learn, just like our patients, to think ahead because you know the food industry is going to offer larger portions of cheaper, tastier carbs than you may be interested in. That's how we build something sustainable; my focus is building your confidence in self-managing your meals for the rest of your life with an expertise only you possess. But are you worried you will feel hungry without your carbs? Want to know my guideline for that?

Find your balance.

Many of us enjoy carbs for pleasure, or mental reasons more than physical ones. Generally staying within 80–100 grams a day, especially in my mostly Indian and South Asian patients (who have a smaller body frame compared to Caucasian counterparts), allows for flexibility and options. You can use this range to keep some carbs that you love (in moderation), while also reaching your health goal. If you are choosing to eat dessert or a favorite savory/salty carb, enjoy it and own it. Please don't put it into your mouth while feeling guilty like a thief, a cheat, or a fraud. Why the split personality?

Are you feeling severe powerlessness around carbs?

Can you permit yourself to enjoy a small amount of carbs while holding yourself accountable?

Mindfulness helps here, because we are building a new lifestyle, not a rigid diet.[44] If these are issues for you, it may help to work with a professional, because emotional eating is a real thing. It can be powerful and unconsciously drive choices that turn these general guidelines into harsh rules you use to judge and critique whether you've been good or bad, right or wrong. We have seen our patients develop deeper awareness around their relationship with their food and their bodies after working with our therapist or on their own to better understand their mind-body connection.

Developing a deeper relationship with food will help you understand the guideline that **no food is wrong.**

Food is food. We can choose to make drama about it in our heads if we're not monitoring our thoughts and are flip-flopping on our beliefs about food based on the external situation. In reality, eating extra carbs today doesn't mean punishing yourself tomorrow.

Cake is cake. If you say cake is good when you are putting a candle into it and smilingly singing to it, only to wake up the next morning and say cake is bad —it's not the cake doing that. Check what is flip-flopping inside your head when you think about your favorite pleasurable carbs. Remember, the most important guideline is that **you get to choose foods** that keep you happy and keep your fasting glucose levels below 100 mg/dL (5.55 mmol/L), and postmeal glucose levels below 140 mg/dL (7.77 mmol/L) after meals with the least medication.

You also get to choose to partake in alcoholic beverages. People often ask me for low-carb alcohol suggestions, but I'm not a fan of implying any form of alcohol is healthy.

Do I have the occasional drink? Yes.

Do I prefer a gin, vodka with lime, or single malt without any mixer or sweetener? Yes.

But I don't choose those drinks because "it's low-carb." I choose to have a rare drink as part of my social life and I don't need alcohol to have fun. Alcohol is not healthy. I have it sparingly, and my Oura ring and body will be sure to tell me the next day how it feels. You might not know, but **alcohol works like sugar and carbohydrates on the liver, and is toxic to the mitochondria our brains rely on.**[45] Again, the choice to drink or not is based on how alcohol and its effects fit into your goals.

Whether you choose alcohol or keto or cake, you can always *also* choose **exercise, as it improves your ability to handle carbs**. Exercise and other **holistic lifestyle changes** go beyond nutrition to reduce insulin resistance (as we will discuss in Parts 3-6).

It's possible that the carbs that spike your glucose today *may spike it less* after six months of investment in sufficient protein intake, better sleep, stress management, exercise, and fasting.

This list of guidelines is available all over the internet. The reason the diabetes epidemic still exists is because we still need to help people change their daily choices and habits in a world where carbohydrates are everywhere. Let's go one step deeper into helping you redefine your relationship with carbs and clear any remaining carb confusion.

2.16: Clearing common carb confusion and the stages of a healthier relationship with carbs

After discussing ways to reduce carbs, I want to be clear that we are not demonizing carbohydrates. We are instead fostering a deeper understanding of carbs and their complexities so that we may have a healthier relationship with carbs than the internet has led us to believe is possible.

To me, there are **four stages** in this journey.

Stage one comes with *the understanding* that even though the ADA doesn't openly say so, carbs are not essential. Keeping carbs in the low-carb range, around 80–100 grams/day, helps lower insulin requirements and insulin resistance, and since you've read Part 1, you're already here–congratulations!

Patients find themselves at **stage two** when they *begin balancing the relationship* with carbs, with flexibility, thus taking care of both types of needs: pleasure and health. This happens when they begin to implement the things that they learned previously in a way that works for them. And then we move into **stage three:** *learning that all the carbs are not equal.*

Carbs from yogurt; dal/legumes; whole, unprocessed grains; fiber; and vegetables are complex, requiring less insulin. Sugars and processed refined carbs cause a higher insulin requirement, and at this stage, patients are gaining expertise with which carbs suit their goals best and in what quantity.

By **stage four**, patients are *focused on upgrading the texture, or quality, of their thoughts and feelings around sugar.* This involves moving from guilt or powerlessness to honoring our deeper needs. Self-leadership then, is a balance between self-understanding and self-accountability, as William Ury, author of *Getting to Yes with Yourself,* puts it. Someone who has moved through all four of these stages is not only making balanced food decisions that make them happy; they feel confident while doing so.

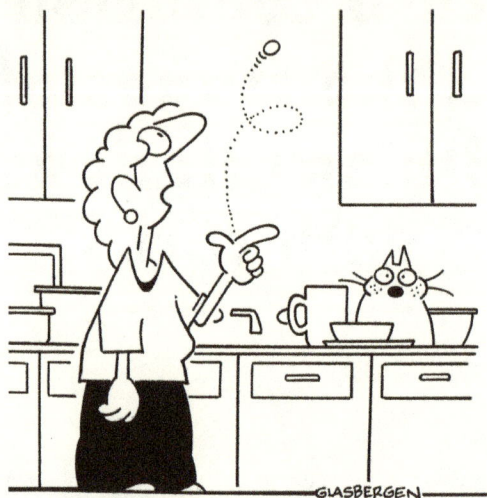

"Heads, I eat what I like and hate myself.
Tails, I eat what I hate and like myself."

At this point, we've discussed a low-carb diet that caters to both health and pleasure, and making sure to choose the right carbs for *you*, or stages one through three. What we haven't touched on, is how to feel confident in these decisions.

The opposite of confidence, in this case, is confusion.

We lack confidence when it comes to carbs and sugars because there is so much conflicting information out there, that even being confident in a "truth" could lead you astray. In order to make it through stage four, *we have to clear up some of the common confusion when it comes to carbs.*

First, people are told **they need carbs for energy and that they should make up 50–60 percent of daily energy intake.** Neither of those things is true. *Eating carbs is not essential for mitochondria to produce energy in the body, and humans can even survive with carbs being zero percent of daily intake.*

Then we are told that **people with diabetes have to eat carbs to prevent low glucose** (hypoglycemia), but that's backward. As we covered in Part 1.1, diabetes is the issue of having high glucose. *You develop a risk of low glucose only if your prescription includes specific tablets or insulin.*[*]

---

[*] We are not discussing insulinoma here, which is a rare insulin-secreting tumor that's outside the scope of this book

But you have to eat glucose for your brain! Nope. Your liver (the glucose provider musketeer from Part 1.7) knows how to maintain stable blood glucose even if you don't eat any carbs, sugar, or glucose. *The body has sophisticated ways to make its own glucose for energy from fat and protein through a process called **gluconeogenesis**, which literally translates to "making new glucose."* You need essential fatty acids and essential amino acids, but again, there are no essential carbs. You don't need glucose to survive, you need gluconeogenesis.

I can't tell you how many people with diabetes think that **if their hemoglobin A1c (HbA1c) is normal with medication and insulin, then they can eat as many carbs as they want**. If this is you, what are your goals? *Insulin resistance will progress anyway* with time on a high-carb diet. If you are looking for a way to turn around diabetes with fewer prescriptions, lowering carbs is your most powerful tool.

When I mention lowering carbs, I often hear "**But carbs are light and easy to digest!**" implying that, therefore, carbs are good for you. My response to that is: what does "light" mean? Processed carbs are known to not make you feel full as they get digested very quickly, releasing glucose into the bloodstream and creating the highest insulin requirement.

More carbs = more insulin = more body fat storage—but, you don't <u>feel</u> heavy or full.

Does that make it good for you?

After that realization, they often ask about snacks, because "**fat-free carbs are good snacks then, right?**" The truth? The low-fat, low-calorie approach has failed to cure obesity globally, and the money food manufacturers spend on creating low-carb snacks is not spent on making them as healthy as possible.

"**What about multigrain snacks or cereals—they're heart-healthy!**" These products are usually ready-to-eat powdered or processed grains. *There is no evidence that carbs from the processed food industry improve cardiac health.* Printing a heart logo on a food package does not equal medical protection, and it does not mean that **"whole-grain" packaged food is better.** If you found an actual unprocessed whole grain inside a packaged food, you would probably spit it out as unchewable. *The slow-absorption benefit of the outer coating of the "whole-grain" structure has been lost, and rapid digestion = rapid glucose rise = maximal insulin requirement. More insulin = more body fat storage = more insulin resistance*, and that's not "better" for anyone.

If low-carb snacks, multigrain cereals, and whole-grain packaged food aren't on the table, many then fall victim to believing **millet or quinoa is better than rice,** but as we covered in Part 2.10, *millet and quinoa are very similar to rice in terms of carbs.* In fact, powdered processed millet snacks have suffered the same changes as "whole grain packaged food" from above, and aren't any healthier.

Well, what **if your oats, rice, or millet are gluten-free—is that better?** The truth is, *avoiding gluten only helps if you have gluten intolerance.* Switching from wheat to gluten-free grains does not reduce your carb intake much. Do it if it makes your body feel better like Kanika did, but still track your carbs!

Patients in India think they should keep other carb sources because they believe that things like **beets, dates, finger millet (ragi/nachni), and jaggery are good sources of iron.*** But if you use these foods to get iron while having uncontrolled diabetes, you will probably spike your blood glucose levels before getting any meaningful iron from them! Why? *Since iron is a micronutrient and these foods have carbs as the predominant macronutrient, you're always going to get more carbs than iron.* It's better to check your glucose levels two hours after eating these and talk to your doctor about an iron supplement.

And please, don't believe that the **"sugar-free" or "diabetes-friendly" labels mean low-carb.** Like I said before, learn to read labels. There are hidden sugars and additives in many of these packaged foods, and just because you may think **sugar substitutes and noncaloric sweeteners are okay**, the facts are that we don't have enough long-term data on what they do for gut health, cravings, insulin resistance, cardiovascular disease, and inflammation.[46] Because they are considered nutrition supplements, *they do not undergo the safety testing that medications do, and therefore, we don't actually know if they are "okay."*

Even after all of the back and forth, some patients will tell me, **"Well, low-carb is just a fad diet!"** But anything can be a fad, depending on how you think about it. *We are focused on trying to find a lifestyle that works for you long term, and that no longer qualifies as a fad.*

"But what about the keto diet? That's a fad, and **ketosis is dangerous!**" The truth? *Nutritional ketosis for people with diabetes is safe under medical supervision.*** Diabetic ketoacidosis (DKA) is completely different and is a rare medical emergency in people with diabetes. You need to consult a qualified medical professional if you are considering a low-carb diet so that you know the difference, especially **if you believe that people with diabetes cannot follow a keto diet.** It can be a very powerful treatment for diabetes and each person responds differently. *People with type 1 or type 2 diabetes considering a keto diet need to work with a well-informed medical professional who can monitor medications and insulin doses as the blood glucose comes down quickly* on a keto or very low-carb diet.

Those who really fight back like to make the point that **"hospital meals serve carbs because you 'need at least 50 percent of your daily fuel from carbs,'** to get better!" Here's what I can tell you—*those food trays are not treating insulin*

---

* Micro means "small," and macro means "large." As the name suggests, iron is a mineral present in tiny quantities (milligrams), and carbs are present in large quantities (grams).

** Nutritional ketosis is achieved by consuming less than 20–50 grams of carbs per day. You can monitor this with a ketone monitor that uses strips to check blood or urine.

resistance! Whenever I have estimated the protein in these trays, it barely reaches 0.8 grams per kilogram of body weight per day. If you are sick enough to be hospitalized, you need *more* protein to fight illness, boost immunity, and repair diseased tissues. People often leave the hospital with more diabetes prescriptions than they were on when they were admitted. I go into more detail about hospital stays in Part 8, but for now, know this: *carbs are not essential for the body to heal.*

So much of the carb confusion comes from confusing the symptoms of insulin resistance with other factors. For example, some people believe that **you should start the day with carbs at breakfast, carbs (and fruits) are best taken before noon or that carbs should be avoided at night;** the messaging is that negative reactions from carbs are because of the time of day, not the carbs themselves. But that theory doesn't hold up against science. *The morning is the most insulin-resistant time of the day because of the normal dawn phenomenon.* This is when the body naturally releases the counter-regulatory growth hormone and stress hormone (cortisol) to counter the effects of insulin; this provides slightly higher glucose levels to start the day. Eating more carbs when insulin-resistant will require higher amounts of insulin to keep the blood glucose normal. A vicious cycle of insulin resistance will be perpetuated by a carb-dominant breakfast.

Some people believe that **religious fasts help diabetes**, but really, *this depends on what your fast looks like*. A pure water fast will lower insulin levels. A Ramadan dry fast may lower insulin requirements but comes with the risks and hormonal implications of dehydration in uncontrolled diabetes. Some Hindu religious fasts rely on protein-deficient and carbohydrate-predominant foods. Some Jains follow time restricted eating and water fasting once a year, and then resume eating a carbohydrate predominant diet. Some people in India give up animal protein during Lent and their diet becomes carbohydrate focussed. We work with our patients who want to fast for their religious beliefs, and we modify their meals to address both needs: health as well as religious faith.

On the other hand, people think that if you aren't fasting, then **people with diabetes have to eat small, frequent meals.** Why would that be true? *Eating all day doesn't cure type 2 diabetes,* because every meal causes an insulin spike. Repeated insulin spikes keep the body exposed to high insulin for longer periods of the day, making insulin resistance worse. The only time someone with diabetes might need to keep eating at regular intervals is when their medication is causing hypoglycemia between meals. The treatment for that should be to work with the doctor to adjust the medication, so you don't have to eat more food.

Some people go out of their way to **switch from genetically modified organisms (GMOs) to organic, ancient, or non-GMO because they believe these might be diabetes-friendly.** Truthfully, making the switch might improve your glucose, but *the only way to really know is by checking your levels two hours* *after any food*, and that's going to hold true for any and all carb confusion you may come across in the future.

2.17: Still feeling addicted to carbs? Like there's always room for dessert?

Yes, our science textbooks say carbs are "energy-giving foods."

Yes, you have heard how the brain requires a constant glucose supply.

Yes, you have experienced instant energy from carbs, especially simple sugars or processed carbs.

Yes, you have been exposed to repeated marketing and advertising messages that promote energy supplements that are mostly carbs.

Yes, you may have been told to eat small meals at frequent intervals for constant energy.

Yes, you might be feeling energy slumps despite snacking throughout the day, with 5:00 p.m. being the worst time.

Yes, you might be experiencing sugar cravings.

These experiences are exactly what keep people addicted to carbs and unnecessarily stuck with uncontrolled diabetes. I'm sorry if any of these have happened to you, but now you know you can change your diabetes experience by working with your doctor to change your diet and improve your addictive relationship with sugar.

Sugar and cravings aside, have you ever wondered why there is always room for dessert?

If you are offered an extra serving of pure vegetables or protein at the end of a meal, you would instinctively refuse. Leptin signaling is what tells you that you are full, but dessert is usually loaded with carbs **and** fat in unnatural ratios, and these combinations don't trigger fullness. Those sugars and processed carbs can instead trigger leptin resistance.

Leptin resistance is a problem where your brain feels hungry all day, even though there is excess body fat on the body. It's stored there, but it's not accessible. The only way to make that stored fat accessible is to have insulin resistance step aside. Reducing carbs reduces insulin requirements, which reduces insulin resistance rapidly—reducing leptin resistance. That's when your hormones are better aligned so that you can start training your body to become that lean, mean, fat-burning machine.

Think of a body that's dependent on carbohydrates as a car that has become dependent on an inefficient fuel. Do you want a fuel that gives you short, jerky, quick bursts of momentum, followed by the bottoming out of speed and energy? Much like that uncomfortable car ride, most people don't enjoy the chaos of an energy roller-coaster ride and want steady, high energy levels throughout the day. Most people also wish they could actually use the fat they are carrying around instead of permanently storing it as excess body fat.

So, how can we achieve both goals—to have consistently high energy all day and also burn excess body fat?

2.18: Fat politics, bad science, and fat burn

The healthcare industry is still making up its mind, and most of us are not on the same page about fats.

From the late 1970s, the world marketed the idea of replacing saturated fat with refined vegetable or seed oils for cardiac health, and now most people are confused about what advice to follow. I don't blame you.

As of 2013, I was still telling people to avoid ghee, fat trimmings of meat, and egg yolks because I thought dietary saturated fat and cholesterol gave people heart attacks. The US government clarified in 2015 that cholesterol is not a nutrient of concern for overconsumption. By 2017, I started softening my stance on natural fats.[47]

The American Heart Association has clarified its position on dietary cholesterol with this statement: *"For both dietary cholesterol and egg consumption, the published literature does not generally support statistically significant associations with cardiovascular disease (CVD) risk."*[48]

But old rumors die hard. Fear around unprocessed dietary fats still persists in circles where people are not updated with the progress in the medical literature.

Some of my old patients noticed my about-face on foods I had discouraged a few years prior. As a person of science, I will always be open to a better idea and better science if it can disprove previous understandings with evidence. That's how medical science evolves.

Now, after questioning the data behind my medical education and reading extensively on this topic, I am telling patients to avoid refined and processed seed oils. For a deeper understanding of the controversy around dietary fat, an easy starting read is *In Defense of Food* by Michael Pollan. A deeper investigation into this controversy is Nina Teicholz's book, *The Big Fat Surprise*.

As of today, the consensus among the metabolic health community is clear, and I can fill a page with the number of scientists and doctors who have changed their definition of healthy fats. For forty years, the world was fed bad science about a heart-healthy diet. The controversy continues even today and has enormous financial, legislative, and political implications beyond the scope of this book. Future nutrition guidelines are still vulnerable to being influenced by the flawed "diet-heart hypothesis" even though clinical trials were *never able to prove that natural saturated fats in the diet cause heart disease.*

Thankfully, public opinion is getting louder, and the investigative process is forcing this conversation into the limelight.[49]

If you do decide to add more fats, here is a list of healthy fats that I recommend to my patients, but it's likely you probably won't need much after protein satiates you.

For those on a plant-based diet, try using more extra-virgin olive oil (avoid using for high-temperature cooking); cold-pressed coconut oil; medium-chain triglyceride (MCT) oil; seeds; nuts and nut butter; avocado and avocado oil; and cacao butter to get more fats.

If you are looking for animal-based options, you can select ghee, butter (not margarine or vegetable oil butter substitutes), full-fat fresh cream, tallow, or lard from grass-fed, free-range animals to round out your healthy fat intake.

However, most of the people I work with have insulin resistance and excess body fat to lose. They don't need to purposely eat more fat. I have seen people who embrace the keto or low-carb diet go overboard with fat bombs, keto desserts, multiple avocados in protein shakes, high-fat snacks, nuts and nut butter, extra cream or butter in their bulletproof coffee, and basically adding fat to everything they eat. Fat improves flavor and mouthfeel. But there is such a thing as too much healthy fat.

Remember, even if we don't count calories, fats are still nutritionally very dense. If you are doing everything right but not seeing results, check if you are overdoing it. If you keep eating fat, why will your body bother to burn the excess body fat?

Fat taken by itself will be easy to self-regulate. Nobody finishes a bottle of coconut oil or a stick of butter in one go. It's when you add fat to protein, artificial sweeteners, salt, and carbs that it becomes easy to overeat. Your way to minimize the risk of overeating is by getting in tune with your body's hunger and fullness signals.

So before you go on the unlimited fat keto diet or add in more fat sources, go through this mindfulness checklist to make sure you are aligned with what your body says is right.

- How quickly are you eating? It takes up to thirty minutes for your stomach and brain to release hormones that signal that you are now full and can stop eating.

- Are you eating with distraction? That can reduce satiety and enjoyment from any meal.

- Are you making the meal multisensory? Focus on the smell, sight, texture, sound, and flavor of taking and chewing each bite.*

In the process of surveying thousands of patients in my practice over the years about their mindful eating habits and digestive symptoms, I noticed the most frequently cited physical symptom was evening hunger and the most common eating habits were that they struggled with cravings; they ate while watching television or consuming content on an electronic device; and they could eat tasty food any time, even if they were not hungry.

By understanding why you may be eating more than your body wants, you can then change your habits and energy intake, and then we can proceed with trying to achieve both of our goals—to have consistently high energy all day and burn excess body fat.

But first, we have to prepare your body to burn fat. How?

Step 1: *Increase your protein intake closer to the target.* This gives you more natural satiety and fullness. Feeling full with more protein makes it easier, in turn, to reduce your dependence on the beloved carbs. By increasing protein from the first meal of the day, you will have fewer energy crashes later in the day. Every single person I have worked with has been pleasantly surprised by how getting enough protein completely takes care of hunger pangs and cravings.

Step 2: *Ensure sufficient hydration.* I advise my patients to aim for at least three to four liters of water a day.

Step 3: *Reduce carbs.* My patients find it much easier to reduce their carbs after increasing protein and water intake to target.

In extreme situations of uncontrolled diabetes and severe insulin resistance with very high insulin levels, the above steps sometimes take very long to create breakthroughs. In those rare cases, I have used Fat Fasting as a very brief nutrition intervention to quickly disrupt the vicious cycle. It's not really a true fast (which we prepare you to get to by Part 6), because you are eating a lot of foods mostly rich in healthy natural fats. My team and I have modified the Fat Fast, described by Megan Ramos of the Intensive Dietary Management Program; and the Fasting Method, which is described on the Diet Doctor website as a way to quickly break through the grip of extreme insulin resistance. Our modifications have worked for vegetarian people of Indian origin and need to be done under strict medical supervision.

---

* Parents, take note. I hope you are not feeding your kids in front of screens where they turn into zombies who open their mouths just so that the show goes on. Let your kids experience their food with their hands and feed themselves until they are full. Otherwise they will need others to prescribe the "right" amount of food to eat when they grow up because they have lost the innate mind–body connection they were born with. I cover this in Part 9.

On to Part 3!

Why do you eat food anyway? As a fuel for energy, right?

Now that you have understood how you can change your nutrition by getting enough protein, reducing carbs, and having a healthy relationship with natural food and fats, you have taken care of fuel.

This brings us to the second wheel of the lifestyle car: sleep. It doesn't matter how balanced or "clean" your diet is if you aren't getting enough good-quality sleep.

Bad sleep can overpower a great diet and leave you feeling exhausted and tired.

Let's read on to understand how to improve sleep to have high energy levels all day, and how this also improves your blood glucose levels with less medication.

Part 2 summary

- Instead of looking for the perfect diet or meal plan, find the way of fixing protein malnutrition that works for you.

- Monitoring your glucose levels in response to different foods helps you decide if going low carb is how you want to have lower glucose levels with less medication.

- Learning to read and see past packaged food labels is a life skill.

- Healing your relationship with food is possible and professional help is available.

- You deserve satisfaction, pleasure, and satiety from your meals.

For Bonus Materials, Visit the Website Here:

PART 3

THE SECOND WHEEL
OF THE LIFESTYLE CAR

SLEEP

3.1: The first two wheels: Eat better so that you can sleep better

We just talked about improving nutrition, and how it's the first step to being able to reduce insulin requirements, feel less hungry and provide enough protein for the body's needs.

Let me explain why I always work with people on nutrition and sleep as the first and second wheels, respectively. Once people get their protein intake to target with intake of high-quality, complete proteins, they report better sleep within as little as two weeks. Two weeks, and they are sleeping better with less reliance on sleeping medication. That means waking up more fresh, and starting the day with more energy and clarity. *People really appreciate their sense of vitality coming back.*

I suspect this is likely due to getting your essential amino acids, like tryptophan, which is a raw material for essential mood and sleep agents in your brain, such as serotonin and melatonin.[1] There seems to be a bidirectional gut-brain component here, too, so a healthier gut means a healthier brain and a healthier brain means a healthier gut. More research is needed on how fixing protein malnutrition improves sleep, but for now, I see them tied together in an energy-boosting way that makes sense for them to be the first two wheels of our lifestyle car.

The intuitive observation that a good night's sleep gives you more energy is supported by new evidence that poor sleep is tied to poor metabolic health through a vital pathway: **having fewer mitochondria.**[2] Remember, mitochondria are the energy powerhouse of each living cell. *Low mitochondrial quantity or quality can cause our cells to age more rapidly.*

That's the opposite of longevity.

Recall our discussion in Part 1 about brown fat being rich in mitochondria. Mitochondria are found in higher concentrations in metabolically active tissues like the brain, heart, healthy active muscle, and brown fat. Your mitochondria are the site where your basic fuel currency of adenosine triphosphate (ATP) is made, and without ATP, we would not survive.

Imagine a sleep-starved person trying to make healthy lifestyle choices. They would be mitochondria starved, which means their brain cells, heart cells, and muscle cells don't have enough baseline battery power to function, and then are exhausted by trying to make healthier food choices or exercise during the day. Their body and brain are overwhelmed—they just don't have the physical or mental energy. This is why fixing your relationship with sleep comes right after your relationship with nutrition when it comes to succeeding at turning around your diabetes.

Sleep: An active process of repair and recovery

The different phases of sleep play different roles in repair and recovery. We are still learning more about the mysterious processes that happen when we sleep.

It's already clear that poor sleep means poor mitochondria, and therefore poor energy. What we also know is that deep sleep is when growth hormone is released, which helps in the growth of muscle and bones, repair of injuries, and maintenance of immunity. Researchers think dream (rapid eye movement [REM]) sleep is when the brain learns, solves problems, regulates pain perception, and consolidates memories; allowing for sharper cognition, concentration, and attention during the day.

Once, a friend told me she was a great sleeper because she could fall asleep anywhere.

Ummm, no, wrong. Try again.

Being unable to stay awake in the middle of a boring meeting or a boring movie without really planning to take a nap is a symptom we call "excessive daytime sleepiness." This is not cute. It's potentially immediately dangerous if sleepiness strikes when operating heavy machinery or driving. It's not a good thing and points to terrible sleep quality at night.

When they were in the younger grades, my daughters would tell me how if the class was really noisy, the teacher would have the entire class put their heads down on the desk for a few minutes till all the children settled down. A handful of their classmates would always fall asleep within this opportunity, which pointed to their very low "sleep latency." It's the same thing as falling asleep as soon as your head hits the pillow. It's a sign we are a sleep-deprived society and are paying the price with metabolic health.

3.2: Sleep deprivation and its signs and symptoms

Falling asleep anywhere, anytime, is a sign of sleep deprivation. Sleep deprivation is not just about the quantity of sleep you get, but also the quality. Knowing that sleep is when the body recovers, and knowing that sleep is tied to metabolic health through mitochondria, it makes sense that a lack of sleep will have negative effects on the body and mind.

When it comes to the **body**, you may find yourself suffering from fatigue or lethargy, low immunity, irregular bowel timings, or unsatisfying evacuation leading to constipation, increased insulin resistance, high blood pressure, and increased blood glucose readings. You may also find that you have poor muscle gain despite exercise, delayed recovery from injuries, and difficulty losing weight in general.

Brain function is affected with symptoms like waking up groggy and unrefreshed, poor memory, brain fog and difficulty solving problems, concentrating, making decisions, or focusing attention. Chronic pain causes poor sleep and poor sleep makes chronic pain worse, setting up a chicken-and-egg situation. There is also daytime sleepiness—falling asleep when not intending to.

Additionally, there are **emotional symptoms** like irritability and impatience, low mood and depression. Anxiety makes sleep quality worse, and poor sleep makes anxiety worse, setting up another chicken-and-egg situation. Not only do the effects on the brain show up in cognitive and emotional ways, but when it comes to urges, the mind starts to feel the effects of sleep deprivation through increased cravings and difficulty resisting temptation.

Just a week of sleep deprivation can make you measurably sick and hungry. A landmark study published in the *Lancet* in 1999 showed that sleep-depriving eleven healthy young men by allowing them to only get four hours of sleep per night, *for just six nights*, made them develop signs of insulin resistance and abnormal glucose metabolism.[3] What's worse is that sleep deprivation reduces leptin levels and raises ghrelin levels. So leptin isn't able to tell the brain you are full, and ghrelin from your growling stomach is telling your brain you are hungry.

It's a double dose of "I want more food," and shows us that sleep deprivation can trigger prediabetes and hunger.

Sleep is so necessary for survival that nature generally wants us to get seven to eight hours of it every night—that's a third of your life!

You can go for three straight days without food, meditation, sex, or exercise, but three whole days without sleep would make you extremely dysfunctional and sick–so fix your sleep to get the return on your health investments. Insufficient sleep predicts lower weight loss and poor maintenance of weight loss; yo-yo dieting is no fun. Nobody likes to put effort into fat loss only to get fewer results or to see the results be reversed within a year.

Sleep deprivation + dieting = weight-loss plateau

Picture this: you and a hypothetical twin go through the same weight-loss efforts. Your twin gets sufficient sleep (seven to eight hours per night), while you get less than five hours.

What if I told you that in this scenario, the research says that your twin will not only lose more body fat than you during the effort but will also keep more of the fat off a year later? What would you do with that information?[4,5]

It may seem crazy that sleep could have that big of an impact on your weight loss goals, but there are three truths that we can't ignore.

1. Only when you are eating and sleeping well will your body have the repair systems working in your favor.

2. Only when you are well rested will you have more bandwidth to find creative solutions to challenges and stressors in your life.

3. Only a good night's rest can prepare you with the energy to exercise and give you the gains you seek from that same exercise.

This essentially means that if you can't get enough sleep to recharge or repair, you won't have the energy to work toward your goals, and any muscle repair or growth will be near impossible. Despite this sleep science being published and available, so many people attempt to invest in their health by cutting carbs or calories without securing those investments by getting enough sleep. You don't deserve to be hungry, sleep-deprived, cranky and frustrated by a slowing metabolism. We can do better.

But what if your sleep deprivation isn't your fault?

3.3: Obstructive Sleep Apnea–What is it?

How Obstructive Sleep Apnea, or OSA, affects us when we sleep by causing an upper airway blockage that allows less air to enter the lungs. To prevent us from choking, the body creates low pressure inside the chest to pull air from the bedroom into the lungs. A quick refresher of physics here: air and liquids move from high pressure to low pressure areas.

The low pressure in the chest helps the lungs achieve ventilation, but it causes a problem for the heart and circulation. The heart is located between both lungs and its job is to pump blood out of the chest to the rest of the body. Low pressure in the chest pulls blood backward into the chest. This sucking force brings more blood into the right side—the receiving chamber—of the heart and increases the cardiac workload.

This low pressure in the chest is *backward for what the heart is trying to do.* So, the heart muscles have to pump harder to get blood out while the chest is trying to suck air into the lungs.

The increased force generated by the heart muscles can show up as high blood pressure. When the right side of the heart stretches as it fills with blood, it generates a hormone signal saying there is too much fluid inside the heart. This sends instructions to the kidney, asking the kidney to offload some extra fluid by throwing out excess water, via extra urine. This explains why **the first signs of OSA are often high blood pressure and waking up to pass large amounts of urine at night,** despite drinking less water before bed.

I *always* think of sleep apnea when I meet someone with daytime fatigue, unrefreshing sleep, morning headaches, nighttime urination and unexplained high blood pressure. OSA can even happen in someone who is not overweight as there can be other causes of the upper airway narrowing.

The catch with OSA is that the clinician has to suspect it to ask about it, and then test for it.

With that in mind, let me tell you about Paul.

My patient Paul was seeing me for diabetes and had recently been started on antidepressants by his family doctor. He reported barely getting any sleep at night because of frequent unexplained night awakenings. As his clinician, I suspected OSA and asked about it. Sometimes he woke up with a choking sensation, and he often had to use the washroom to urinate multiple times a night. He woke up exhausted and unrefreshed, dragging himself through his workday. I asked about his sleep in more detail, and he confirmed that he had been snoring heavily for 20 years, even before he developed high blood pressure or diabetes. Nobody in his family would share the room with him because the snoring was so loud.

What does that sound like to you? Untreated obstructive sleep apnea (OSA) is linked with progression to type 2 diabetes, and treating OSA can yield better results in your efforts to turn around diabetes, so I pressed him to get an urgent sleep study, and referred him to a sleep specialist.[67] You see, doctors often miss diagnosing obstructive sleep apnea *because they usually assess you when you're awake.*

What's a sleep study, and do you need one?

A home sleep study or polysomnogram (PSG) gives an apnea-hypopnea index (AHI), which reflects the number of apneas and hypopneas (complete and partial airway obstructions) that occur in the night. The experience is a bit disorienting because you will be hooked up to multiple wires and probes in your home before you go to sleep. It's a lot of gadgets and will feel unnatural. Many people feel weirded out by the science-fiction feel of it all, and report difficulty falling or staying asleep just because of the equipment. That's okay and expected. The test still manages to catch sleep apnea pretty accurately.

When Paul had his sleep study, they found that **his AHI was thirty**. A *normal score is supposed to be below five*—and an **AHI above fifteen is considered to be severe sleep apnea.**

His AHI doubled to almost seventy in his dream (REM) sleep. If you regularly drink alcohol at night, your doctor may want you to continue as usual to see how it affects your REM sleep, so check with them regarding alcohol intake. In this case, his sleep physician advised him to continue his daily alcohol on the night of the study to see the impact of alcohol on his sleep, particularly in his dream sleep. When you dream, you shouldn't be enacting those dreams in bed, so the brain prevents the muscles from moving while you "watch" the dream. This muscle block also inhibits the airway muscles to an extent and makes the airway lining more floppy in REM sleep, and it makes untreated sleep apnea worse. A problematic side effect of OSA can be that the body gets less REM sleep, which seems to play an important role in learning and memory, and so people with untreated OSA struggle to function during the day.

The study showed that as a result of his airway obstructions going untreated throughout the night, Paul was spending almost fifteen minutes below an oxygen saturation of 90 percent, and it was 81 percent at its lowest. After the COVID pandemic, we all learned that an oxygen saturation below 95 percent is not acceptable.

Paul's severe sleep apnea was probably at the root of his insulin resistance, diabetes, obesity, hypertension, fatigue, and depression. The *diagnosis of sleep apnea is often delayed by many years* because nobody is watching people sleep. Vague symptoms like low mood, weight gain, and fatigue are blamed on their lifestyle. The OSA diagnosis explained why Paul was feeling so low, and proved that his brain fog was real.

When it comes to a sleep study, there are three main levels to choose from. The doctor will need to do their initial assessment and may ask you to continue your nightly routine, much like Paul. Then you can choose between a hospital sleep study, where you check into a hospital room that will generate more detailed reports; or the home study, which is cheaper and usually sufficient to make a diagnosis.

I recommend a level 2 study for all of my patients, with or without a sitter. Some people find it creepy to know a stranger is in their room to watch them snore, which makes sense as being asleep is a vulnerable state anyway. You can always opt for the unobserved study, and I have included a chart explaining different sleep study levels in your bonus materials to help you know your options. The chart can help you discuss with your doctor what is best for you once you know you need a sleep study–but how do you know if you need one?

The **STOP-BANG** questionnaire has been found to be a good self-rating score you can take to your next doctor's appointment. It asks the following questions:

S–Do you **snore** loudly, louder than talking, or loud enough to be heard through closed doors?

T–Do you often feel **tired**, fatigued, or sleepy during the daytime?

O–Has anyone **observed** you stop breathing during sleep?

P–Do you have or are being treated for high blood **pressure**?

B–Is your **body mass index (BMI)** more than thirty-five?

A–Is your **age** above fifty?

N–Is your **neck circumference** more than forty centimeters?

G–Is your **gender** male?

If your answer is '**YES**' to three or more of these questions, then you should consider getting tested for sleep apnea. Having multiple of these findings suggests that your sleep apnea might be severe enough that you are unable to move air through your upper airway, even though your chest and heart are trying desperately to get you to breathe. Individuals with undiagnosed OSA are at extremely high risk for cardiometabolic complications and events.

Here's a pro tip: Don't just rely on your family's version of how badly you snore. According to Dr. Chris Winter, the more severe sleep apnea becomes, the less noise you might make, so be sure to listen to your body, not just your family.[8]

3.4: How to treat sleep apnea so you can lose the fat and start learning again

If your OSA is due to obesity and fat accumulation around the airway, then your doctor will tell you to lose weight to reverse the problem.

The catch is that severe sleep apnea can prevent you from losing weight because of the insulin resistance it causes.

With our modern soft-food diets (overcooked food, smoothies, and ready-to-eat snacks), the muscles lining our mouth, upper airway, and jaw become floppy because they barely get the exercise that used to come from chewing raw, hard food. Because of this, your doctor may prescribe **oral myofunctional exercise** to strengthen the muscles that line the mouth and upper airway. Strengthening these muscles when we are awake can keep the upper airway more open when we are asleep.

Normal-weight individuals with a smaller lower jaw or those with more severe cases of OSA will also be advised to **use continuous positive airway pressure** (CPAP) to force the air past the blockade so that it reaches the lungs without the negative-pressure compensations inside the chest. That way, you fix your breathing and allow insulin resistance to start improving before waiting for the weight loss.

Paul started oral myofunctional exercise and CPAP therapy. He traveled a lot for work and realized the impact of wearing his CPAP machine immediately. He had forgotten what it felt like to wake up fresh after a good night's sleep. Before starting CPAP, when he was prescribed antidepressants, he had started to think he was losing his mind. Now, he felt like himself again and could think clearly. His diabetes management became much easier after addressing the sleep apnea and changing his sleep routine. He had stopped driving because he almost fell asleep at the wheel after being sleep-deprived one night, and he was able to resume driving after his OSA was treated.[9] His mood improved, his weight-loss efforts started to pay off, his blood pressure normalized, and his psychiatrist was able to stop the antidepressants.

Not only do you need the improved energy from more restful sleep to feel like exercising, but you also need that energy so that your brain can learn again, and have new experiences. Imagine trying to learn new recipes, new stress management responses, and new workouts—but the brain is so sleep-deprived that overnight learning and daytime problem-solving are compromised. Nothing actually becomes a new habit! By addressing OSA, you have more energy to do things and a higher ability to learn from the things you do: two for the price of one!

3.5: Screen time is breaking your body's internal clock

© Glasbergen/ glasbergen.com

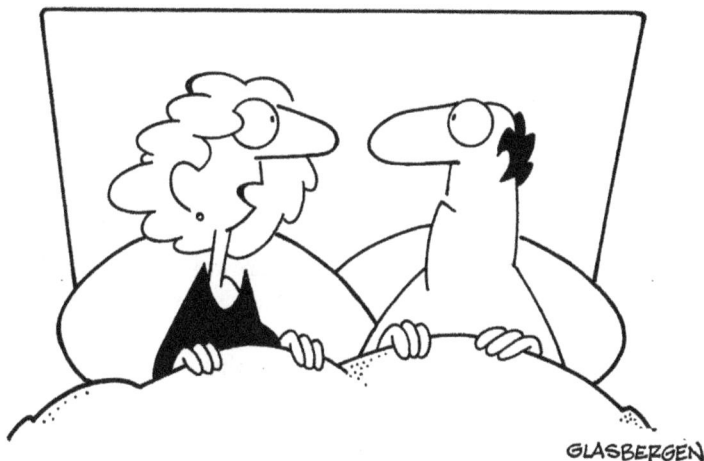

GLASBERGEN

"When you have a great dream, click Share so your friends can watch it on Netflix too."

Do you use your TV, mobile phone, digital tablet, or computer to watch content and unwind at the end of a long day? Does it relax you because you finally get time away from the world and nobody interrupts you?

Are you watching till your eyes can't stay open?

Falling asleep while trying to watch TV is the same thing as falling asleep while trying to drive, although one feels cozy and the other is life-threatening!* In

---

* In fact, drowsy driving is probably responsible for more accidents than drunk driving. Matthew Walker, *Why We Sleep* (New York: Scribner, 2017).

both situations, the homeostatic sleep pressure and sleep debt finally become so intense that you just can't maintain wakefulness.[10]

I have patients who will spend two to three hours on their light-emitting diode (LED) screens before bed as their way to fall asleep. They watch something to take their mind off things—till their eyelids come down like curtains. They are even willing to push bedtime by a few hours, just for the sense of reclaiming their "me time" after feeling like the world has demanded too much from them all day. This paradox is also called **revenge sleep procrastination**, where *we take revenge on our busy calendars by staying awake to do what we "want."*[11]

If you are consuming content to relax, Eckhart Tolle compares that to consuming alcohol.[12] In both situations, you feel "relaxed" because you get a break from hearing your own mind and your own thoughts.

Would any parent help their child fall asleep by making them staring at a screen?

Although well-meaning parents may try to feed their kids while using screen time as a distraction thankfully, very few use a screen to try to make the baby go to sleep.* Caregivers know that the baby needs a dark, quiet room to fall into a natural, deep sleep, so, why use a brightly lit screen to fall asleep yourself? Not only is this illogical, but it's outright harmful to your hormones.

Remember Paul? Well, after a few months of CPAP therapy, Paul realized he didn't want to spend any time on his screen anymore. The content now felt too stimulating right before bed. He looked forward to a restorative night of good-quality sleep. Looking back, he realized that he was probably resisting sleep and preferring to stay upright on the sofa. Lying down was physically dangerous every night due to the untreated airway blockage that had taken so long to diagnose.

It turns out, maybe **he wasn't completely addicted to Netflix after all**. He was *unknowingly avoiding the danger of choking in his bed every night.*

During the time that he was obsessed with every new thriller series on Netflix, he also never realized that this crutch was demolishing his body's internal clock. Your body's clock is more commonly known as the "**circadian rhythm**," which is maintained by exposure to natural cycles of light and dark. The term *circadian* comes from the Latin phrase *circa diem*, which means "around a day."

Staring at an LED screen after sunset disconnects your natural body clock from its most powerful stimulus to prepare for sleep: the onset of darkness in the environment. Normally, your eyes are constantly sending brightness or darkness updates so the body clock can maintain homeostasis – via the suprachiasmatic nucleus (SCN) – to the pineal gland in the brain, which releases melatonin around **two to three hours after darkness**. But in today's modern habitats, you experi-

---

* I cover this in more detail under the section on adolescent type 2 diabetes in Part 9.

ence constant artificially controlled brightness for the whole day, the same way you have artificially controlled indoor temperatures.

This natural experience of nightfall as a gradual process over a few hours is replaced by an abrupt switching off of LED screen gadgets and bedroom lights when you suddenly opt to go to sleep.

Sadly, the brain now needs a few hours of *low light exposure* before it will release melatonin, and melatonin needs a few more hours to create drowsiness. Deep sleep kicks in, and that alarm clock goes off when you are in the middle of that last stretch of sleep, often rudely pulling you midway out of either deep sleep or a dream.

This leaves you feeling cranky, hitting the snooze button, and chugging coffee to try to wake up and start the morning.* Compare this to a gradually brightening sky sending natural morning twilight gently filtering through your eyelids—the natural stimulus that told your ancestors' pineal gland it was time to switch off the melatonin supply so that they could wake up. If you are trying to increase productivity by setting an alarm to wake up, what you really need to do is reset the body clock by setting an alarm for when you should begin *preparing for bed*, at night.

---

* According to an Ethiopian legend, over 1,000 years ago, a goatherder named Kaldi noticed his goats stayed up energized late into the night after chewing the berries of a local tree. The berries were later brewed into what we now know as coffee.

3.6: Solutions for night-shift workers

Speaking of productivity and sleeping at night, our modern world needs night-shift workers who provide essential services in hospitals, ambulance services, fire departments, police stations, and various other industries—transportation, aviation, information, manufacturing, and more.

Before the 1870s, all human-made light came from burning something and generating a flame. It's hard to imagine life relying on just fire and flames to stay productive after sunset, but that is how humans lived until just three to four generations ago.

Light bulbs became common in the 1870s. LED bulbs penetrated homes after the year 2000. Smartphones brought the LED source within 12 inches of our faces just over 20 years ago. LED technology emits blue-wavelength light that is particularly powerful at blocking melatonin release from the pineal gland. Matthew Walker explains how this probably has something to do with the fact that all life on Earth originated underwater, where there are only two colors to experience: blue means day, and black means night. The technology supporting your life has evolved, but your body has not caught up.[13]

Night shift is not going away, even though it has been linked with increased instances of heart attacks and diabetes, and is also recognized by the World Health Organization (WHO) as a probable carcinogen—linked to chronic inflammation and reduced immunity through disruption of the natural light-dark schedule.[14,15]

If the technological advancements we've made have surpassed the evolution of our homeostatic systems, then how can a night-shift worker reduce their risk of metabolic harm from their job?[16,17]

There are ways to leverage technology to support your natural rhythms. Using blue-light-blocking glasses or blackout curtains when off duty can help you time the exposure to bright light and dim light. There is **chronotherapy** in its many forms, where you can aim for basically resetting the body clock. This includes *chrono-phototherapy, chrono-diet, time-restricted feeding for metabolic and gut health, chrono-exercise*, and more.[18] Additionally, research is currently underway regarding the benefits of *red-light therapy*.

We don't have to overcome the technology of lights with more gadgets. Life-style solutions can include dedicating time for sleep when you are off duty, wearing an eye mask (if it helps), maintaining consistency, and limiting the number of night shifts – by talking to your employer. Request that the night-shift dates be grouped together so that you complete them back to back to establish a predictable schedule for those days. For example, if you have to do ten shifts in a month, doing all ten nights together with the same sleep-wake time is less confusing for your body than different timings every single day of the month. A frequently changing sleep schedule is like never-ending jetlag; it makes it even harder for your body to adjust. By consistently following a dedicated sleep schedule regardless of your shift, you can give your body clock predictability as close to its natural 24-hour rhythm as possible. These things are more about being mindful of what your body needs so you can minimize the stress it goes through.

Too many night shift workers try to burn the candle at both ends, staying awake during the daytime to take care of household responsibilities, and if you find yourself there even after remaining consistent, you can try talking to your doctor to know if you have shift-work disorder, and whether melatonin may help.

3.7: Too busy? The vicious cycle of poor sleep

"I'm too busy!"

We've all said it, and sure, we live in a world that celebrates productivity, even if it might border on toxic levels of workaholism.

But what does productivity mean to you? What are the goals of your longer working hours?

What is required to get more work done? If you need mental efficiency, a sharp memory, accurate decision-making, learning, resilience and overall confidence, is staying up longer helping you see it through?

What if I told you that all of those mental superpowers are gifted to you by restorative sleep?[19,20]

Kids who stay up late the night before a test, cramming at the last minute, have been shown to have poorer performance than the ones who got a good night's rest. On the contrary, good sleep duration, quality, and consistency in the week and month before exams have been correlated with higher grades in college kids.[21] Sleep allows the running engine of the brain to switch gears and go into learning, memory consolidation, cleanup, and repair mode. Running awake all day accumulates waste material that needs to be cleared by the brain's glymphatic system during sleep.

What we often fail to acknowledge, is that these memory and cleanup benefits matter beyond the college years. Considering that diabetes is strongly associated with an increased risk of cognitive decline and dementia, it makes sense to invest early in sleep to improve brain health—never mind that there is growing interest in the idea that sleep deprivation could cause memory and brain cleanup problems later in life, too. Things like the reduced ability to prevent accumulation of beta-amyloid in the brain and the lack of enough good-quality sleep has been associated with Alzheimer's dementia.[22,23]

Some people aren't telling me that they are busy, but that they are stuck in their heads all night instead of falling asleep.

If you notice your thoughts playing on loop all day and night, chances are, your body awareness might be low. Low body awareness can show up as problems with falling or staying asleep. If the self-help tips from this book don't help you achieve rejuvenating sleep, work with your healthcare professional to consider a sleep study, and cognitive-behavioral therapy for improving sleep.

If, instead, you are the type to use alcohol, food, and sedatives to "fall asleep," then let me tell you about Sean. Sean was using bedtime whiskey and carbohydrate-rich snacks to *feel like he slept*. Otherwise, he would be tossing and turning all night. Alcohol works very similarly to a sedative tablet.[*]

When alcohol was not available, he would take an antihistamine to knock himself out from the drowsiness side effects instead.

Neither alcohol or sedatives give you natural sleep; they both give you unconsciousness.

Both of them reduce REM sleep, which is important for memory and learning. Losing REM sleep has been linked to struggles with handling stress and solving problems. Sedatives are used intravenously by anesthetists to make patients stay unconscious during surgery; patients are not sleeping on the operating table; nobody "sleeps" through a knife running through their skin. They are chemically sedated.

Sean realized he had a drinking problem. The daily drinking was affecting his family life. He was drinking more than sixty milliliters of whiskey every night and not spending any time with his family after getting home from work. This was affecting his sleep, and I told him that the quantity of liquor qualified as high-risk drinking, and was directly working like glucose on his liver, worsening insulin resistance and diabetes.[24]

I asked him what he wanted to do about his health. His business was under financial pressure, and he wanted to numb himself so that he could fall asleep. His glucose levels were not coming down, he was gaining weight, and he could not stop drinking on his own. He accepted that he needed help to get sober. So he did.

With this in mind, I want you to note that **chronic sleep loss** is not only determined by the *absence of sleep, short duration,* or *infrequency*, but also by the *quality* of the sleep. By self-medicating, remaining distracted by technology, or becoming inconsistent with your sleep, you can begin to slide down a slippery slope where multiple vicious cause–effect cycles are set up against you.[25]

When it comes to sleep deprivation, two big things happen:

---

[*] My favorite book on sleep is The Sleep Solution by Dr. Chris Winter, a neurologist and sleep specialist who consults professional sports players and the US military. Matthew Walker's book Why We Sleep is great and is written by someone who has dedicated their life to researching sleep. I found Dr. Winter's book had more relevance to my medical practice and gave me a clearer understanding of the clinical implications of sleep. Chris Winter, The Sleep Solution: Why Your Sleep Is Broken and How to Fix It (New York: Penguin, 2017); Matthew Walker, Why We Sleep (New York: Scribner, 2017).

- Sleep deprivation → worse glucose metabolism and difficulty losing fat → worse insulin resistance.

- Sleep deprivation → hormone changes increase hunger → eat more high carb comfort food → worse insulin resistance.

Both of those introduce a plateau in weight loss, and eventually, weight gain.

- Weight gain → risk of obstructive sleep apnea → worse sleep quality → worse insulin resistance.[26]

Isn't it interesting how sleep deprivation can lead to weight gain, leading to sleep apnea? And isn't it interesting that sleep apnea, going untreated, leads to sleep deprivation? It's easy to see how these cycles can make the root causes even more confusing to find. But now we know: ***getting seven to eight hours of good sleep is better for your metabolic health, and increases your ability to learn and come up with creative alternatives to decisions that fed your insulin resistance.***
But how?

3.8: If you struggle to wake up: A checklist for sleep hygiene and body-clock reset

The following habits have helped most of my patients reset their sleep rhythms and wake up fresh and recharged to take on the new day, without needing prescriptions for sleep. As an unintended side benefit of fixing sleep rhythms, people's bowel movements (regarding regularity and constipation) have also been corrected, because bowel activity is cyclic and gets reset by the day-night cycle.

A benefit of wearable technology is that it gives you feedback on how soon your heart rate settled overnight and how consistent you were with your bedtimes and wake-up times. Using the Oura ring or Apple watch can also give you insights about how a late night or alcohol before bed affects your sleep quality.[27] I have been using an Oura ring for close to two years now, and I love the insights it gives me. Personally, I prefer the ring over the watch due to its unobtrusive design and lack of a screen. For me, the less distractions and lights, the better, though you're free to choose what works for you.

The sleep hygiene practice I share with my patients starts with the question: what do you feed your mind at night?

For many of us, it's screen time. Whether it's an e-reader, a tablet, or a television, check the effect of feeding your mind with stimulating content like a thrilling mini-series, negative news, or graphic social media feeds. Passively watching a screen seems to have less impact than actively interacting with the content, and I personally suffered from disturbed sleep when watching the gripping series Narcos.[28] It was part of my "me time" with my husband, but my heart was jumping out of my chest multiple times per episode—and then I was on high alert at bedtime.

Many people struggle with waking up and think they need to adjust their wake time or morning routine.

I'm here to say: **work on bedtime first.**

We start here because fixing bedtime is more powerful than trying to force a different wake-up time. *Set a fixed bedtime, not a fixed wake-up time.* Forcing a wake-up time risks the alarm catching you in the middle of a sleep cycle, and coming out of a half-finished sleep cycle makes you feel unrested and groggy. As you achieve healthier sleep, your brain will naturally start waking up on its own. Your eyes will open, and you will emerge from light sleep without an alarm. Your brain will be fully alert without needing caffeine to kickstart your day. (Not that caffeine is bad. I love my black coffee. You just don't deserve to feel like a zombie without it.)

Once you're up, a morning walk in natural sunlight helps reset all of your body clocks. You will still benefit even if it's cloudy outside. Even if it's sunny, skip the sunglasses because the ultraviolet light is what resets the clock. All you need is a few minutes after waking up.[29] Many successful people start the day with five minutes of journaling and report better clarity throughout the day.

But waking up is after.

First, let's go through a sleep hygiene checklist with custom wind-down rituals so that your mind can predict what it has to do next: sleep.

How?

Through creating your nighttime sleep routine, learning mind-body-awareness techniques, and reducing light pollution, you can work towards the sleep of your dreams. I always give my patients these suggestions on how to **build a bedtime routine** as a starting point, but as always, feel free to do what works for you.

Create a calm, cool sleeping environment, then *stay out of bed* until you are drowsy. This allows the mind to learn that the bed is for sleeping, not for insomnia. In the meantime, you can try using *lavender aromatherapy* or take a *relaxing bath*, as lowering the body temperature helps sleep. You can opt for an *Epsom salt soak* that provides magnesium sulfate, or even discuss taking a *magnesium glycinate supplement* with your doctor.

Changing into *cotton pajamas* that keep the hands and feet cool can also help. Have you ever noticed that kids keep sticking their hands outside their blankies? It helps!

If you don't have time to soak every night, you can try listening to relaxing music, maybe even while *journaling before bed. Dumping the next day's work into a to-do list* using a pen and paper before bed has been shown to reduce the time taken to fall asleep, and a *two-week gratitude practice* has been shown to improve sleep and blood pressure.[30,31]

No matter what routine you build, it's ideal to *keep the same bedtime*, even on weekends. When changing sleep times by three hours, it can take up to three days to recover (roughly one day per one-hour time zone shift) and can have effects on the body similar to flying from the United Kingdom to the United States. One time zone at the equator is 1,665 kilometers wide. It would take you 333 hours to *walk* through one time zone if you walked at five kilometers per hour. Even if you walked for twelve hours a day, it would take you *four weeks* to cover that distance by foot, plenty of time for your brain to deal with the one-hour time change. A flight gets you there in less than three hours, so if you fly often, try reducing flights that cross multiple time zones.

The human body has not yet evolved to such rapid changes in time zones or fluctuating bedtimes. Most people don't recover lost sleep, and the debt is not repaid. This catches up with us, even if we don't catch up on the lost sleep. This "social jetlag" is associated with a higher hemoglobin A1c (HbA1c) in metabolically unhealthy people with obesity.[32]

Once you have your nightly routine set, you can begin learning about the different ways that **mind-body awareness techniques** can help you. It really comes down to meditation of any kind that works for you.

If you are new to meditation, it may be helpful to start with breathing techniques like *Yoga Nidra*, an ancient practice that has been proven to improve sleep.[33] There is also 4-7-8 breathing, which has foundations in pranayama and activates the parasympathetic system. The 4-7-8 method can cause some light-headedness, so it's best done lying down.

It involves placing your tongue on the roof of the mouth, with the top of the tongue behind the front teeth. Inhale for four counts of easy breathing, hold the breath for seven, and slowly exhale over eight counts. Repeat this for three to four cycles twice a day.

Mindfulness-based stress reduction (MBSR) techniques, and *progressive muscle relaxation* are also available options.[34]

For me, I find the *emotional freedom technique* quite useful.[35] This self-help tapping technique has always helped me fall asleep when I am tossing and turning—but everything depends on what feels good to you. It might help to reduce caffeine intake after 2:00 p.m. because it can last for up to seven hours and impact your sleep. Like with everything, some people might be blessed with different metabolisms of caffeine, so check what works for your body.

When you have a routine to stick to and you know how to step into your body so your mind doesn't keep you up all night, the last thing to do is **reduce light pollution.**

The easiest place to start is *mood lighting*. By shifting the color of light sources away from the blue (cool) end of the light spectrum and toward the warm end, we can change the entire environment going forward. Think about it: a candlelight dinner feels relaxing because of the effect this has on our mood; a fast-food restaurant is brightly lit, inducing us to eat quickly and leave!

Adding blackout curtains to prevent light from filtering through your window until you wake, can support your natural rhythm without too many changes to your daily routine. More ways that you can actively support your body include *dimming the lights* in your home after sunset–especially a few hours before bed, and wearing *blue-light-blocking glasses* for any unavoidable screen time after sunset. If you are using an e-reader, *try switching to a paperback book.*

When it comes to the bedroom and bedtime specifically, I recommend applying *"screen-free" bedroom rules*, this applies to your bed partner, too! Keep *mobile phones away* from the bedroom or in sleep mode so that they don't light up with notifications, and *cover the glowing lights* on air conditioners or other gadgets. *Remove backlit alarm clocks* from the bedroom; you don't need to know that it's 3:00 a.m. when it's 3:00 a.m. You need to go back to sleep if you're to get enough sleep before starting the day. *An eye mask* will help block out all of those sources, if that's easier for you.

Improving your sleep, and by proxy, your partner's, you may find that your overall mood and relationships improve. Much like Sean, many people realize that their nightly routines have affected more than just their sleep and health. Seeing how Sean's sleep was affected by financial pressures from work, alcohol and strained relationships, it makes sense how we end up at the third wheel of your lifestyle car: stress management.

Part 3 summary

- Falling asleep during the day without planning to is a sign of poor sleep.

- Poor sleep quality and quantity are associated with worse insulin resistance and more difficulty losing body fat.

- Sleep apnea needs to be suspected and tested for when relevant.

- Fix bedtime and get early morning sunlight to reset your body clock before forcing an earlier wake up time.

- Sleep helps your brain learn, heal and solve complex problems. Do you want to respond to external situations in more creative, productive ways?

For Bonus Materials, Visit the Website Here:

PART 4

THE THIRD WHEEL OF THE LIFESTYLE CAR:

STRESS MANAGEMENT

4.1: The stress management skills you need

There is a specific reason that I have placed stress management as the third wheel, only after fixing nutrition and sleep. High glucose levels have been proven to increase sadness and anxiety, with impaired processing speed, memory, and attention and lower energy levels.[1]

It gets even harder to observe your own thinking patterns when your glucose levels are high.

The good news is that both reducing carbs and getting better sleep will help your glucose levels come down quickly, and you will see your brain function improve automatically. The mechanism might partly be through the gut-brain axis, improving mitochondrial health in nerve cells, and also partly through reduced insulin resistance, but truly, this area needs more research.[2] While we await more scientific insight, the best part is that my patients have often noticed better moods. They are surprised by how it's easier to respond to stressful life events with more creative solutions, simply by changing their nutrition and sleep habits.

But what about when you fix your relationships with food and sleep—and you're still stressed?

At a certain point, it may help to examine your coping mechanisms and determine how to handle stress in a way that is better for your health and your life. I am here to share what I tell my patients, but first, let's make sure we understand stress in the same way.

Perhaps the simplest definition of stress could be *"the loss or absence of desired experiences and the presence of unwanted experiences in life."* With that definition in mind, what areas of life cause you the most stress?

If you are anything like most people I know, stress usually falls under some major categories. I find that the biggest stressors fall somewhere along the lines of **relationships, finances, sense of purpose, or undesirable events outside of our control.** There are so many things out of our control, like war, global politics, natural disasters, climate and weather changes, and even circumstances affecting other people or topics we care about. Many people will report stress from things like "career" or "health," but career stress is related to finances and sense of purpose at its core, and stressing about your health is connected to its impact on all of the above.

Because all of these points seem to be part of daily life for all of us, there are plenty of opportunities to become stressed. Because of this, situations like Priti's make a lot of sense.

Priti was thirty-four when we first met to discuss her uncontrolled glucose levels. Her hemoglobin A1c (HbA1c) was 9 percent, which meant we had to act urgently. Her diabetes had started in her late twenties when she had started gaining weight during a hectic job that required long working hours. She was ambitious, was quickly promoted within her company, and then met the love of her life right there, in that office. Six years flew by. A marriage and two children later, they were trying to make ends meet. On the surface, her life looked great—a husband, two kids, a stable job, and smiley photos on her Instagram page.

When we started talking, I enquired about her stress. On the questionnaire I have all patients fill out, she indicated her stress levels as ten . . . out of ten. I never let it slide when someone selects a ten.

She mentioned how her workplace had become toxic after some reorganization due to an abusive boss. If that wasn't bad enough, her husband had lost his job in recent layoffs. Now, as the sole provider, she put her health last while working two jobs to pay their bills.

She stopped spending money on her diabetes testing strips and was skipping medication. She would sometimes eat a few donuts after work to feel better before getting home.

She sometimes lost her patience with her young children, who had been waiting all day to see her. Her husband would intervene, which often resulted in an argument between them.

She was feeling like a mess.

At that appointment, the latest HbA1c result of 9 percent came as a shock. When I asked what she wanted to do next, she put her face into her hands and burst into tears.

Why am I telling you her story? Because while her struggle was especially difficult and she was doing the very best she could, there are common patterns in how she was coping that I have seen while working with thousands of people on diabetes self-management over the years.

It's true. Chronic stress can raise your glucose levels and reduce your ability to manage diabetes. It's also true that nobody *likes* having diabetes. I haven't met anyone who looks back with joy at the day they found out they had diabetes.

When you were told you have diabetes or prediabetes, your response may have fluctuated on a broad spectrum: from taking it as a wake-up call to empower yourself to get better, to the other extreme of denial, inertia, and avoidance. Over time, maybe you grew resentful of all the restrictive rules you were expected to follow and the shaming that occurred from loved ones at home or doctors who tried (albeit with good intentions) to police your diet and force you to exercise. If each doctor's visit results in more prescriptions and increased doses, you may have found any effort to be pointless, and you might even feel afraid, alone, misunderstood, judged, unsupported, anxious, rebellious, angry, sad, helpless, or hopeless.

You already know the solution isn't to run off to some cave in the mountains where stress can't find you. Everyone wants a vibrant life full of experiences. You probably also wish for a more stable, calm, and peaceful *inner* state–regardless of the constant *outer* changes and events around you. In reality, we all share the universal human need to experience joy, true happiness, kindness, connection, love, gratitude, and abundance. That's what we all want, so let's talk about how to get there—and don't forget about Priti, we'll come back to her later.

4.2: Psychology, behavior, the body-and diabetes distress

If we are trying to move from stressed to unstressed, it helps to start by acknowledging that thoughts lead to emotions. Scientifically the transition from thoughts to emotions and stressed to unstressed is experienced through the release of neurotransmitters and hormones.*

These biochemical signals carry messages in the brain, and this complex phenomenon is now studied in an emerging field of medicine called *psycho-neuro-immuno-endocrinology*, which links the phenomenon of thoughts to brain effects, the immune system, and hormonal responses.

Our conscious or unconscious decisions lead to actions. Repeated actions become habits, which form our lifestyle. Positive or negative, our thoughts and emotions about diabetes lead to certain daily actions and habits. Based on these, we get certain health results.

While this is an oversimplification of the complexity of human behavior, it's not intended to blame anyone for poor health, but rather, to empower you.

Behavioral dynamics often go unaddressed by overburdened healthcare systems, despite their best intentions. What's worse, the health system might make you experience guilt, shame, or blame for your reality. The good news? If you can catch a negative, self-limiting thought, you can find the power to change it—and potentially change your results. Awareness is the first step, and this realization was a life-changing one for me.

If you are experiencing large amounts of stress, or have reached the point of diabetes distress, you can still take charge of your life and your health. You may be experiencing diabetes distress if you relate to any of these statements:

- I ignored my diabetes/I went into denial/I pretended I didn't have diabetes.

---

* The Greek word hormao means "excite" or "arouse."

- I couldn't keep up with the sugar monitoring/The medication was getting to be too much.
- I am failing in my diabetes management.
- I am always anxious about getting sick from diabetes/what will happen to my family.
- I lost my loved one to diabetes, and it's a matter of time till I get sick from it myself.
- Everyone is disappointed in my habits.
- I hate not being able to eat what I want without worrying about my sugar.
- I can't talk to anyone in my family about diabetes because they don't understand.

Diabetes distress is not the same as depression, but it can be powerful enough to alter your ability to practice diabetes self-care. There is an online questionnaire to know if you are experiencing diabetes distress. You can find the updated and validated Diabetes Distress Scale for type 2 diabetes (T2-DDAS) and type 1 diabetes (T1-DDAS) – developed by Lawrence Fisher, PhD, and William Polonsky, PhD – on the website of the Behavioural Diabetes Institute.[3]

Research has shown that although diabetes distress affects self-management skills, it is also very responsive to intervention through diabetes self-management education (DSME) and diabetes self-management support (DSMS). *Put simply, if your healthcare team and community help reduce your diabetes distress, you will be more likely to adopt healthier diabetes self-management habits.* This has been shown to improve overall diabetes control.[4]

Whether it's diabetes distress or typical stress from life's responsibilities, it is possible to lighten the load. Stress has many physical ramifications, but managing it effectively starts with your mindset. When it comes to shifting how you think about stress, there are three things I want you to adopt as truth, first.

One, no rational person is intentionally trying to harm themselves or stay sick, and people who are uninterested in their health don't keep taking medications and visiting doctors. You are reading this book because you want to thrive. You may have been made to believe that uncontrolled diabetes is because of some character flaw, but that's not true. But it's difficult to imagine remission of type 2 diabetes, or having better health with less medication if nobody tells you about it. It's difficult to imagine having type 1 diabetes with stable glucose levels and minimal insulin requirements–where you are safely doing everything your heart desires–if nobody tells you it's possible. Which, of course, leads me to the **second truth.**

To turn diabetes around, you first need to know it's possible. Maybe you were never told that the C-peptide test will tell you how much insulin your pancreas is making and whether your diabetes is due to insulin resistance (prediabetes or type 2) or insulin deficiency (type 1 or burned-out type 2). Maybe no one told you that turning your diabetes around, having more energy, and reclaiming your health with less medication are not only possible—but that *remission* of prediabetes and type 2 diabetes and getting off or reducing medication is possible, and it's also possible to achieve stable glucose levels with lower insulin doses in type 1 diabetes. Maybe you didn't know any of that, but if you adopt it as a known truth, it makes the journey to service your lifestyle car *that* much easier. Why?

Because the third truth is that **giving people the information and support they need reduces diabetes distress**, improves habits, and lowers HbA1c.[5] I have seen it happen again and again. When you feel stuck or feel like giving up, you *deserve to know* that information and support are non-negotiable. If you seek help, you might be surprised at how many people want to see you succeed. You were never meant to do this alone—you deserve to have a health team and community that supports and helps you.

4.3: Chronic stress, chronic diabetes

We already covered how being human comes with a myriad of stressors about money, purpose, and relationships—even if you don't have diabetes.

Our hunter-gatherer ancestors also had stress, but their stress came from living in the wild. Missing a meal (fasting) or hunting the next meal (exercise) were some of the brief (acute) stresses they faced. The stress hormone, cortisol, would briefly spike up to activate the fight-flight-fright response, then come back down to baseline for the person to rest, repair, and digest.

The stress response system is largely run by the sympathetic nervous system (SNS), and the relaxation system is governed by the parasympathetic nervous system (PNS). Of course, they cooperate in many functions together, but they manage different sides of the balance.

Follow the work of Dr. Stephen Porges, psychologist, neuroscientist, and professor of psychiatry, who has described the *polyvagal theory* as a conceptualization of the many effects of the vagus nerve. Chronic sensations of fight-flight-fright can also lead to a sense of "no escape ," with the only option being a freeze response with shutdown and dissociation. Although the theory is not widely accepted in mainstream health care, it offers a concept of healing that has been endorsed by trauma experts like physician Gabor Maté and psychiatrist Bessel van der Kolk.[6]

Nowadays, we don't run from hungry tigers but have daily worries about diabetes plus managing economic hardship, family, pets, responsibilities, relationships, and more. The stress hormone cortisol stays high for longer because the same person you find annoying is still there to deal with tomorrow. That promotion is still waiting to happen, and that loan is not getting approved. The problems don't go away, and we carry them in our thoughts. The body stays on high alert, and this long-term, high-cortisol state can worsen insulin resistance and diabetes via the hypothalamus–pituitary–adrenal axis, the gut–brain axis, and the immune system. This long-term, high-cortisol state, is the scientific way to describe the effect of chronic stress on the body.

The never-ending nature of the stressors is what classifies it as chronic. Since many people experience diabetes over an extended period, it too, is considered to be chronic.

But remember the second truth? That you first have to believe that it is possible to heal?

Diabetes is chronic and progressive only if you don't change the habits that made it so. Before we continue, let me clarify: *This statement is not to blame people for diabetes or obesity–it is meant to empower people.* Getting metabolically sick is not your fault, but there is plenty you can do about it. Everyone with diabetes deserves and benefits from the support of their care team so that they can do what it takes to turn things around.

Science has known since 2002 that lifestyle change is more powerful than metformin, or just "doing nothing," in preventing the progression of insulin resistance.[7] Although there are endocrine disruptors and obesogens in the environment, I have seen people turn around diabetes while living in their exact same environment. Sure, we absolutely need the world to make better policies that protect us from harmful foods and toxins. We have champions like Dr. Robert Lustig, Nina Teicholz, Gary Taubes, and many others calling out for policy reform. While that economic and political battle happens and must continue, this book tells you what you can do for yourself today.

Despite the power of lifestyle changes being proven over 20 years ago, the common (but incomplete) prediction of a person's future with diabetes is bleak. It carries the image of unwanted long-term suffering, marching on like a relentless enemy that will win in the end, no matter what. This naturally comes with an emotional burden for many, which often stays outside of the doctor–patient interaction–but is very much woven into the fabric of a patient's daily life as soon as they leave the clinic.

I have had patients with diabetes from all walks of life, including doctors, psychotherapists, and surgeons with diabetes themselves, who were silently and unknowingly in diabetes distress—drowning in resignation and belief that losing to diabetes was an inevitable part of their story. Life itself has so many chronic stressors that nobody needs the added weight of constantly feeling like you're fighting a losing battle. I have seen firsthand what people can do for their health with the power of lifestyle change. I've also seen what people can save.

4.4: Uncontrolled stress and diabetes are more expensive than you think

Stress doesn't just increase blood glucose. It affects every cell. Do you recall from Part 1.4, the role of long-distance messaging that hormones carry out, making sure all the organ systems are on the same page?

Well, the same goes for cortisol.

Acute spikes in cortisol mobilize the whole body to fight for survival. Chronically high cortisol levels keep the sympathetic nervous system on full throttle, forcing the body into survival mode all the time. Think psycho-neuro-immuno-endocrinology on steroids, literally—cortisol is a *steroid* hormone. Chronic stress and higher cortisol levels have been correlated with more cravings, increased intake of sweet foods, and weight gain, which as we know, can lead back to the cycle of insulin resistance.[8,9]

Every medical specialist will tell you that a large percentage of the people they see every day have illnesses that are worsened by or directly caused by chronic stress. Each doctor can write prescriptions that manage symptoms but don't cure the root problem.

Diabetes costs us. Psychologically, physically, and financially.

Type 2 diabetes used to be a condition of the wealthy, but it is now highly prevalent across all socioeconomic groups around the world, tending to impact lower-income groups more severely.[10] Besides the expensive medication and direct devastation of diabetes complications, uncontrolled diabetes sets up a vicious cycle dragging people further into financial distress. This is especially visible in low-income groups across India, where the loss of daily wages and year-on-year expenses from diabetes complications can accelerate a family's decline into poverty.[11] Even in the United States, people with diabetes who have a family income below the federal poverty level have twice the risk of diabetes-related death compared to their highest-income counterparts.[12]

In spite of innovation adding more technology and prescription options to manage diabetes, the epidemic is getting worse. Diabetes and obesity are affecting more and more people, including children, costing society more every year. Are we really getting better at treating diabetes?

With type 2 diabetes for example, doctors are more likely to treat the high glucose initially with pills and later, injections. Some prescriptions lower glucose by improving insulin sensitivity. Some raise insulin levels or include insulin injections, making insulin resistance worse.

Prescriptions alone don't address nutrition, sleep, stress, or exercise–the root lifestyle drivers of insulin resistance. The truth is, diabetes isn't the only illness that chronic stress can trigger. Still, healthcare systems may not treat stress as a root cause, focussing instead on reducing the symptoms.

If you suffer from **chronic aches and pains**, you get painkillers and anti-inflammatory drugs. Suffering from **allergies**? You need antihistamines, medicines that cause narrowing of blood vessels, immune response modulators, or steroids. **Asthma**? Bronchial muscle wall relaxants, immune response modulators, and steroids for you.

Acid reflux and peptic ulcers are treated with antacids and acid suppressants, while **irritable bowel syndrome** (IBS) gets you laxatives, antispasmodics, and gas-absorbing agents. **Inflammatory bowel disease** (Crohn's or ulcerative colitis)? There's anti-inflammatory drugs, immunosuppressants, biologics, antibiotics, antidiarrheal treatment, and painkillers for that. If you suffer from **small intestinal bacterial overgrowth** (SIBO), you might get antibiotics. For those whose chronic stress led to obesity–you get drugs that block fat absorption, antimigraine medication, opioid blocker–antidepressant combination, and diabetes drugs that cause weight loss.[*13]

For **insomnia**, you get sedatives, sleeping pills, antidepressants, and melatonin; for **migraines**, you're given pain prevention, antinausea medications, and antiseizure medications. Prescriptions for **depression, anxiety, bipolar disorders, psychotic disorders, autism spectrum, attention deficit disorders, mood disorders, and neurodegenerative disorders like dementia or Parkinson's** include antidepressants, sedatives, anxiolytics, mood stabilizers, neurotransmitter agonists, and receptor blockers. We see herbal supplements, vitamins or repeated antibiotic courses to combat **recurrent infections**.

It has become so common to accept medication for every symptom, because that's how we see the big health issues being treated.

We see illnesses like **cancer** being treated aggressively with drugs that destroy rapidly dividing cancer cells; receptor blockers, and biologics are given to modulate the immune response.

---

* Personality, anxiety and stress in patients with small intestinal bacterial overgrowth syndrome. See the Polish preliminary study: Kossewska, Joanna, Karolina Bierlit, and Vladimir Trajkovski.

The symptoms of **neuropathy** are often treated with antidepressants, antiseizure medications, counterirritant creams or balms (that make you feel heat instead of pain), or painkillers. Things like **atherosclerosis, coronary artery disease**, and **strokes** are given cholesterol-lowering medications (statins) and blood thinners, and it makes it easy to accept that the treatment for **high blood pressure** is simply to administer blood-pressure-lowering medications.

Not only can these examples all be *directly worsened by chronic stress*, but many also have root causes based on nutrition and sleep as well–the wheels we've already discussed. Three wheels, three potential root causes, and yet, I've listed more medications than any one person would want to be on in their lifetime. This is why so many people with uncontrolled diabetes and high levels of stress end up taking more than ten different medications every day, like Dinesh. Sadly, many of them don't feel normal or healthy even after taking so many prescriptions.

Stress is expensive. Not only are you paying in suffering, you're paying to see the doctors, paying to take the medications, and it continues to cost you physically and emotionally when you still don't feel like yourself. That's how to consider the true toll that chronic stress can take on your life. Knowing all this, it might be best to consider that a fragmented healthcare system might not be helping you address the root causes of certain underlying problems, and maybe, you deserve better. You can save your health, save your relationships, save your future, *and* save money by digging for root causes and addressing the stress in your life.

4.5: We start with thinking versus feeling

Managing stress starts with recognizing that you are stressed in the first place. It sounds easy, but most of us are irrational when stressed. You probably know every "correct" behavior you "should" be doing, but maybe you tend to experience **emotional eating** or **eat junk** every day. You could be choosing to **skip exercise, binge-watch TV, or escape on the internet.** Maybe there are times that you **don't check your glucose readings**, you **don't visit the doctor**, you **don't get regular blood tests done**, and **you don't get your feet or eyes checked.**

Your mind and intellect have various complex needs. These needs drive your behaviors. What might look like repeated self-destructive behavior has a deeper explanation.

This tendency towards irrationality is what makes it so hard to recognize that we are stressed. It's almost engrained, so much so that I learned how to recognize my own stress in my mid-thirties—*for the first time.**

My own personal stress crisis hit a climax between 2011 and 2013. Moving to India from the United States with a young family and setting up a new career was extremely challenging. I ended up developing prediabetes during that time, and had the highest number of physical health complaints of my life through that same phase. I was miserable, and I wanted everything outside of me (people, situations, unwanted problems) to *just change* so that I could be happy. The more I wanted the outside to be different, the more miserable and powerless I felt. Everything was closing in around me.

On the outside, I had an enviable life.

But I still felt hollow inside.

At some point I admitted to myself, my ego crushed, that I was exhausted from futile efforts to control, manipulate, cajole, and bend the world to give me what I wanted. My racing mind was not helping me find peace, and my heart was

---

* I could take off on how early schooling doesn't teach us how to manage health, relationships, or finances, but that's a different conversation.

constantly throwing palpitations. Defeated and tired of being unhappy, I realized all I wanted was happiness–regardless of what the world was doing. I was tired of outsourcing my happiness to external circumstances outside my control. I wanted the keys back.

At that darkest moment in my life, I turned to a friend, who guided me, saying I was ready for a spiritual journey. I was all in. I did whatever I could to change my thinking patterns and unhealed negative emotions so that happiness could become my default state of being. Imagine being a highly qualified diabetes doctor and having to learn how to consciously chill out!

Over a decade later, I am still a very messy work in progress. I have not attained nirvana, and I have my crazy days. But they are much fewer and further apart.

Pro tip: I still slip into thought loops sometimes, and one of the ways I have learned to catch myself sooner and snap out of it is to notice if my *need to use lots of words* has increased. Sometimes the stressed-out state causes some of us to overthink, overstep, or overexplain. See, words and speech are generated by the thinking region of the brain, which is a relatively new upgrade in human evolution. But a lot of our *emotional distress is processed in a totally different location* in more primitive brain centers. **To put the science simply, feelings can be very difficult to verbalize**. Those who are body-aware notice how they feel in the body (racing heart rate, sweating, anxiety, shallow breathing, churning in the pit of the stomach). Some of us just loop in our thoughts in a slightly dissociated way and shut down, silently internalizing our thought chains, unable to effectively express ourselves.

We often think or talk about our feelings without feeling them.

So, I do a quick self-assessment to notice if I am doing a lot of high-pressure talking or high-speed thinking, because let's face it—feeling unheard, misunderstood, blamed, alone, unsupported, betrayed, unworthy, or unloved are uncomfortable things we'd much rather not feel. I remind myself,

> *The more I am talking, explaining, thinking, and analyzing, the less happy I'm feeling.*

> *The more I am breathing, listening, observing, and watching, the calmer I am feeling.*

I know we'd rather talk, deflect, debate, or rationalize to get away from those nasty feelings. But how can we change that? How can we get comfortable doing the self-assessments and change our relationship with stress?

4.6: Changing the stress response

Stress becomes a distressing experience when you, the experiencer, struggle with what is being experienced, which could be a person, thing, situation, or event. Said mathematically,

experience = the experiencer + that which is experienced

Looking at that expression, it becomes clear that you can't change "that which is experienced." People try, but that's what we might refer to as "projecting", "controlling" or "running away from their problems." Because you can't change what is being experienced (it's essentially out of your control), the only way to change the entire experience you are having is by changing *yourself* so that you can approach what is being experienced in a different way.[14]

How?

The first step is knowing what to do—then actually doing it. Let's see how this can be applied to diabetes.

When it comes to knowing what you "should do" for diabetes, versus *actually doing it*—how can you bridge the gap between the two? It can seem difficult to navigate if you don't know where to start. It helps to start by **comparing your current diabetes self-management habits** to *what you know they "should" be*. GPS navigation can't get you anywhere without knowing your current location and where you want to go.

Second, ask yourself: "Is there a **disconnect** between what I do and what I want in the future?" If yes, please know that it's completely normal to feel two different ways about something. We call it ambivalence in motivational interviewing. *It's what can keep us stuck.* The good news is that you can get unstuck.

Once you're aware that you are stuck, **list out the opposite, conflicting pairs** of habits: *what you do now* for short-term, immediate reward and gratification–and what you want in the future. The lazy mind prefers instant rewards that can be obtained effortlessly and that immediately take care of an emotional need (whether conscious or unconscious).[15] Most of us have plenty of internal conflicts at any given point in time.

What you do now	What you want in the future
Immediate goals	Distant goals
React to emotional needs	Plan for logical needs
Short-term need (urgent)	Long-term need (important)
Effortless, automatic	Analytical, deliberate

For me, in 2013, as I was learning about the power of self-talk, I started paying attention to my internal rationalization for not exercising. Of course I knew that exercise was good for me–I had just come out of prediabetes! But I told myself I *couldn't* exercise because there wasn't enough time. I was a young doctor building my reputation in a new professional environment and also a mother of two young daughters–*clearly* I was too busy to exercise.

So, what were the valid needs that were opposing each other?

My **short-term/urgent need** was to s*ave time by skipping exercise* so that I could focus on my work and my kids.

My **long-term/important need** was that *exercise would eventually make me a fit doctor* and a fit mother. I would take pride in walking the talk for my patients. I wanted to be a role model to my daughters.

This leads into the next step—**check for commonalities between the opposite pairs.** For example, my love for my kids and my work was *relevant to my current actions and my long-term goals.*

Once that is clear, be sure to **check how the self-talk makes you feel** on both sides. Not having enough time *made me feel constricted*, with a sense of scarcity and limitation. There was some *guilt*, too. If I could be a role model in the future for my kids and patients, that would be incredible. I would feel confident and happy when that future moment would arrive. I would feel better about myself as a person.

Then ask yourself, **which person do you want to be? Which version of you resonates more strongly?** For example, did I relate to the person who felt rushed, short on time, and guilty for not doing what I should? Or did I *identify with the fit and busy* woman who was a role model for her daughters and patients?

Now take this one step further. If you want to be that future version of yourself, **what needs to change now** so that you start moving toward there?

Finally, **add sustainability:** If you are looking to make a long-term change, love is a *stronger long-term motivator than fear or guilt.*

Like I said, from my journey, you can see that the first step is to know what you want, so that you can *decide* what to do, then you can act on what you know, and *make the changes* needed for your diabetes and your life.

So, what was I to do?

I knew what I wanted and why, so **I changed the limiting statement** in my head about exercise. My previous self-talk was about me not taking action.

It went from **"I am too busy to exercise because of my work and kids"** to *"I am a busy and fit doctor because I inspire my work and kids."*

And a few days later, just like magic, as I was waiting in the hospital for the elevator so I could start morning rounds, something changed. The staircase seemed to emerge out of nowhere with an opportunity. I was a busy fit doctor who didn't have time to wait for a silly elevator.

The staircase, kids or hours in my day didn't change.

I did.

I *started noticing opportunities* for movement and activity within my busy day and started feeling consistent with who I wanted to be.

My patients are living proof that knowing what to do and then actually doing it, can be revolutionary for your diabetes and your health. By changing the self-talk, you can change the way you approach everything, even stress.

4.7: From powerless to empowered thinking

What if I told you turning around diabetes was about reclaiming your power, and the first step of self-care is to check if your thoughts are supporting that goal?

© Glasbergen/ glasbergen.com

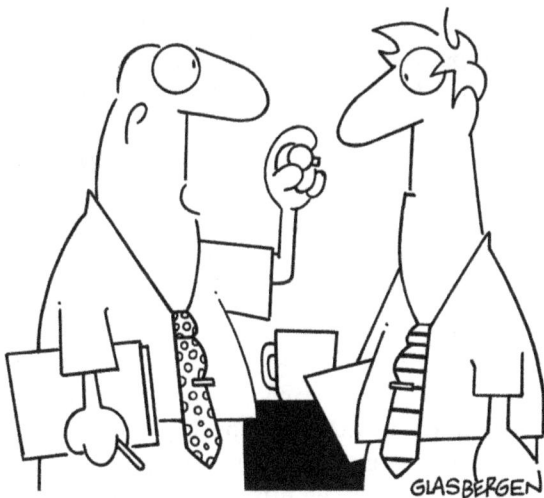

"It's a special hearing aid. It filters out criticism and amplifies compliments."

What if I asked you: **"How clean is your thought diet?"** That might seem like a crazy question, but hear me out.

In Part 2, you started paying attention to the food you put in your mouth (*a nutritional diet*, the first wheel) and in Part 3, you started reducing the artificial light you put in your eyes (*an environmental diet*, the second wheel). Now in Part 4, I want to ask, do you monitor your thought diet, or what you put in your head?

Do you need to clean up your self-talk?

Through working with people on behavior change to turn around diabetes, I have seen them *gradually shift* their thinking patterns in baby steps.

Don't wait for motivation or inspiration to magically strike with a burst of rainbows and butterflies, giving you "happy ever after" endings. Behavior change happens along zigzag, circular, or meandering bumpy paths, not perfectly straight racetracks. People succeed in changing their self-talk by identifying what they value in terms of *emotional or functional beliefs*.

There are quite a few common disempowering thoughts people with diabetes can pick up without even consciously noticing. While these examples are an oversimplification of how people's thoughts have evolved over months and years of introspection, coaching, education, and sometimes therapy, I still want you to see if any of these resonate.

The good news is that if you relate to any of these, you can shift the direction of these thoughts by consciously deciding to. You are in charge of your thoughts. You can change them.

Here are some examples of changing your mindset about food. Maybe you think **"I can't cook separately for myself."** You can see two valid needs here: planning your healthy meals and feeding your family. To honor both needs, you might instead tell yourself *"reducing carbs and getting more protein is good for the whole family. I can change my portions from the existing family menu, and that might inspire my family, too."*

Ideas like **"my diet goes for a toss when I travel. I gain weight on every holiday,"** don't have to be your story. The two valid needs here? To enjoy new food and stay healthy. How about *"I plan ahead when traveling to new places and enjoy new foods while getting enough protein. I enjoy some carbs for pleasure and check my glucose levels to monitor the effect. I carry my protein options when I know the place I am visiting won't be able to cover my nutrition needs."*

If you're the type who falls victim to believing that **having a sweet tooth**, or **feeling like food is your weakness**, you're not alone.[*,16] The same goes for those who say, **"I'm a foodie,"** or **"I'm on a 'see-food' diet. I see food and eat it,"**

---

[*] Did you know that the link between sugar and dental health was the first time sugar was pointed out as a nutrient of concern? Prior to 1960, the term sweet tooth was probably used by dentists to describe the link between sugar and cavities. John Yudkin pointed out the link between sugar and systemic disease in his 1972 book Pure, White and Deadly (London: Davis-Poynter). See also P. Hujoel, "Dietary Carbohydrates and Dental-Systemic Diseases," Journal of Dental Research 88, no. 6 (2009): 490–502, https://journals.sagepub.com/doi/abs/10.1177/0022034509337700.

or simply **"cheat" on a diet and then feel guilty.** Is that your truth? Or does *"I know how to lower my glucose by lowering my carb intake. I am learning how to balance my food intake for pleasure as well as health, and I observe the feedback from my body when I eat high-carb foods versus getting enough protein,"* sound more like who you'd like to be? This book has discussed ways to improve your relationship with food. Is it fair to say that you're somewhere on the journey to become the best version of yourself? Is it more empowering?

The same can be said for sleep. We discussed your sleep hygiene, or "environmental diet," and now you can change your "thought diet" about it! Instead of being the person who says **"binge-watching till 2:00 a.m. is my me-time,"** you can be the person who believes that *"I invest in a good night's rest and wake up ready to face the day."* It's more empowering to be an investor in your health, than a passive actor, and we can apply that to stress, too.

One of the main disempowering thoughts that causes stress, specifically as it pertains to diabetes, is that **"nobody understands me."** It makes it hard to change how you live your life, eat, and turn the lights off earlier in your home, if we think the people around us won't understand us, or worse–will judge us. Instead of worrying about whether they understand you or not, you have the option to change what you do to improve understanding with others. This could be self-talk like *"I am learning to communicate my needs to my loved ones and get the support I need. I am taking responsibility for my experiences and accept that I cannot change things outside of me. I can only change myself. I am learning to walk away from unhealthy patterns."* We are all works in progress, and we can give each other a little grace, but in the meantime–start with you.

When it comes to exercise, we'll be sure to get into it in Part 5, but the mindset is still a big part. Like in my case, I made a lot of excuses regarding time. You might be saying things like **"I'm lazy—or I'm too busy,"** whereas, instead, you could be saying to yourself *"I invest in nutrition and sleep so that I have more energy. I find time to move my body and enjoy feeling more alive."*

Some people are different. Some people are past the point of trying to get fit and have resigned themselves to **"I hate what I see in the mirror."** While that may be true, this could also be true *"This body is my permanent address for this lifetime. I keep it fit and strong."* Is it possible to change from self-hate to self-love?

Some people are fed up with exercise because they genuinely believe that **"nothing works for me."** Not every exercise routine works for everyone, and that's okay! As long as you know that *"I invest in my fitness and strength, and every time I show up is another small win. I trust my body's intelligence and know it will respond to my efforts,"* your exercise doesn't need to match what anyone else is doing!

No matter what, you deserve to be doing what feels good and right for you. If you go through all this and you find yourself struggling with repetitive negative thought loops, then here's my pro tip: seek professional help. Taking help is a sign of strength, not weakness, and it's the reason people like me have jobs. The only thing that matters is you getting better, and there are people who want to help.

Your long-term mental health can improve greatly with the act of being kind to yourself. If it's too scary or too much of a struggle to be kind to yourself, again, that's what the professionals are for. We are here to be kind to you through this journey, and to help you be kind to yourself because truly: **kindness makes a difference.**

In one study, an eight-week mindful self-compassion program in people with type 1 and type 2 diabetes showed improvement in diabetes distress, depressive symptoms, and HbA1c, so kindness now has scientific proof backing it![17] You can learn self-compassion yourself or from a professional—and as soon as you learn it, your mind will thank you.

By choosing to change your self-talk so that it aligns with who you are and what you want, you will end up being kind to yourself on the journey. This act of self-care can help you make great changes in the ways you handle stress. To take it to the next level, you can integrate mindfulness practices with your positive self-talk, the first being "present-moment thinking."

4.8: How does present-moment thinking apply to diabetes and stress?

Have you ever planned an amazing holiday and filled the preceding weeks, days, and minutes with excitement leading up to the actual event? And then the time arrives, the future event happens, and then it goes into the rearview mirror. If you are looking forward to something wonderful tomorrow, you have to wait until tomorrow becomes today.

You only experience the future, when it becomes now.

You have no guarantee what tomorrow will finally be, and your mind fills that void with projections of what similar days in the past have been like. That's the experience of being influenced by the past in the present moment as you imagine future events unfolding in the mind. Now let's apply that to diabetes.

Let's say a friend has invited you to dinner tomorrow.

You could start thinking to yourself for the next twenty-four hours, *"Gosh, that host is so pushy—she won't take no for an answer. She doesn't know I am working on my health, and she's such a socialite, she won't understand. Besides, I don't want to sit and explain my diabetes to people at her party and attract unnecessary attention. Carbs will be unavoidable over there. She will be offended if I act fussy about my diet. My diet might just go for a toss. I always get overwhelmed at parties and stop paying attention to my diabetes. I will deal with that next week."*

Now you have filled your present moment with a sense of powerlessness about your diabetes. This feeling is based on you recalling past experiences and feelings, and in turn having a future imaginary conversation with your friend where you accumulate a hint of resentment and aversion toward the host! What's worse is that this isn't simply a projection—you've also potentially lied to yourself by saying you "always get overwhelmed!" By using the word "always", you are speaking for tomorrow. You don't know for a fact that tomorrow will be exactly the same as last time, and you just might surprise yourself.

Much like changing your self-talk, consider this response to the invitation instead: *"Oh, nice! I am looking forward to seeing her tomorrow. There is lots to catch up on. I will ensure I get enough protein during the day so that I am not too hungry and can still try the new food there. I am learning ways to balance my meals so that I can enjoy my social life. By checking my glucose levels after the party, I can learn from each experience. I am open to new possibilities."*

Do you see the difference in both responses to the invitation? In the first, your mind is running through the past and predicting what could happen in the future; while in the second, we only addressed what we have control over in the present, in order to influence the future. Staying in the present moment minimizes the amount of stress you put on yourself, and you can fully embody the moment.

As you are reading this book, your body is what allows you to **physically** experience—touch, smell, feel, and breathe—*in this present moment right now.* Monitor whether your thoughts are holding you in this present reality, or are they bouncing back and forth between the past and future?

I ask this, because I want to point out that your *body* doesn't time travel; your mind does.*

All. The. Time. (Pun intended!)

If you want diabetes to turn around in the future, you can't really experience that turnaround until the future becomes now. In fact, *where* you reach in the future is all about what steps you take right now. Just like driving from your city to the next might be a twelve-hour drive, and you know you will get there as long as you monitor your navigation and keep driving in the right direction.

With that, which way are you headed right now; **are you staying in the now?**

Much like those disempowering thoughts from the previous chapter, it's possible for conflations of the past and future to contaminate our present-moment awareness. This is relevant to how you self-manage diabetes. The trick is to remember that *always/never language* means we are copying and pasting the past into the future, therefore disconnecting from present-moment reality. Maybe the truth is slightly different.

If you believe that you are living in the present moment, but think to yourself **"My family *always* forces me to eat food that doesn't help my diabetes,"** is that maybe because *that happened in the past?* The truth is that whether it happens in the future or not depends on how you communicate with them.

But **"I'm an emotional eater!"** You are saying that like it's your name. You are making it your identity. *Maybe food helped you manage emotions in the past.* How do you want to handle food and emotions now and going forward?

---

* Maybe in the movie Interstellar and the book Autobiography of a Yogi by Paramahansa Yogananda (Los Angeles: Self-Realization Fellowship, 2007), but that's outside the scope of this book.

Some people say **"My workouts *never* help. Everything hurts."** They don't realize that *future workout experiences* depend on figuring out (with professional help) what needs to change to improve the return on your exercise investments. Maybe your nutrition lacks protein or magnesium; maybe insufficient sleep is preventing muscle growth; or maybe the workouts need modification.

Maybe you don't check your readings, because **"it's too scary to see the glucose levels."** It could be that *in the past, you didn't know what to do* when you saw the high numbers. What do you think about self-monitoring now that you are reading this book? You probably have more ideas about how to work with your healthcare provider on turning diabetes around. Are you getting curious to learn something new from the information the glucometer provides?

Some people come to me saying **"I can focus on my health after __[insert life event]__."** This tells me their *mind* doesn't feel equipped to handle their health while that life event happens. They sometimes ask me to give them more time, or to cut them more slack, both of which are departures from reality. As their doctor, I tell them I have no control over anyone's diabetes timeline or slack. The real conversation needs to happen between this person's mind and *body, because no matter the life event, their body shows up every moment of every day*, regardless of Sundays and public holidays. It is witnessing and participating in glucose management every moment; whether your mind is engaged or not. The body is never waiting until "the right time."

Stay present, stay true to the now. If you plan to be kind to yourself *later* on this journey, you can only act on that later time, when it becomes now.

4.9: If self-help isn't working

You don't have to battle stress and life alone. Dealing with diabetes is hard enough. I know I didn't have the bandwidth in 2013 to just pick myself up and get my act together. I needed help and was at my wits' end. It is alright to reach out for help, and nobody deserves to suffer alone.

Having lost a classmate to suicide, I always hope that we as a society can let each other know that each of us is valued and has a place to make a unique contribution in this life. You are not alone–it happens to all of us, so I want to talk about what else might help, if you feel like you can't help yourself.

First, **talk to someone**—anyone. A friend, a helpline, or anyone you trust. *Feeling heard can be immensely therapeutic* because of the basic human need for connection. A video call works better than texting, and meeting in person is better than video because it allows for a hug, although some people may not want to be hugged. *Self-soothing touch and receiving a hug have both been researched and shown to improve cortisol responses to stress.*[18]

That doesn't work for everyone, and if that's you; **move beyond talk therapy**. Though I'm not a therapist, I have worked on my own stress responses and benefitted from "alternative" approaches that went beyond talk therapy. Talking helps up to a point. Talking to my friends and family helped me feel loved and accepted. When I tried talk therapy, I found myself repeating thoughts out loud that I had been saying inside my head for a while. There was very little new content or perspective. Why? I think because words can express what you currently know consciously, but *so many of our emotions are unconsciously running the show* when we're completely unaware.

When it comes to any sort of therapy, know that **professionals can make it safe to feel the feeling**. When you talk about stressful things, remembering or re-experiencing an upsetting event can trigger physical sensations in the body: a racing heart; a tightening of the chest; shallow, jerky breathing; vertigo; a churning in the stomach; a flip-flop, hollow feeling in the belly; diarrhea; stomach cramps; shaking fingertips; sweaty palms; headaches and migraines; neck pain—you name it. Does this happen to you? You might not have words for what you are experiencing, but they are *felt senses*. This is where *a concerned friend or relative* *may not have the professional tools* to help you unpack or work through whatever is coming up to the surface.

Talking to someone, moving beyond that talk therapy, and working with professionals are things that many doctors would recommend, but I want to also be clear that **alternative therapy is an alternative**. I always tell my patients that considering a form of *therapy is like visiting an ice cream shop, there can be more than one right answer, just pick what works for you.* So work with a trusted professional, remain open to clear whatever negative emotions surface, and trust that you can overcome past hurts and come out stronger, happier, and clearer than before.

4.10: Alternative therapy is an alternative.

Like I said, therapy is like visiting an ice cream shop.
Some people like vanilla, some like chocolate, and some like a combination of flavors. Therapy that worked for you may not work for someone else, or perhaps their journey is completely different from yours.

In my case, I made much more rapid progress in my stress management skills when I used modalities that helped me get in touch with the unconscious or subconscious negative emotions that were stored in my psyche and body at a nonverbal level. The symptoms did not make complete medical sense, but the experiences were real. And frankly, none of us are born with an instruction manual from the manufacturer.

Whether I know that I had a past life or negative karma to clear in this life or not, as long as the story in my head empowers me to take positive steps in my life–I'm fine rolling with it.

Why? Because my alternative is to run with narratives that would keep me victimized and powerless–and that's not fun. Whatever helps me achieve peace, acceptance, connection, compassion, unconditional love: give it to me, because I am no longer willing to compromise on happiness.

Don't believe in God?

No problem. I believe in whatever or whoever makes sure we have a sunrise every day. Some intelligent phenomenon invented black holes and put the rings of Saturn and the Milky Way out there. Something smarter than me created the reality of the universe and also created the reality inside the human body that was given to me. I was willing to pay homage to that and surrendered that I wasn't the smartest thing around. Continuously attempting to crush the ego to powder also helped.

I share this because not only is alternative healing an option, but various types of healing have helped me over the years. What needs to be healed also changes over time. Who you are today is not the same as last year, nor will you be exactly the same person next year. It makes sense that your path to healing might not always look the same. To use the lifestyle car analogy, the rearview mirror tells you what happened in the past. As you are driving in the present moment, the future path will open and unfold in front of you, bringing new experiences. The terrain will change. Navigating the present moment with whatever technique helps you can fill the journey with more happiness.

Personally, I have discovered that breathwork and meditation play a large role in many different alternative practices.

Meditation is not just chants, mats, and yoga pants

By reading up until this point in the book, if you have already started observing your thoughts and their effect on your feelings and body responses, you are already practicing an advanced form of "open-eye meditation." Congratulations!

Meditation is not just for religious or mystical people. Prayer and surrender to a higher power or a spiritual notion of the universe can be powerful, but they are not necessary to turn around diabetes. By developing awareness of your thoughts and releasing your attachment to outdated thoughts that no longer serve you, you can experience more mental calm and clarity to turn around your diabetes.

There are documented benefits of meditation in diabetes.[19]

While alcohol or sedatives can numb anxiety or stress, they are addictive and don't address what's going on in the mind. *Meditation, on the other hand, helps you rewire the stress response, upregulate the relaxing parasympathetic nervous system, increase heart rate variability (HRV, a marker of nervous system balance), and provide alternate ways of dealing with stressful external circumstances.*

People who meditate experience more positive emotions, perhaps initiated by an attitude of acceptance of present-moment experiences.[20] In essence, meditation has the potential to help you use the natural pharmacy inside your body to calm the nervous system, tune in, and reduce feelings of anxiety and depression.[21,*]

---

* For severe symptoms of anxiety or depression, always work with a healthcare professional. This book does not replace medical advice or consultation from your doctor.

Breathing: Where science and spirituality converge

If you venture to learn more about meditation and becoming aware of your thought patterns, you'll end up coming across **breathwork**.

Deep breathing and observing the breath help reduce our stress levels through activation of the parasympathetic nervous system. Scientifically, they both work similar to meditation. Wearable devices can show you if there is too much sympathetic activation without enough parasympathetic activation, which is reported as HRV. The higher your stress levels and sympathetic activation, the lower your HRV, so we want to have more parasympathetic activation and a higher HRV.

From time-tested breathing techniques to new meditation apps entering the market, there are many ways to increase parasympathetic activation and the relaxing properties of the vagus nerve. After a meditation or focussed breathing session, most people report a sense of peace and quieting of the mind.

Spiritually, the universal comforting truths can be exchanged in silence. Love, safety, connection, trust—these are experienced. They don't demand to be spoken about. You just feel them, you just know. They just are–in silence. This is why I sometimes have to catch myself and tell my own chattering mind, "Your chaos is not helping. I allow you to move on." That helps me come back to quiet in the center. Later on, I can do some deeper work to see what threw me off.

I continue my spiritual practice and introspection every day, and recently started studying Kriya Yoga to strengthen my mind–body connection. The physical movement of the body is married with gaining mental control over your breathing in order to get the mind and body on the same page. It makes sense as the word yoga comes from the Sanskrit root yug, which means to "unite," after all.

Different modalities of alternative healing all seem to build on this mind-body connection, but getting into alternative healing itself can seem daunting if you don't know where to start. In the event that some of the different self-help methods I've tried can help you, I wanted to share some of the options I've worked with. There are certainly more that I've not tried yet, so this is by no means the one and only list.

I have found great success in things like **dance movement therapy, art therapy, transpersonal therapy, craniosacral therapy, transactional analysis, hypnotherapy,** really just **psychotherapy** in various forms. Other forms include **reparenting** or **inner child healing and integration, trauma work,** or even things like **forgiveness techniques** and **tapping or emotional freedom technique (EFT). Neurofeedback** or **biofeedback equipment** work directly with the body using feedback signals.

If you have a spiritual practice, **reading spiritual books, visiting spiritual sites or places of worship, prayer,** and **participating in spiritual discussions and learning groups** are all considered methods of growth and healing.

Modalities such as **Magnified Healing** or **Akasha healings, reiki, matrix reimprinting, journey workshops,** and **access consciousness** are included in alternative healing. These are joined by different types of meditation, like **Vipassana, guided meditation,** and **quantum meditation**. Add in **holotropic breathwork** and **progressive muscle relaxation and mindfulness,** and you've got a pretty good list of options available to you.

These techniques all helped me peel back more layers of myself so that I could get to know myself better. Some helped me more than others, and some helped only at certain stages of my life.

Now I have reached a point where I am far from nirvana, but most of my days are happy, creative, and abundant; filled with love, gratitude, and purpose. I get to choose how to respond to life. Sure, I have some crazy days, but I recognize that as the universal human experience of being a work-in-progress.

We all face unique stressors in life, but we are united in our humanity. We are also united by our common desire to thrive. It is possible to suffer less and experience more happiness. Recognizing my own imperfections took off some filters at work, and I saw that the people who sought my advice were experiencing their own authentic versions of imperfection, too. Consultations moved from doctor–patient to human–human interactions and became more deeply enriching.

4.11: Remember Priti?

Earlier, I discussed how she came to me at a ten on the stress scale, to the point where she felt her life was falling apart. Changing the way you show up in life is tough, especially when it knocks you down, but she was committed.

So what happened to Priti?

Priti knew she was stressed, and she knew it was making her diabetes worse. She felt the responsibility of the world on her shoulders. Along with her worsening health, there was a strain on her marriage, financial burden, the need to grow in her career, and worry for the future of her two children if she fell sick. Her toxic boss at work was causing her the most stress because she felt powerless about the situation.

All I did was listen to her share her worries, and explain the Karpman Drama Triangle to her.[22] This triangle is made of three roles: victim, aggressor, and rescuer. Personally, what I love most about the Drama Triangle is that once you can identify it and see how it makes relationships toxic, there is a way out of it. Priti felt like she was the victim when she put up with her boss's behavior and was the aggressor when she yelled at her kids. She wanted out of the drama.

I asked her how she wanted to change the situation. She said she would think about it.

We went on to her diabetes management plan. Of course, I'm not a therapist, but our consultations go thirty minutes each, and sometimes they stretch longer if required. I understand most people don't get this type of healthcare experience, but it's the only way I know how to connect with the person across from me.

I saw Priti a month later. She looked different. She was sitting up straighter and had a much less harrowed look than before. She had reduced her carbs, and her glucose levels were better. I asked how her work stress was. She told me how she had decided that she was done being the victim. She knew she was a valued employee at her workplace, and she decided she needed to have a frank conversation with her boss. She negotiated a paid sabbatical with the firm because she realized she had never used up her sick days or vacation days. She had banked a month of unused time off and needed it to focus on her health. As soon as she did that, she started getting clarity on what mattered most.

She reconnected with the strong woman that she always had been, the one who excelled in her work, loved her kids, and wanted to build a rewarding family life with her husband. She was creating the environment that she hadn't experienced as a child in her parents' home. She needed her physical health to be in order so that she could do all these things, and she was grateful for the time I had given her that day a month ago when she broke down.

I asked her what helped her turn things around.

In the rearview mirror, she made it look easy. In truth, it was messy—but beautiful. She started with the Drama Triangle steps I am about to share with you. Over the coming year, she extended her sabbatical, spent some of her savings, and found a better job with a healthier work culture. Her health improved, her husband found a job, and she overcame the darkest years of her life. She still does self-work; she found an eye movement desensitization and reprocessing (EMDR) therapist and keeps working on her issues as a work in progress. Self-love and a sense of purpose are what keeps her going.

I hope you, too, can find ways that work for you. I hope that noticing negative emotion, negative thought loops, the tendency to over explain or to feel stress move through the body can serve as a warning light on your dashboard, indicating that self-care is in order and that servicing is needed for healthier flow.

Everyone's stress management journey looks different. I was lucky to have learned about the steps of the Drama Triangle from a gifted inner child integration therapist, Trisha Caetano. Knowing how much it helped Priti, I want to share the steps I learned with you.

Six steps to exiting the Drama Triangle

As I mentioned before, the Karpman Drama Triangle is made of three roles at the three corners of the triangle: victim, aggressor, and rescuer. These roles are important, but what's more important is getting out.

The first step to exiting the Drama Triangle is **awareness**. You might be in a Drama Triangle if you hear words or thoughts like *"I always/never," "You always/never,"* or *"They always/never"*—for example, "I always give into sugar," or "He always makes me do things against my will." According to Dr. Karpman, these absolute statements are at least 10 percent untrue. Don't underestimate yourself or others. Nobody is "always" or "never" anything. People can change. You can change.

You might be in a Drama Triangle when *there are exchanges that cause guilt, shame, or blame. Gaslighting* is a hallmark of toxic communication. It could be a good relationship with unintentional, unconscious, manipulative ways of communicating. Either way, these are red flags that something needs to improve. As soon as you realize you are stuck in a Drama Triangle, breathe a sigh of relief. That means you have a way out.

Now that you know what you're dealing with, step two is to **make an appointment with the person** you are in drama with.

It sounds weird, but if we make appointments for haircuts and manicures–why not this? This is an important conversation and *the other person deserves a heads-up* that you want to discuss something important. Jumping right in because you have just made a discovery might not go so well if they are not ready. That's why *it's in your best interest that they come to the conversation ready to communicate.* You could say: I want to discuss something important with you. When is a good time?

Once you've got your time and date, you can move on to step three: **create a safe space.**

When the conversation starts, *start with something positive and true.* Why? You are being constructive. It could be something simple—for example, for a boss at work, "I understand you want the best for the company," or for a partner whom you raise kids with, "I know you want what's best for the kids." No need to flatter or butter people up here. They will see through it and might get defensive. Be genuine. If you can't find anything positive to say to them, you may want to work on yourself first. Starting the conversation with blame or pointed fingers will put them on the defensive, and the conversation will probably not go too well. The whole point of this is to give them a chance to hear you out.

If you have successfully created a safe space where no one is on the defensive, then it's time for step four, **speaking your truth**.

Tell them what is going on with you. Be careful here to *take ownership of your feelings.* It's often easier to blame others for how you feel. The little child in us wants the people in our immediate lives to make our problems go away. It's the mature adult in us that recognizes that change starts from within—and that is the only way toward less stress.

Avoid words like "always" or "never." We now know that is the sign of a Drama Triangle, and we want to exit it. Instead, *use phrases like "I feel __."* For example, you could say to a boss, "When you give me an overnight work deadline and raise your voice in front of my colleagues, I feel disrespected and undervalued." This is much more effective than, for example, "You always insult me and throw last-minute work at me without understanding what is already on my plate." To a spouse, you might say, "When you disagree with me in front of the kids, I feel undermined," rather than, "You never stand by me in front of the kids, and it's your fault that they don't take me seriously." Do you see how the toxic way of communication includes assumptions and accusations about what is going on inside the *other* person's head? Most of us can barely keep track of what is going on in our own heads!

So if this is a relationship that actually matters to you, *it's your responsibility to let people know how you feel* and what is going on with you. Just like you can't know their reality, they can't know yours unless you speak your truth in a way that allows them to listen. Screaming your truth with grenades flying out from both of your hands will probably not work. How can people sit still and listen if you throw stuff at them? They will duck, hide, or counterattack.

Neither of you will hear anything when a grenade goes off. The victim/aggressor dynamic might be the familiar default, and you will both get sucked right in. *This step is quite difficult to do in intimate relationships without getting in touch with your deeper needs beforehand.* Professional help will make the process easier, but know that it's alright to give yourself some time. You may want to give yourself space to build up your bandwidth so you can enter this work with some stability, as there may be unconscious triggers inside you that could get in the way.

Once you speak your truth and get it all out there without the conversation escalating, that is when you can focus on step five. If you've made it this far, it's time to **tell them what you want.**

To the boss, you might say, *"What I want is that we find a more organized way to deliver expectations and work deadlines. I want to be given my targets in writing with at least two days' notice so that I can organize my schedule to work toward what the company needs. That would help me bring my best to the workplace."* To the spouse, you might say, "I want us to be able to disagree in private so that we can be a more unified team in front of the kids. That would help our kids learn healthier communication from us."

Now this is where *you will need some patience.* See, you may have had your blinders pulled off. You suddenly wanted to change, and decided to communicate this new information.

The other person has no idea what you are talking about.

Status quo is easier initially, even if it's toxic, because change takes effort. People sometimes get used to abusive communication without noticing its effect. The victim and rescuer roles remain magnetic and hypnotic, until emotionally mature people realize that *victimhood equals unhappiness*. You will need to use the previous steps at least a few times on a few separate incidents between you both so that you give the other person time to recognize that you are consistently using a new form of communication. If you don't get a ticket every time you break a red traffic light, you will probably keep breaking it. *Consistent feedback helps emotionally mature people get the message*, and healthy relationships benefit and evolve from this because the other person values the relationship enough to listen. Give yourself and them the chance to grow. People do change for the better when given a chance.

If we know that change takes time, and we know we have to be patient, there is still one thing left to do. When it comes to the final step, step six, it's time to **set a boundary.**

If you have tried the previous step multiple times in the best way you possibly can, then you will need to *introspect on whether you are done trying. If so, let them know what you will do* if you don't get what you want. To the boss, you might say, "If we can't find a way to agree on work deadlines that give me at least a few days to prepare, then I will _[consequence]_." To the spouse, you might say, "If we can't find a way to take our disagreements up privately, then I will _[consequence]_."

You decide what the consequence needs to be, and be sure to follow through on it. That is the only way for you to honor your truth. If we can't honor what matters to us, how can we expect anyone else to? Healthy relationships will grow through this difficult phase and come out stronger. I have seen it time and again. The process will be an ongoing one that keeps upgrading itself over time. The connection gets stronger and more authentic. Relationships that are meant to end will end. *The other person's truth is not in your hands.*

If a negative event taught you something you needed to learn about yourself, *find some gratitude for what the experience did for you.* It probably made you stronger and got you in touch with a deeper, more authentic version of yourself.

Part 4 summary

- Diabetes distress can get better with support and education, and this can improve your ability to self-manage diabetes.

- Chronic stress can wear you out physically and mentally, causing a disconnect between knowing what is good for you and actually doing it.

- Mindfulness of thought and connecting to the body through breath can help you return to present moment awareness.

- Identifying the Drama Triangle, self-help and professional therapy to address stored negative emotions can be powerful and life-changing.

- It is possible to move from victim thinking to an empowered growth mindset.

For Bonus Materials, Visit the Website Here:

PART 5

THE FOURTH WHEEL OF THE LIFESTYLE CAR:

EXERCISE

5.1: Why exercise is the fourth wheel

Although everyone with diabetes and excess body fat is told to "eat less and move more," or to simply "lose weight," those two-word phrases are not enough to get the job done. Besides being unhelpful, vague, and insufficient, they risk placing blame on the person struggling with the condition, as if they are not moving because they are lazy or don't want to be fit.

Everyone wants to have a strong, active body.

Everyone.

I intentionally keep exercise as the fourth lifestyle wheel in my practice because addressing the first three wheels of nutrition, sleep, and stress management (in that order) will automatically **give you more energy, lift your mood, and help you come up with new ideas about movement.**

I approached the wheels of the lifestyle car in this sequence around 2016 after listening to my patients and personalizing their lifestyle changes. By the time my patients have addressed the first three wheels, they spontaneously tell me they are ready to take their fitness to the next level because they instinctively feel their body moving differently. When they service the fourth wheel, their car really starts to move.

They become unstoppable.

This sense of feeling alive doesn't come in a bottle—it's something they experience because their mitochondria are healthier and insulin resistance is lower. What I was seeing in clinical practice was confirmed by others' research. The fact that exercise can make your health worse if you don't use the first three wheels to improve insulin resistance was scientifically published in 2020. Elegant investigation showed how most of the thousands of molecular beneficial changes that happen after exercise were reduced and sometimes reversed in people with insulin resistance.[1]

Having more energy will make you want to exercise, too.

Many people think that they would never *want* to partake in strenuous exercise. That is only because we are designed to move–yet forced to sit.

Humans have 360 joints in the body so that we can jump, dance, twirl, dive, twist, climb, flip, and more. Babies try to move as much as they can. Toddlers explore. Children play. Somewhere along the way, we adults lock them down within typical classrooms, making them sit for more than eight hours a day. At adolescence, unless the teenager is involved in some form of sport or dance, they copy the grown-ups and become sedentary.

If we lose our natural inclination toward movement—then exercise has to be prescribed.

Exercise increases life span and health span

The whole point of turning around diabetes is so that you can live a longer, healthier, more vibrant life. Exercise plays a massive role in longevity and is even more powerful than quitting smoking in terms of adding years to your life expectancy. Having higher muscle mass not only improves your daily quality of life, but it also appears to be linked to your ability to survive an intensive care unit (ICU) stay.[2] The best thing about exercise is that it not only increases your lifespan but more importantly, your health span.

The idea of a health span is laid out by Peter Attia in a concept he has named the Centenarian Decathlon™. He invites you to consider what activity levels you want to be enjoying in your final decade of life, then work backward from there while accounting for age-related muscle losses. Read his book to be convinced. Fitter, stronger people have about half the risk of death than their least fit counterparts.

The best time to work toward that is now. Muscle loss, or **sarcopenia**, in diabetes patients can have long-reaching effects.

We discussed the role of muscles in the development of insulin resistance and worsening diabetes in Part 1.5, where I described that about 60–90 percent of postmeal glucose is expected to be taken up by your muscles.[3] That explains why exercise reduces postmeal blood glucose in people with obesity and diabetes. Remember muscle is the glucose taker among the musketeers? Activated muscles consume more glucose, as we will cover later in this chapter.

Have you ever wondered why some of our grandparents dodged diabetes their whole lives, only to develop it in old age, even though their habits stayed the same? Age-related muscle loss accelerates after the age of sixty-five.[4] This contributes to the loss of our biggest glucose-disposal system and influences new-onset diabetes in the elderly.

Diabetes itself is toxic to muscle tissue. This toxicity is also called **diabetic myopathy**, with high glucose levels causing muscle loss. This in turn results in *chronic overactivity of the mechanistic target of rapamycin* (mTOR), *oxidative stress, reactive oxygen species* (ROS), *chronic inflammation,* and *toxic fat accu-*

mulation inside the muscle.[5,6,*] This fat accumulation inside the muscle (myosteatosis) sets up toxic hormonal cross-talk between muscle and fat tissue, and sets up a vicious metabolic cycle:[7]

muscle loss → higher glucose → insulin resistance → muscle loss → higher glucose

This cycle will send the patient into an endless battle. The metabolic changes are a clear trap for anyone–old or young. The patients trapped in this metabolic cycle tend to notice other physical changes, too.

Diabetic neuropathy makes your feet and fingertips numb and *affects your ability to safely exercise* due to the loss of sensory input. You become unsteady on your feet because you cannot normally feel the ground underneath you or your position in space. Burning pain at night may ruin your sleep, making you less willing to try new things or exert yourself during the day.

This is understandable.

When you see the doctor with these symptoms, they may prescribe approved medications (covered in Part 7) to reduce the symptoms of neuropathic pain. These drugs don't increase your fitness or strength, and they come with side effects. In fact, some make you drowsy, less coordinated, and more prone to falls! The good news is that exercise can improve muscle activation, nerve function, balance, and pain, even in people with diabetic neuropathy.[8,9]

People may excuse themselves from exercise for a while because of neuropathy, travel or a busy schedule. When it comes to **muscle loss in the elderly, a prolonged break in exercise is known to accelerate aging**—both metabolically as we discussed above and physically.

Muscle loss in the elderly has physical implications in terms of *function and stability*.[10] *Frailty* from muscle *loss of aging is due to loss of mostly Type II muscle fibers* (which we will discuss in upcoming sections). This is associated with a loss of strength, quality of life, falls, and fractures. A fracture in a frail elderly grandparent after falling in the house often becomes a terminal event, with a five-year survival rate worse than many cancers.[11]

The good news is that addressing sarcopenia and frailty has been shown to improve functional independence, self-esteem, quality of life, and glucose control.[12] We need to get our parents to invest in strength training and aerobic exercise and join them in getting stronger. It's unacceptable for us to discourage our elders from building muscle because they don't plan to be in the Olympics or

---

* Mechanistic target of rapamycin (mTOR) is needed for muscle synthesis from dietary protein, but overactivity is thought to be central to aging. This explains the growing research interest in rapamycin, an mTOR inhibitor, as an antiaging molecule. See: David Papadopoli, Karine Boulay, Lawrence Kazak, Michael Pollak, Frédérick A. Mallette, Ivan Topisirovic, and Laura Hulea, "mTOR as a Central Regulator of Lifespan and Aging," F1000Research 8 (2019), https://www.ncbi.nlm.nih.gov/pmc/articles/PMC6611156/.

become competitive bodybuilders. Perhaps people say this because they don't know it is possible to gain muscle at any age.

Frailty is not the only way to age.

You don't have to struggle with diabetic neuropathy or sarcopenia. You deserve to use your body to move in the way it was designed to.

But what if you feel like you can't "move more?"

Patients tell me things like this. Take Jayesh, the real estate developer, for example.

Jayesh first saw me when his diabetes was in its early stages, although the insulin resistance had been around for much longer. He had developed high blood pressure in his thirties that he'd attributed to work stress. His hemoglobin A1c (HbA1c) had gradually crept up from prediabetes into the diabetes range of 6.9 percent. Having always been slightly overweight, he had put on an additional twenty kilograms (forty four pounds), mostly around his waist, after he stopped casually playing sports in college. Most successful people he knew also had a paunch.

In the real estate world, "throwing your weight around" and having stature had literal meaning. The most influential builders were not petite. Strangely, his arms and legs were skinny, and people around him said he looked "weak." While the paunch made him look prosperous, the wasting arms and legs made him look frail. Now in his mid-fifties, he felt like age had taken over and he was always too tired to exercise even though he knew it was "good for him." He was tired of hearing his wife and doctor telling him to "lose weight," mentioning the phrase as though he *wanted* to be fat. He held multiple gym memberships, but had stopped going because he was always huffing and puffing as soon as he got on the treadmill. Seeing young, fit people in the gym made him feel like he didn't belong there.

On the other hand, I've also had patients like Tina tell me they feel like they can't move more. In Tina's case, she was a floor salesperson at a busy retail store in the new mall in the city. Her day started at 5:00 a.m. since she had an hour and a half commute, one-way, which included standing in a crowded train and switching between two different forms of public transport. After getting home, she had domestic chores waiting that would keep her up until midnight.

All she craved was crashing into bed, but her feet had started tingling and burning recently. That was keeping her up at night. She had no plans to bulk up in the gym because "that was for the guys." Her smartwatch kept congratulating her for steps walked and calories burned. She figured this should have caused some weight loss, but she was noticing the inches going up on her midsection. By the time she saw me her HbA1c was 8.8 percent–despite taking two diabetes medications and walking so much.

Whether it's your schedule, breathlessness, or tingly toes that make it so there's no time, space, or energy to move more–you can change it. I worked with Jayesh and Tina to change how they approach movement, but before we discuss what they chose to do, let's go through all of the steps. As I told them at the beginning of their journey, the first step when getting started with exercise is to get to the point where you want to add movement to your lifestyle car.

5.2: Getting started with exercise

Of course, we have covered the first three wheels of the lifestyle car. We have addressed **nutrition** and getting enough protein to provide the raw material in Part 2.4; **sleep** and getting enough to release maximum growth hormone at night to do the repairing and building while allowing the brain to recharge, learn, and solve problems in Part 3.2; and managing **stress** that stalls long term planning and the chronic high cortisol that causes muscle breakdown in Part 4.2. Much like three great wheels and one flat won't get your car too far, just eating, sleeping, and meditating doesn't give you stronger muscles.

When you're ready to begin exercising and have thought about how to create time for it, then you can start with figuring out the basics. In my practice, I tell my patients that the basics are learning **how to stimulate your brain to build muscle, how much and how often to exercise, and how to jump in if you're starting from a sedentary lifestyle.**

Regarding **how to stimulate your brain to build muscle**, the truth is that the only real stimulus to grow muscle size, strength, or mass is for the brain to have an "aha" moment. *The brain needs to be put in a situation where it realizes, "Oops, I am not strong enough.* I barely survived today, so I'd better make bigger muscles tonight so that I don't get eaten by that predator tomorrow. I need to be fast enough to complete my hunt and strong enough to forage in the wild to get some nutrition." When the muscle fails to complete a movement, it releases **myokines** that stimulate the brain to build muscle. The different stimuli tell your brain that it needs to *improve the brain-muscle connection, recruit more muscle fibers, and build more muscle* (hypertrophy). If you want to build muscle, you're going to have to get moving first!

But **how much, how often?**

Before we go further, there's a **disclaimer**: *This book does not replace a medical evaluation or medication review.* Assess your cardiac and musculoskeletal health before getting started with a new exercise program in the context of uncontrolled diabetes, and get your medical clearance to exercise.

Initially, an exercise program could be a mix of light weights with more repetitions; *later on, the resistance needs to get heavier.* As you gain fitness over the years, you will need to push each muscle group until technical failure. Although we still need more research on the best ways to build muscle in trained versus untrained people, failure means continuing until you reach the point where you cannot complete another repetition without compromising safety or form.[13]

Muscle gains are typically seen when you target each muscle group twice a week, so doing isolated upper-body and lower-body once a week each is not enough. That puts seven days between two experiences. When you have gaps longer than 4 days between stimulation, you end up losing what you built up. A strength training workout twice a week focused on the full-body gets the job done and leaves enough time on the other days for cardio, mobility, and recovery.

With that said, if you have struggled with keeping exercise as a part of your routine, there are some ways to help you build consistency.

To make exercise a part of life and push yourself hard enough to accumulate long-term benefits, there are six steps I recommend patients take to help them create their own exercise plan.

Step one is *obviously* the most important, and it's to **start with something you enjoy**. *If you like it, you will show up*. Thinking "I hate walking" will make you consistent with not walking. Check if your self-talk can improve in this regard, like we covered in Part 4.7. Once you figure out what you like to do, then you can do step two, which is to **promise yourself two to five minutes a day**.

When twenty-four hours in a day don't feel like enough, it's tough to carve out time for a sixty-minute workout. Imagining a full workout feels like too much, it's too daunting; zero feels safer– and you don't get started! A five-minute commitment, on the other hand, might seem manageable enough. After five minutes– stop! Leaving a workout incomplete may just give you enough FOMO that you will want to come back tomorrow with more time on hand.*

That brings us to step three: **extract short-term rewards** from each workout. Your mind craves instant gratification, but visible abs and biceps only come after years of workouts done in anonymity. Some people that we've worked with have come up with creative ways to derive immediate rewards that make them want to keep showing up, and you can, too. If you need some inspiration first, you can borrow some of the ideas they had.

Some chose to use accountability as a mechanism, where they would *send a selfie to a workout buddy* or accountability partner or *share the workout on social media* so others knew they were showing up.

Some made decisions that made exercise feel like a reward! They got excited to start the workout by *wearing new socks or workout clothes they liked* instead of clothes they didn't want to be seen in.

---

* Learned this term from my teenagers. "Fear of missing out".

Some chose to give their bodies a little treat after a workout. In many cases, that looked like *enjoying some fresh new deodorant, enjoying a cold shower after a sweaty session, or eating a fulfilling and healthy meal.*

I want to point out that none of these reward methods include junk food as a "treat" to be earned after "burning calories."

Take a look at that contradiction. Healthy food can be pleasurable–but it depends on your mindset. If you are exercising for health, what food would give you the highest return on your exercise investment? Remember from Part 4.6: punishing yourself in the gym so that you can overeat at the table would be a battle of you versus you; that becomes difficult to sustain.

The first three steps are about getting comfortable with exercising. Once you've found what you like to do, committed to showing up for short intervals, and figured out how to best reward yourself, you can look to steps four through six and begin to get serious about your fitness and movement goals.

When you're ready to get more technical with your training, you can move to step four, **learning to engage the core and including some compound movements.**

Imagine your core is like a **six-sided rectangular box**, made of twenty-nine pairs of muscles that are responsible for the structure and movement of your torso. When I say muscles, however, I want to be clear that it also includes things that go beyond what you may consider to be "the core."

Starting with the **obliques** on the *sides* of the trunk and the **rectus abdominis**, or the abs, in the front, nothing seems new–you've likely heard of these muscles before. While you've also likely heard of the diaphragm and the pelvic floor, these are what people typically think of when we say to "focus on your core." The **diaphragm** takes the *top* position, while the **pelvic floor** forms the *bottom*, contributing to the structure and movement of that rectangular box.

And it doesn't stop there.

There's a deep muscle that wraps around the abdomen or trunk called the **transversus abdominis**. This muscle runs *horizontally around your trunk* like a brace to support you in addition to the **muscles that run alongside the spine and back.**

Have you ever heard the phrase "sitting is the new smoking?" Even though our core has muscles spanning on all six sides of this box, sitting all day causes those different parts of our core to disengage or hibernate. This leads to the upper- and lower-body to become uncoordinated and tight. Prolonged sitting makes the body forget how to function as a whole; this can set you up for injury. Since many of us have this risk, you just may have to work with a fitness professional to **learn cues and techniques to activate your core before you try to strengthen it.** They may have you start with *focused abdominal engagement and breathing,* and simple drills like *dead bugs, toe taps, modified planks, bird-dog, and hollow-hold* to get you acquainted.

These practices make you more aware of your core, improve the overall mind-body coordination and support compound exercises in the gym; this carries over into functional movements in your daily life. After a while, you will find that your body is more coordinated overall.

Compound movements are movements that involve more than one joint. A whole-body workout can be made quite intense using compound movements that coordinate the upper body, lower body, and deep core muscles. This is how you gain overall *strength, stability, and agility.*

An oversimplified way to start thinking about compound movements is by comparing pushing, pulling, lifting, twisting, and dragging heavy things; versus sitting down. The first examples listed are day-to-day functional movements—chair sitting, however, is not.

After spending hours in a chair hunched over a desk, muscles become increasingly tight and uncoordinated. Suddenly spending chest day on push ups without a healthy core can trigger shoulder, neck, and rotator cuff issues. You can prevent injuries like this by paying attention to the invisible shoulder joint and shoulder blade stabilizers, in addition to strengthening the upper back muscles.

Functional training and **pilates** exercises are options to *improve your overall body awareness when done under skilled supervision.*

Once you're comfortable with the previous steps, you're ready for step five. At this point, you have an activity you like, a time commitment, and a reward system that works for you. You've added in deep core activation to get the most of your workouts and now, it's time to **track your strength gained**–not calories burnt. *Monitoring your workout performance over time becomes a self-sustaining way to keep coming back*, and there is a certain joy from seeing yourself getting faster and stronger.

When it comes to **cardio**, for example, you can see your aerobic fitness improve as you *cover more distance* and *generate more power* in the same time commitment. This is a sign of healthier mitochondria in your Type I muscle fibers.

For **strength training**, target each muscle group until failure–where you can't complete another proper repetition without compromising safety or form– and perform each movement twice a week. Track your ability to *lift heavier weights, perform more repetitions, or achieve longer isometric holds.* You can avoid stagnation by periodization of your workouts and **progressively overloading** the system, where the muscles send myokine signals to the entire body saying: we need to be stronger and faster! The brain responds by growing muscle, especially Type II muscle fibers, helping you minimize the risk of plateauing. Not only will you get stronger, your glucose levels will improve, too. Muscle gains help improve diabetes control with less medication in both type 1 and type 2 diabetes.[14,15]

This may seem like all you need to get started with exercise, but there is a sixth step.

Step six is to **celebrate and be grateful for your functional fitness in daily life.**

When you almost trip on an uneven surface but hop back to balance without spraining your ankle, buckling, or crumbling like a house of cards—thank your reflexes and stability. If you lunge to pick up something heavy from the floor without back pain, be grateful for the successful weight transfer.

When you lift a backpack, suitcase, or young child above your shoulders, celebrate how hard you've worked for that *upper body strength*, and when you squat down Indian style or sit on the floor and get up unassisted, you can appreciate your *lower body strength*. You can delight in the strength of your *core* when you hold a plank longer than your colleagues or juniors, and cherish how working on *cardio* makes it so you can run for the bus or walk briskly up a slope without losing your breath.

When you are at a meeting maintaining confident body language, give credit, not just to your state of mind, but to the muscles that give you great *posture*. If you recover from an illness or injury faster than expected, thank your *body wisdom*.

And finally, there is *the infinite game*, as described by Steven Kotler in his book, The Art of Impossible. When you get fitter with each passing birthday, you know you are competing with yourself on the path to longevity.

How to get started if you are sedentary

We all want to be on that path to longevity, but let's be realistic: many of us accumulate nearly sixteen hours of sedentary time every day. Many people with uncontrolled diabetes have not been active or athletic for a while, but that's okay. To turn around diabetes, you can only start from where you are, not from some ideal, perfect hypothetical place. It's more about small lifestyle changes that support the process and the journey. The destination will come.

If you are super sedentary, there are still different types of movement that you can choose from before exploring traditional exercise. A clever starting point is to **alternate sitting and standing at your desk.** Sedentary, overweight office workers with desk jobs participated in a trial to look at the effect of using an electric height-adjustable workstation to change from sitting to standing posture every thirty minutes. This simple change had a beneficial effect on postmeal glucose levels.[16]

If a height-adjustable desk is not an option, or if you just want to go a little further, you can try to **break up the sedentary time.** If you know you have a long day of sitting at your desk, try getting up and pacing a few rounds back and forth in the room every thirty minutes. This activity is correlated with better triglyceride levels (according to observational data) and better postmeal glucose, insulin, and triglyceride levels (according to a clinical trial).[17,18]

In addition to making changes regarding how long you sit at your desk, you can also leverage fidgeting. This is commonly seen as tapping your fingers, bobbing or nodding your head, or bouncing your knee wherever you are sitting, but some experts call it increasing nonexercise activity thermogenesis (NEAT). Instead of counting the calories you are burning by doing this, remind yourself how it's keeping the mitochondria inside your muscles busy. The person sitting next to you might find it rude, but a study done on people with obesity showed improvement in glucose and insulin levels after consuming a glucose load just by fidgeting their legs intermittently (2.5 minutes on, 2.5 minutes off).[19]

This may seem like a sneaky little trick, but it works. When it comes to moving from a sedentary lifestyle to one full of movement, we want as many tips and secrets as we can get.

5.3: The secret golden key to make you a fat-burning machine

In cases of type 2 diabetes, people start with insulin resistance which causes weight gain; while in type 1 diabetes, people start storing excess fat in the body if they've been exposed to excess insulin. Up to this point in the book, we have articulated the importance of food as fuel that gets converted to energy. That final energy generation happens inside the mitochondria.

Think of carbohydrates as the matchsticks, dry grass, and small twigs you would use to start a campfire. They ignite fast, bursting forth a flame for a few moments, and then the flame dies down momentarily. To sustain the fire, you would have to keep putting lots of grass into the firepit every few minutes. On the other hand, if you were hoping for a steady flame that burns reliably through the night, you'd need thicker logs.

That is the kind of enduring energy supply available in your fat stores. If high insulin leads to an insulin-resistant state, it means the mitochondria have become unhealthy and will keep demanding carbohydrates for instant energy, instead of building the metabolic machinery to burn fat. Even though there is excess fat available, the mitochondria are not efficient enough at switching gears to burn it, so they keep burning carbs and signaling low energy levels to your brain. This is what keeps you hooked on carbs for short-lived bursts of energy.

While we briefly discussed mitochondria in Part 1.6 when describing brown fat, this is a good place to dive deeper into an understanding of mitochondria since they are the power plants that produce energy for the body.

You guessed it—**the secret to turning you into a fat-burning machine is to focus on healthy mitochondria.**

Healthy mitochondria make all the difference when you want consistently steady energy levels instead of swinging between high and low energy states.

If you have unhealthy mitochondria due to insulin resistance and try to run a marathon, you'd likely want a carb source midcompetition in order to prevent "bonking," or "hitting the wall" when your glycogen (stored carbs) runs low. Yes, you have body fat, but you haven't built enough fat-burning (aerobic) flexibility in your mitochondria to switch fuel sources.

If an untrained person attempts a sprint, the rapid burn of carbs generates lactic acid through anaerobic metabolism. Your heart rate jumps up to zone 4 or zone 5, and you are huffing and puffing to blow off carbon dioxide. You're burning mostly carbs for energy and lactic acid is accumulating in your muscles, creating an acidic environment that limits performance and forces you to stop.[*] Your workout intensity can't progress simply because you lack the aerobic base. The pain and suffering for an untrained athlete going into zone 5 are real. This may make you want to avoid exercise like the plague.

Zone 5 can be very uncomfortable even for elite athletes, but they have conditioned their minds and bodies to go longer distances despite rising lactate levels.[**]

If you've ever noticed how long-distance runners have very little visible body fat, it has a lot to do with having a fat-burning metabolism through lots of healthy mitochondria. In terms of approximate numbers, even a very lean elite endurance athlete with 10 percent body fat still has around 2,000 kilocalories available as stored carbs and more than 40,000 kilocalories available in body fat; they've just trained their bodies and mitochondria to be more efficient at burning fat.[20]

You can **build your mitochondrial ability** to burn fat and improve aerobic and cardio (endurance) fitness by *spending more time in the lower heart rate range of zone 2*. The easiest way to know if you are in zone 2 is if you are able to carry on a conversation with slightly faster breathing and are able to complete short sentences without gasping.

But how?

First, you have to see whether your mitochondria are burning carbohydrates or fat.

---

[*] Zone 4 or 5 is when you are gasping for air, unable to speak more than a few words because you are breathing so hard. Average people cannot sustain zone 4 or 5 for more than a few minutes. You can work with your healthcare professional to calculate your target heart rate to improve your aerobic base. Wearing a heart-rate monitor allows you to modify exercise intensity to stay in the target zone. Again, you need to consult your doctor before trying out any new exercise routine, especially with uncontrolled diabetes. See: Phil Maffetone, "The MAF 180 Formula: Heart-Rate Monitoring for Real Aerobic Training," May 6, 2015, https://philmaffetone.com/180-formula/.

[**] Elite endurance athletes measure their lactate levels.

Are your mitochondria preferring to burn carbs or fat?

The application of sports physiology helps us get an understanding of whether you are burning more fat or carbs by performing a VO_2 max test, which is used to measure your cardiorespiratory (heart and lung) fitness under the supervision of an exercise physiologist.

A VO_2 max test is where you are monitored as you are pushed into the uncomfortable range of zone 4 or 5. For the test, you'll run on a treadmill wearing a mask that measures the amount of carbon dioxide produced, relative to the oxygen consumed in the air you breathe out (respiratory exchange ratio [RER]). The RER and pulse is tracked as the treadmill gets more challenging in terms of metabolic equivalents (METs) using the standardized Bruce protocol, and the test ends when you just can't run anymore. How long it takes you to reach exhaustion depends on how rapidly you've jumped into carbohydrate burn. That's the stage when you struggle to exhale carbon dioxide fast enough. This is reflected in the rising RER and heart rate recorded when the discomfort and breathlessness are no longer bearable. A higher RER is reached when carbohydrates are the predominant fuel being burned, while a lower RER is maintained when fat is the primary fuel.

Your VO_2 max score tells you the maximum aerobic capacity you were able to achieve just before you had to stop on the treadmill; this is an indicator of your body's oxygen consumption and cardio (aerobic) fitness.

If you're having difficulty finding a physiologist to administer the test, there are handheld RER meters available. The handheld RER does not tell you your aerobic fitness but people can measure the amount of carbon dioxide they're producing relative to the amount of oxygen they're consuming, in order to observe how lifestyle changes affect their predominant fuel source. **Full disclosure:** I have an affiliate partnership with Lumen because I believe in the power of technology when it comes to receiving actionable feedback. Personally, I enjoy waking up in the morning and blowing into my Lumen to see whether I am burning mostly fat, then tracking how my fuel burn shifts after a workout, a low-carb home-cooked meal, a late dinner, a fast or an occasional night out with a small drink and some tasty carbs.[21] Everyone wants to burn fat efficiently, right? I'm no different.

If your RER indicates that you're burning fat, congratulations! If not, don't worry. Athletes may want to burn carbs for performance in certain sports. If you find out that you are unable to switch fuels to burn fat, don't worry–your mitochondria can be trained.

How to train your mitochondria to burn fat for fuel

Zone 2 training is aerobic (cardio) training, and engaging in aerobic endurance exercise trains your body to shift to fat metabolism. "Shifting to fat metabolism" basically means your body is predominantly burning fat to fuel your energy requirements at that moment.

To do this, we have to better understand the difference between fat-burning mitochondria, and their carb/glycogen/sugar-burning mitochondria counterpart.

When it comes to **carb-burning mitochondria**, they predominate where there is a *high-carb diet* made of *small, frequent carb-based meals* every few hours. There are *high insulin requirements* due to insulin resistance, and it's *common to need a carbohydrate snack* in order to workout after glycogen runs out. These mitochondria are *predominantly located in the white fast-twitch muscle fibers, also known as "Type II" fibers.* Fast twitch fibers, and therefore carb-burning mitochondria, generate energy through **glycolysis**; they *support bursts of high-power, high strength and high-intensity exercise like sprints.* Unhealthy mitochondria that are burning through carbs and sugars for energy *will push an untrained sedentary person into heart rate zone 4 or 5 with minimal exercise; their respiratory exchange ratio (RER) quickly approaches 1.*

Fat-burning mitochondria, on the other hand, are *increased by low-carb diets, when you consume below fifty to one hundred grams of carbs a day.* In this situation, energy is generated through fat burn (nutritional ketosis).* Fat burn *can be bolstered by fasting beyond twenty-four hours;* this depletes most glycogen, leading to a switch to fat burn. At that point, there are low *insulin requirements* due to insulin sensitivity; this *allows for fasted workouts* where body fat is burned as fuel to support exercising muscles once glycogen runs out. This is healthy and desirable when done intermittently; it's the opposite of the insulin resistant situation we discussed in Part 1.5, where high insulin levels prevent stored fat from being used. I will come to this again in Part 6. Fat burning mitochondria are *primarily located in the red slow-twitch muscle fibers, also known as "Type I"*

---

* As a reminder, ketosis from a low-carb diet (safe) or fasting (safe) is completely different from diabetic ketoacidosis (dangerous). Work with a qualified healthcare professional to understand how this applies to you.

muscle fibers; these support endurance exercise.[*,22] Slow-twitch fibers *get their red color by having more mitochondria.*[**] Healthy mitochondria that burn through fat for energy will *keep a trained person comfortable in heart rate zone 2 during endurance exercise*, and will usually produce a *respiratory exchange ratio (RER) closer to 0.7 once glycogen is depleted.*[23]

In technical terms, if you want to train your mitochondria to burn fat, then expect to train the red muscle fibers that are denser in mitochondria.

Pro tip: If you use a cardio machine or wear a smartwatch, instead of focusing on calories or grams of fat burned, visualize your body gaining more metabolically healthy mitochondria. Picture yourself building a healthier aerobic base as you spend more time in zone 2, and remember that you are cardio training to improve your metabolism–not to burn calories from something you "indulged in" at the last meal.

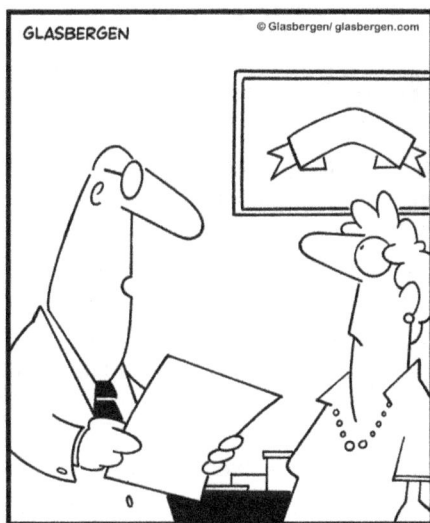

"To break through a weight-loss plateau, increase your walking to 40 hours a day, 9 days a week."

---

* Some of the Ironman and Iron woman triathlon records have been broken by athletes using a very low-carb approach. Tour de France athletes need a combination of endurance plus brief sprint performance. One of the worldwide experts on mitochondrial metabolism and respiration is researcher and cyclist Inigo San Millan, who also consults some of the top endurance cyclists of the world. Their exact pre-race and mid-race fueling strategies remain proprietary for obvious reasons. See: "Interview with Tadej Pogačar and Dr. Inigo San Milan," NiceHumanBeing, 2022, https://www.reddit.com/r/pelotonmemes/comments/v94naa/interview_with_tadej_poga%C4%8Dar_and_dr_inigo_san/?rdt=40479.

** Interesting coincidence: Brown fat and red muscle fibers owe their color to higher mitochondrial density and correlate with fat burn. Hello, mitochondria!

If calories were all there was to burning fat, then salads and treadmills would have cured the world of obesity and type 2 diabetes by now.

The word *calories* doesn't have a role here.

Calories are what scientists measure by burning food in labs, and they have no place in assessing fat loss from my standpoint.

They don't matter because we know that simply doing more cardio or burning more calories doesn't mean more fat *loss*.

It's why we look to exercise physiology, the study of how the body tissues and systems respond to exercise. Cardio training means more healthy mitochondria, greater aerobic capacity, and increased metabolic flexibility to burn fat. By pairing exercise physiology with endocrinology–the study of hormones and what your mitochondria do to energize life (whether feeding or fasting)–we can improve metabolic health without focusing on calories.

We start by building up our aerobic base.

Building your aerobic base

Remember, motivation is one thing. Showing up is another thing. You don't reach a life of regular training by thinking about it. You reach there by showing up, one five minute commitment at a time.

By building your aerobic base, you are setting yourself up for long-term success. By making exercise less miserable, you will actually enjoy different workouts and start seeking more movement instead of mentally running from it.

To get *excited* about the power of an aerobic base, I can recommend the work of Dr. Mark Cucuzzella, a professor of family medicine and an endurance athlete himself. Dr. Cucuzzella has an excellent presentation on zone 2 training that's freely available on the Low-Carb Denver 2023 YouTube channel.

Aim to spend thirty to forty-five minutes in zone 2–twice a week to start with, then up to four times a week. Remember, zone 2 is when you can carry on a conversation and speak full sentences while exercising, but your breathing is a bit heavier than resting, and the person you are talking to knows you are exerting yourself. This is also described as the *rate of perceived exertion* (RPE) or the "talk test." Even when focusing on improving the health of the mitochondria, exercising can feel like a drag when you can't see the results. While you can't see it, there is good news! **After six months of consistent zone 2 training**, your aerobic base will have increased, and *exercise will not feel as miserable*.

Additionally, Peter Attia, in his book *Outlive*, outlines a cardio exercise protocol that helps you build your aerobic base and then **add bursts of maximum effort once a week to improve VO$_2$ max**. A higher VO$_2$ max is associated with longevity. Similarly, Tabata workouts have also been shown to improve VO$_2$ max.[24]

But as always–we want to find an option that works best for you.

If you want better postmeal glucose levels, you need to build more efficient carbohydrate metabolism in your mitochondria. It sounds like a complicated thing to do, and yet the solution is shockingly simple. Activate your muscles.

Research has shown that **walking for thirty minutes immediately after a meal** *has a beneficial impact on postmeal glucose, regardless of carbohydrate load.*[25,26]

Remember how we described muscle as the "glucose taker" among the three musketeers? This means that if you are looking for ways to reduce that postmeal glucose spike without needing more medication, triggering the "glucose taker" with a walk may help. As always, only do this under medical supervision so your doctor can adjust your medication safely.

Walking is something we can easily work into our daily lives, but because I work mostly with Indians, many people ask me if yoga can be their preferred form of exercise.

The meaning of *yoga* is "yog," or "union of mind and body," and yoga itself is a very powerful science when used properly. Ancient pranayama breathing techniques derived from yoga are associated with spiritual growth and enhanced mental functioning, but unfortunately, most people I work with use yoga in its oversimplified form without a specified dose in mind.

Some use yoga as a basic warm-up and stretch session, holding some basic poses. It's better than nothing. I've witnessed practitioners of advanced forms of yoga turn around low back pain and disc injuries in ways that Western medicine hasn't been able to do. I've also seen other forms of yoga that focus on the mind-body-spirit connection and are less physically intense. To gain muscle, you really need to follow the principles of progressive overload.

We need more high-quality research to establish how yoga can help people with diabetes; we know yoga generally helps in multifactorial ways such as reduced sympathetic activity, increased parasympathetic activity, reduced perceived stress, improved sleep and mood, and improved physical function.[27] **So when it comes to those benefits, keep yoga in your life if you enjoy it,** *but be sure to focus on building muscle and getting stronger along the way.* I recommend that you work with a professional if you have osteoporosis, osteopenia, any heart condition, or high blood pressure; and remember that more intense forms of yoga may need to be modified for certain clinical diagnoses.

By fixing nutrition, as discussed in Part 2; working on our muscles to gain strength and training our mitochondria to burn fat, as explored here, you set yourself up to succeed if you choose to burn excess fat through fasting, which we'll cover in Part 6. You may have noticed the term fasted workouts a little earlier. The reason we are covering *nutrition, sleep, stress management and exercise before fasting* is that we want to give your brain and body a very specific metabolic message: **build muscle while burning fat.** I get into a lot of detail here with my patients so that they are protecting muscle at all costs.

5.4: Overcoming obstacles to resistance training

We've discussed how strength training to build muscle and protect your Type II muscle fibers is beneficial to both your mitochondria and your diabetes. We haven't discussed all the reasons people have for why they don't engage in muscle-building exercise. Time and time again, patients start with reasonable explanations for what is getting in their way, only to eventually surprise themselves. They have shown me that no obstacle is impossible to overcome. If you have ever felt like you don't engage in exercise because you feel like you *can't*, then let's address those concerns so that you can make an informed decision for yourself.

A common fear I've encountered among people is being too scared to get started with exercise, because they already **feel out of breath with minimal effort.** You might be surprised to know that most of us might not be breathing properly.[28]

In terms of breathing, there are two ways to think about it. There is breathing as you know it, inhaling oxygen and exhaling carbon dioxide, and then there is deep breathing. You have probably heard advice to "take a deep breath," but many people don't know how to do that properly. I didn't know how to take a deep breath either, until I started paying attention.

When I tell patients to demonstrate how they take a deep breath, they hunch up their shoulders, crunch their necks, puff up their chests, wrinkle their noses, and screw up their eyes. School sat us at desks to teach history and geography. I suspect that sitting in those classrooms from childhood onward is what disengages our core; we stop using our abdominal muscles to assist in deep breaths. We also forget about *diaphragmatic breathing.*

Watch a baby breathe.

Their belly rises when they take air in and falls as they exhale. Ideally, a deep breath causes your diaphragm to move down, pulling air into your lung bases and bringing a rich oxygen supply to your bloodstream. Your belly popping *out* during a deep breath is a visible sign that your in-breath is moving properly. *Yoga and pranayama are powerful ways to relearn how to breathe* in a way that aligns your cardiovascular system with your parasympathetic nervous system.

Learning how to take deep breaths correctly helps, but it's also important to make sure the way you breathe during everyday life is correct. Those are all the breaths you take when you aren't even paying attention. The easiest way to know if you need to fix your usual breathing patterns is to check whether you're a *chronic mouth breather.*

If so, the air you breathe doesn't pass through your nostrils to get warmed, filtered, and moisturized before hitting your lower airways; you just gulp large amounts of air through your mouth instead. This can trigger all kinds of breathing reactions, depending on the ambient temperature, air quality, and moisture levels. I've seen this happen, and it reminds me of a patient I had who moved from New Delhi to London.

He was a former marathon runner and wondered why walking or running by the River Thames was triggering asthma. He was much slower than his former cardio personal bests, but couldn't figure out why. Being a busy man, he made the most of his time by taking work calls during his brisk walks.

We realized he was multitasking—he was mouth breathing and taking cold, moist air straight into his chest. Nobody had ever asked him about his breathing technique! By training himself to breathe through his nose, his asthma symptoms improved, and he was able to run again. *Having large tonsils, adenoids, a deviated septum, or obstructive sleep apnea can all cause mouth breathing.* Paying more attention to how you take air into your chest (through your nostrils versus your mouth), and consulting with your health team can help you get back to breathing correctly.

You should definitely consult your health team or a professional if **you stopped exercising because something hurts.**

Knee pain, low back pain, arthritis, frozen shoulder pain, plantar fasciitis, and so many other aches and pains have kept people on a sedentary path. You, like them, might have been put off the idea of working out because you are afraid of injuring yourself and making the pain worse—and that makes sense. Resting an injured body part helps the body heal. Unfortunately, sometimes this goes on for too long and we stop exercising indefinitely. That costs us more than it helps us.

When it comes down to it, *exercise is about "use it or lose it."* You would not leave the air-conditioning on full blast when you leave the house, and similarly, your body will downregulate your metabolically demanding muscles if you are not working them. For every two weeks the body goes without stimulus, you can begin seeing a loss of muscle. Not only is muscle the "glucose taker" among the musketeers, but muscle mass is also a key contributor to life span and health span because *gravity still exists.* For as long as you live, your muscles will be responsible for holding your body upright against gravity. If you don't address the cause of the pain early on, your joints will wear out even faster because your muscles are doing less antigravity work to hold the joint in alignment.

Nobody gets rid of pain by sitting on the sofa or lying around permanently, *so when in pain, go up the chain.* If your ankle is hurting, you might have gotten some fancy shoe or insole to support a flat foot–but the cause of the flat foot starts much higher up in the skeleton. Your entire weight-bearing chain and posture need to be assessed by a qualified physiotherapist who understands how to help you strengthen the entire muscle system from top to bottom. Only treating the site of the pain is like seeing water leaking through your ceiling–and just putting fresh paint over the wet patch without checking to see where the water is coming from. The opposite would be working with a good physical therapist who can teach you correct exercise form, technique, and breathing.

The difference between a physiotherapist and a personal trainer or chiropractor is the type and duration of medical education that a doctor of physical therapy has at the start of their career. When selecting an experienced professional, you want to ensure that they will not only focus on *functionally strengthening the entire kinetic chain* (both anterior and posterior) instead of just isolated "mirror muscles," but will also *address posture checkpoints from head to toe in order to fix pelvic tilt,* ensure *proper hip hinge and a neutral spine.* Sometimes they need to figure out which muscles are sleeping on the job and causing other muscles to become overactive. This helps to determine *the right sequence of therapy* to address tight spots and weak spots safely.

This sequence should include *engaging the deep muscles of the entire core* as a functional compartment, not just the superficial six-pack. They need to help you *engage the stronger, larger muscles* (like the lats and back) before loading the smaller, weaker muscles (like the rotator-cuff stabilizers), and *strengthen the glutes before attempting high impact explosive movements.* An experienced professional will focus on *fixing mobility and strength through the entire range of motion* of a muscle while also working on *stability training* to prevent falls; they will design workouts that *balance push and pull movements* while incorporating a *warm-up and cooldown* to prevent injury. They can also incorporate functional *training involving all three planes of movement*: forward/backward, sideways, and rotational.

While there is a difference between the training of orthopedic surgeons, physiotherapists, personal trainers, and chiropractors, I say "experienced professionals" because some prescribe exercise more effectively than others. I have seen gifted personal trainers and sports orthopedic doctors who know more about rehabilitation than physiotherapists; and I have seen physiotherapists and chiropractors who know more about optimal movement than some orthopedic surgeons. If you have pain, I always recommend starting with a medical professional. It's perfectly fine to switch to a personal trainer once you know how to safely strengthen your body, but I believe it's best to start by getting a documented baseline from your clinical care team. Ultimately, you'll have to do your research to find someone who understands the human body well. There are excellent and average professionals in every field–and healthcare is no exception.

If you're the type who enjoys research and has already looked into exercising more, but all the talk of building muscle has scared you off because **you don't want to get bulky or be a bodybuilder**—trust me, you won't.

According to Dr. Ted Naiman, a low-carb family physician, everyone is already a bodybuilder. The only difference between someone with insulin resistance and a professional athlete–is what type of body they're building.[29] But just because everyone is technically a bodybuilder, that doesn't mean everyone will end up big and bulky. For everyone who would prefer a toned, lean look–that's exactly what you get from strength training. This is true for both men and women, and if you don't believe me, just ask anyone who exercises regularly how difficult it is to get bulging muscles.

Things like a creatine supplement can help you increase what you are capable of lifting during a workout. You still have to put in the work. Creatine supplements are safe to take under professional supervision, but again, your muscles won't be bursting out of your clothes just by taking it. Besides the proven benefits of creatine in sports science, there is growing interest in what creatine might do for brain health and metabolism.[30] Talk to your health professional before adding it to your strength training and recovery plans.

Maybe you feel there's no point in making those plans because **you can't go to a gym**—guess what—you don't have to. All you need to do to grow muscle is push each muscle group. As long as you understand the correct exercise form and technique to prevent injury, *you only need your body weight and gravity to get started at home*, and you can even get a pretty challenging workout done with just resistance bands and dumbbells.

Initially, this could be a mix of light weights with more repetitions; later on, the resistance needs to get heavier. Like we said earlier, pushing each muscle group until technical failure is what tells your brain that it needs to recruit more muscle fibers and build more muscle (hypertrophy). Home workouts can be made progressively more difficult with modifications of your strength training routine.

The options range from simple tweaks to your usual movements to different training protocols entirely, all of which can be done from home. Things like carrying a load on your back when walking (rucking), gradually *increasing the load* with adjustable dumbbells, or *increasing the time spent doing antigravity and eccentric* movements can help you get more impact from the home workout routine you're already comfortable with.

If you're ready to add in different types of training, you can try adding in asymmetric (one-sided) training. *Super-slow repetitions and isometric holds* increase time under tension to fatigue the fast-twitch, glycolytic type II muscle fibers.[31] *Instability training* can be introduced to your routine by working with a BOSU® ball, Pilates ball, stability ball, wobble board, sliders, or TRX® bands. Resistance bands are also an option as I mentioned before; *many physiotherapists and trainers swear by resistance bands* and how they change the challenge for the muscle fibers as the resistance gets tougher toward the end range of a movement. You can progress up the bands to increase resistance as you get stronger.

No matter what you choose to implement, a home workout is a valid way to exercise. I've exclusively done home workouts for over ten years and I have gotten fitter and stronger, and I even gained four kilograms of lean muscle (confirmed on dual X-ray absorptiometry [DEXA], see Part 7) despite accumulating a whole decade of birthdays. Building muscle helps you delay the slowdown that comes with physical aging by improving body composition. By doing nothing about it, people can lose 8–17 percent of their strength per decade after the age of thirty.

But what if **you have a condition?**

Are you sure your doctor has actually told you "never" to exercise versus recommending exercise with certain precautions before progressing the intensity? An umbilical hernia, history of cesarean section, cervical spondylosis, diastasis recti, osteoarthritis, osteoporosis, slipped intervertebral disc, history of lymph node resection, and other diagnoses *may create a need for you to modify your workout,* but in most cases you don't need to stop exercising forever. Some patients have misunderstood that their condition means they can never exercise again. Not true. *Talk to your healthcare professional and tell them you want to build muscle for better diabetes with less medication.*

Maybe your obstacle isn't a condition, but rather, **you think you can't exercise because you had a joint replacement.**

This is the most paradoxical one! Not exercising because you have an artificial joint?

What?

The joint was replaced so that you could move again! The piece of metal or ceramic is designed to outlive you, so double-check with your physiotherapist and your orthopedic doctor about what modifications are needed. Doctors sometimes misunderstand or mistakenly assume that the patient is just trying to find an "excuse" and isn't interested in exercise.

The biggest piece of clarity I can give you is that *it's your job to let your doctor know that you want to get stronger.* Let them know what fitness goals you have for yourself so that they put more thought into your exercise prescription, because the success of joint replacement surgery goes far beyond getting stitches removed. Having a new joint gives you a better chance at building muscle that can help you improve glucose levels with less medication. Are you moving and living better with that new joint?

If you're just living the good life in general, maybe the biggest obstacle in the way of building muscle is that **you travel a lot and you are busy with "life."** The good news is *that gravity is available at all locations you plan to visit on Earth.* This is helpful, especially since we've already established that *doing antigravity movements without a gym is a valid form of exercise.* Additionally, we previously discussed what happens when you don't stimulate your muscles: Do you really want to come back from a two-week vacation or business trip having gained fat and lost muscle?

All that money, effort, and time spent on travel to enrich your mind–but not your body? Your scale might show the same number when you return, but it won't tell you how your body composition changed. Only you can check in with your body to know if you are losing muscle. Getting busy with life happens to all of us. I get it. I lost two kilograms of lean muscle, which took me a year to build, just because I stopped exercising regularly in the last two months of getting this book written.

Don't do that. I mean, yes, finish your book. Don't lose muscle doing it! You wouldn't be happy with a retirement plan that was causing you to lose money, so why settle for muscle loss instead of gain, especially now that you know muscle loss worsens your diabetes like we discussed earlier. The good news is that *you can keep your muscles stimulated even with shorter, intense workouts when you are traveling or super busy.* Perfection might cause you to skip the full workout, but perfection is rarely necessary or helpful when building a sustainable relationship with exercise.

And perhaps this has happened to you in the past. **You tried exercising before, but you didn't get stronger,** and now you don't think there's a point to exercising at all, much less on vacation. It happens, but there are reasons to explore before deciding your body is defective. If you were exercising, but *your workout intensity wasn't increasing,* you could've hit a plateau in gains. Your body is not plotting against you by purposely holding on to fat and refusing to cooperate. If you are not getting stronger, something needs to change.

Maybe it's not about the exercise at all, maybe we have to go back to the second wheel because *your sleep was not restorative.* As we covered in Part 3.2, sleep is when your body repairs itself with growth hormone. Without enough restorative sleep, you won't have enough of an overnight response to recover and build more muscle.

It's possible the issue is even further back, in the first wheel of the lifestyle car. When it comes to nutrition, *maybe there wasn't enough protein in your diet.* You can go from 1.2 to 1.6 grams per kilogram of body weight (BW) per day, divided evenly across three to four meals (Part 2.5)–yes, four meals. Some of my detail-oriented clients realize that I may encourage them to take a fourth meal beyond just breakfast, lunch, and dinner, so that they get their protein target. Because those clients are working on reversing insulin resistance, they're concerned about the metabolic impact of adding a fourth insulin spike in the eating window.

It's a reasonable response, but if you struggle to decide between being protein deficient while trying to build muscle or adding the fourth insulin spike, choose the fourth meal.

Why?

Because if you *get enough protein to stay in an anabolic state* to build muscle, that net muscle gain can help you reverse insulin resistance more than just avoiding a fourth spike. Insulin is not evil in itself. Insulin has anabolic effects. We'll address the tool of time-restricted eating as a way to lower insulin resistance in Part 6, but restricting yourself to three meals and exercising with a protein deficiency or while underfeeding yourself can cause a stagnation of muscle gains and lead to a plateau in the reversal of insulin resistance.

You could have seen no muscle growth previously for any of these reasons, but maybe that wasn't the real obstacle for you. Maybe for you, your past experiences with exercise have **caused you to become demotivated, so you quit.**

Referring back to Part 5.2, my questions to you are: *What is your exercise mindset? What metric were you using to assess "results?"*

If you were relying on the weighing scale, remember that it has no idea <u>what</u> you are gaining or losing. Ask yourself: Is a kilogram of gold worth the same as a kilogram of sand? Why would a kilogram of muscle be the same as a kilogram of fat?

Exercise causes healthy weight gain on the scale if you're adding lean muscle because muscle is heavier than fat.

So how will you know if you are making progress? How soon will you see results? Exercise takes at least three to six months of consistent work, two to four times a week, before you will see meaningful strength gains. Your six-pack exists, but is hidden under a layer of fat, and a million crunches alone can't make your six-pack visible. Ultimately, losing body fat percentage involves a combination of reducing carbohydrate intake and intermittently fasting to burn fat because you can't out-exercise an imbalanced diet. Instead, you have to reflect and ask yourself: *Are your expectations realistic or fair?*

There are *earlier, non-scale victories that aren't reflected initially on the weighing scale.* It takes years of training and changes in your diet before your muscles become visible through your clothing, so you may notice inch loss, improved glucose levels and increased fitness first. Celebrate it! A win is a win, right?

5.5: So, what happened to Jayesh and Tina?

The approach to exercising and overcoming obstacles that I've shared here is about finding what works for you, and then setting yourself up to consistently win. This is the advice I give all my clients, including Jayesh and Tina.

In Jayesh's case, he wanted to avoid being dependent on his family in his retirement. He had cared for his mother, who had gotten so frail and weak in her final years that she was bedbound; he could see himself heading there physically. While his blood tests were a wake-up call, as a successful real estate businessman, one of his strengths was his ability to think long-term.

Once he realized that his current **fitness** was out of sync with his long-term goals, he decided to make a change. Real estate had taught him how things are built one brick at a time, so he focused on small changes, step by step. The first change he made was to *break up his sedentary time* like we mentioned earlier—he started using an adjustable desk so that he could raise and lower it to alternate between sitting and standing, taking breaks and sitting whenever he wanted.

He wanted to reduce his carb intake, but his family worried about reducing carbs when he already looked so "weak." Once he realized his biggest reason for thin limbs was muscle loss, he explained to his family members why he wanted more protein to support his muscle tissues. The carbs were not strengthening his body. If anything, he was always exhausted.

As his *food habits changed* and his nutrition improved, his energy levels automatically improved. He wore a continuous glucose monitor (CGM) to observe his glucose trends. *He started sleeping better* and his body felt better than it had in years. He started adding brisk walks and started seeing his postmeal glucose levels stabilize; he was encouraged to do even more.

Over the span of a few months, he found a nearby gym and started waking his muscles up one day at a time. The trainer in the gym pointed out how years of sitting had made his glutes go to sleep and how his reflexes had gotten slow. Jayesh wanted to change this and was encouraged to know that it was possible to start exercising later in life and still achieve high levels of fitness.[32]

He started building muscle because he wanted to be able to lift his grand-children up and put his luggage into the overhead compartment when he traveled. These were goals that resonated with the stage of life that he was in, and he realized he didn't need to consider himself old. He started feeling younger as he resumed moving the way he had before. Maybe that's why we call it **muscle memory**. The competitive nature of his sports days in college started coming back, but this time, *he was competing with himself.* By getting serious about what he considered a "win," he was able to get the four wheels of his lifestyle car recalibrated and turning in sync.

Tina, on the other hand, is an example of why my team and I spend three to six months working with people.

In her case, her **nutrition, sleep, stress, and exercise were all off**—all four wheels needed attention. She picked a few easy ways to increase protein from her existing food options. She was exhausted, burning the candle at both ends. Being chronically sleep-deprived was taking a toll on every system, so asking her to "do more self-care" was not helpful.

What we could ask her to do, however, was *introspect* as to why she expected herself to do everything after she got home. When she took a hard look at how she spent her time after getting home at 7:30 p.m., not only did she recognize that she was putting in an additional hour and a half of physical labor every night, but she also realized there was another ninety minutes of screen time after she closed the kitchen.

Tina knew she needed rest, but only she could figure out how to *add higher-quality sleep* to her twenty-four-hour day. She found that sharing the responsibility of preparing and cleaning up after dinner with her family not only saved her forty-five minutes every day, but the family effort and teamwork took care of her social connection needs; this helped her feel less resentful and stressed about housework.

Then, by skipping the screen time, she saved another ninety minutes of her night. Instead of pushing herself until 9:45 p.m. every night, she could finish addressing the needs of her family and herself by 8:15 p.m., and then focus on getting better sleep.

Her brain needed enough restorative sleep to learn, build neural connections, and come up with creative solutions to her problems. With better sleep, she had more mental bandwidth available. She then spent a few months getting her head around how to get enough protein and came up with creative ways to *add more protein to each meal.*

These changes took around three months to align with her life, after which they started giving exponential results. She was finally able to plan her meals to *reduce the carbs* so that her mitochondria could switch metabolic gears. Her movement was already in place because she was running around on her feet all day between the commute and being on the retail floor. With more pep in her stride, her glucose levels got better, further improving her energy levels. Her mitochondria were happily humming along now instead of sputtering and choking through the day.

Eventually, she was able to consider strength training. We knew she wouldn't have the time to go to a gym, *so she started body-weight movements at home.*

Like all of us, she is a work in progress, and she is enjoying better diabetes levels now with less medication, thanks to giving her four wheels the attention they deserve.

But what happens then? When you've aligned the wheels of your lifestyle car to your goals and have gotten comfortable behind the wheel, you will start feeling much better about the progress you are making.

The alignment of the four wheels are what make the car go in the right direction, but what additional effort might help you on the trip?

Part 5 summary

- Even if you are sedentary, you can train your muscles to burn more glucose through movement.

- You can train your mitochondria to burn fat for energy through endurance, Zone 2, and aerobic training.

- Increased cardio fitness measured as VO_2 max strongly correlates with longevity.

- Increasing muscle mass through progressive strength training improves your glucose levels and correlates with longer, healthier lifespan.

For Bonus Materials, Visit the Website Here:

PART 6

TAKING YOUR LIFESTYLE CAR THE EXTRA MILE:

FASTING

6.1: Going beyond the four wheels

Having a car is great. The driving experience is made better if you know about some of the cool features your car has. While nutrition, sleep, stress management, and exercise will take you far on this journey, you may want to utilize the storage space available to make sure you are prepared for the long haul.

Let me explain.

Thousands of years ago, our primitive lifestyle in the wild included opportunities to feast by hunting and gathering unprocessed whole food. Excess food was stored as fat. This informed the first wheel of the lifestyle car. The second wheel looks at our ancestor's sleep habits, and how they fall asleep in accordance with the rhythm of the sun. Back then, humans faced physical and mental stressors of their own. Perhaps they didn't have to worry about college loans, a failing marriage, or retirement; but they experienced stress due to harsh weather, warring tribes, food hardship, and infectious disease. These stressors may be different, but it shows that the third wheel and the stress hormone cortisol apply in both scenarios. Additionally, needing physical prowess, agility, strength, and speed to survive daily life shows that— though the fourth wheel may come last—it's just as important as nutrition and sleep when it comes down to life or death in the wild.

Perhaps one of the biggest nutrition-related stressors our ancestors dealt with was food scarcity. Navigating this was so critical to survival that the human body evolved to withstand periods of food unavailability by storing and burning fat. This is called **fasting** and historically helped the body regulate energy during food shortages. For hundreds of thousands of years, *Homo sapiens* evolved while eating unprocessed food, slept in tune with the rising and setting sun, handled occasional stress, used strength and agility to survive, and spent chunks of time in a fasted state. Even after they tamed fire, they needed to gather fuel to cook, it was hard to keep food preserved, and food sometimes was not available. Since we were built to adapt to periods without food through fasting back then, there's a way it can become a treatment strategy for us today.

The wheels of the lifestyle car were founded on four of the most powerful biological mechanisms you can control when it comes to turning around your diabetes. By investing in nutrition, sleep, stress management, and exercise you can begin driving in the right direction. There's one more thing that can be done.

Whether you have a special luggage carrier atop your car or just a roomy trunk, you have another option to support a long road trip. Specifically, you could pack some luggage with things you may need along the journey.

Knowing how to safely fast in a way that effectively burns excess fat while maintaining muscle and keeping your metabolism up is a powerful strategy to master if you want to reverse insulin resistance and put type 2 diabetes into remission. I've even closely monitored people with type 1 diabetes as we worked toward better glucose levels with lower insulin requirements using intermittent fasting. Let me tell you the compelling story of Mr. Shanti so you can decide if you want to use this tool.

Mr. Shanti was referred to me by his chest physician after being placed on the lung transplant waiting list. He was only forty-eight, and his doctors could not explain why his lungs were inflamed and being replaced by scar tissue. They thought perhaps it was local air pollution, aggravated by obesity. He weighed 110 kilograms (242 pounds), which was too much for his heart and lungs to support. The lungs were so inflamed that he was unable to maintain stable oxygen levels. He was put on steroids to reduce the inflammation in his lungs while awaiting a donor. He also had diabetes, and the steroids were expected to cause more weight gain and higher blood glucose levels.

So he was sent to me. He would get breathless just walking from his sofa to the bed because his oxygen saturation would fall below 90 percent, and he was dependent on oxygen twenty-four hours a day. Together, we worked on whatever lifestyle change could help him achieve better health despite his condition.

He was so motivated to fight his illness that he was exercising with his oxygen cylinder in the pulmonary rehab department. He reduced his carbohydrates, had surprisingly good improvements in sleep quality, and maintained a positive outlook toward his prognosis. He had faith that he was in good hands. At that point, he had optimized all four of his lifestyle wheels as best he could, and now, he was interested in fasting.

6.2: Why is fasting an option for treating diabetes?

In a dysfunctional relationship, people yell louder to feel heard. The communication doesn't get better, and screaming just makes it worse. The inspiration for this book came when I started to question whether any of my patients came back feeling better after I had "treated" their insulin resistance with more insulin, because in all honesty, they hadn't. "Treating" insulin resistance with more insulin and food all day only made things worse.

Diet and exercise are by no means groundbreaking when it comes to taking care of your health. I knew that reducing the snacking made things better, but after stumbling across a video by Dr. Jason Fung at a diabetes-reversal conference in 2017, I was shocked that the power of fasting had not been tapped in clinical practice.[1] I felt like I had just found the missing piece in the puzzle of progressive metabolic diseases fueled by chronically high insulin levels. It all made sense, and it changed my practice forever.

A bit of backstory here. From 2013 to 2017, I had gone from talking only about nutrition with patients to spending twenty to thirty minutes covering all four aspects of their lifestyle so that I could deprescribe medication as their health improved. My initial analogy was not a car, in fact I used to sketch out a table with four legs on the back of my prescriptions. I would explain to patients how even 3 great legs on the table would not create stability if any one leg was wobbly. Coincidentally, I had a makeshift flimsy folding table for a while in that office, so I would theatrically shake the table we were sitting across to show my patient how important each component was. This analogy suited me for a bit, but I gradually realized that lifestyles were far from static like the table I was drawing. People's daily decisions about food, sleep, stressful events and exercise were dynamic responses to complex, rich lives. Even shaking the table was too static, rigid and unrealistic. The lifestyle car emerged as a more fitting analogy, allowing me to acknowledge the person in the driver's seat, facing external challenges like bumps in the road and ups and downs in the journey. Needing to service the car as a whole became obvious. The lifestyle car was already a part of my storytelling with patients when I discovered how Dr Jason Fung was using fasting to complete the journey for people with type 2 diabetes. This made sense, because although I had been deprescribing and seeing people achieve better diabetes results with less medication, I had not been able to get everyone's type 2 diabetes into remission. There were always a handful of people who would hit a plateau in their efforts to completely reverse things like fatty liver, PCOS, high blood pressure and excess belly fat. As soon as I understood the science of how fasting reduced insulin requirements, I was all in. So how did fasting add onto my lifestyle car analogy? I knew the four wheels were absolutely essential before fasting because the biggest psychological barrier people have to fasting is they are worried about feeling hungry or low on energy. I knew our lifestyle car was correcting for those symptoms. Getting enough protein was providing satiety all day. Going low carb was reducing insulin levels, so people were experiencing less hunger and cravings. Waking up fresh in the morning was giving people the mental and physical bandwidth to face new challenges, and think of new solutions to old problems. Having more stress management skills was helping people become mindful of their emotional needs, and this was reducing the extremes of their love-hate relationship with their food and their body. From there, their newfound energy was being channeled into more movement and exercise. I knew that these four elements were essential foundations upon which I could talk to my patients about fasting. I don't like asking people to do things for their health that I can't imagine doing myself, so I started fasting to see what it felt like. I had never intentionally skipped a meal in my life, so the first day of not eating breakfast mentally felt like I was coming to work missing a shoe. I knew I couldn't possibly fast if I was hungry, sleep deprived, stressed or feeling weak. I also didn't want to do anything that might cause muscle losses. So the lifestyle car would stay and I started adding fasting for those who were still a few miles from their destination, and needed something beyond the lifestyle car we have covered already. Perhaps their journey was longer and they needed to pack some bags. Since Jason Fung seemed to be helping people complete their remission journeys, fasting seemed to be the missing link to address the last traces of insulin resistance that I had not been able to eradicate using my lifestyle car. Incorporating fasting in my own life and my clinical practice taught me many things. I already felt like a car mechanic at times, running diagnostic checks on people's lifestyles to see why their body wasn't functioning optimally. As fasting grew in popularity, some new patients would see me and describe how fasting "didn't work" for them. When I ran through my mechanic's checklist, I was able to explain to them which of their lifestyle wheels were out of order, causing fasting to not only fail to give them results, but even worse, it was becoming an unhealthy experience for them. This confirmed my analogy; no matter what luggage you take for a long drive, you don't reach your destination with a flat tire.

You may have noticed that every step of this book has started with assessing yourself and becoming aware of your patterns and preferences, because self-awareness is a powerful tool. Some people start fasting without checking their deeper thoughts and beliefs around dieting. It's difficult to keep up with a habit that makes you feel bad. Since yo-yo diets start as thought patterns and beliefs in the head, the ability to catch them is key. To do so, it helps to **be aware of some red-flag thoughts that can trigger a "dieting" mindset** that negatively affects your relationship with feeding and fasting.

If, on your fasting journey, you find yourself thinking in black-and-white terms, you may have slipped into dieting thinking. Black-and-white thinking can *look like labeling every decision as either right or wrong; good or bad; something you have to or can't do; is allowed or not allowed; or is a should versus a should not.* This is "to help" you make the right decisions, but if the way you set up the choices is so that one decision always makes you the villain, or a failure, that's a red flag, too.

A dieting mindset is one where you tell yourself that the only options are *on-track or off-track; on or off the wagon; cheating or clean eating; or doing a no-sugar challenge versus giving in to a sweet tooth.* By not giving yourself any flexibility or balance, you continue a cycle of *giving in to temptation, weakness, or cravings, only to return to a "detox" option based on depriving, avoiding, and resisting the things you want.* As the cycle continues, you'll see that you've boxed yourself into another either/or situation—you are always ricocheting *from the pleasure of indulging, to guilt and disappointment. You then make "corrections" driven by remorse or repentance.*

This is where the red flags escalate. *If you are experiencing deep guilt and disappointment with yourself—how is that going to be sustainable?*

When you begin feeling this low, you might start to punish yourself. This can look like *declaring that your diet went for a toss—but you're back now.* This time, you can overeat like it's the last supper but then you're going on a serious detox and *since you can't be trusted, you need someone to police you. Fasting to compensate for calories, is also punishing yourself.* By *binging before fasting*, you set yourself up to be miserable throughout the fast. You end up waiting for the fast to end, just to repeat the cycle all over again. So if you are fasting as a way to trap or force yourself into making the right decision, it may be time to reassess.

These dualing options and mindsets create a psychological yo-yo effect. Recall how the lazy mind is wired for instant, short-term rewards from Part 4. If your conflicting thoughts keep feeding negative emotions, it makes sense that you're likely to stop fasting soon and seek something immediately pleasurable instead. It doesn't need to be that way.

You could make a 180 degree hairpin turn to reach the top of a steep mountain. You might get to the top with less motion sickness if you take slow gradual turns around it. It would take longer, but drastic changes make things unnecessarily more difficult. Instead of giving yourself unsustainable choices, you have the option of taking the long way around to see how you can incorporate fasting into your life through a gradual, manageable process instead of a full abrupt u-turn. I want to show you how because I am interested in your long-term success.

Remember, you are fasting by choice. Earth is a free will zone—you are in charge.

You drive.

Even if you are in control of your "thinking" in regards to fasting, we still must address the "dieting," as well. In Part 2 regarding dieting and nutrition, we focussed on the macronutrients, going so far as to say we don't need to count the calories if everything else fits our guidelines. I made a point to say that a caloric deficit means nothing if you are still protein deficient. I say this not just because it's true, but because I've seen people try to use fasting to maintain a calorie deficit, only to still overeat during the eating window and feel miserable for the duration of the fast.

What they were failing to understand is that **a calorie deficit is not the same as fasting.**

The **"diabetic calorie-restricted diet"** is *focused on calorie-counting* to achieve a *deficit through low-calorie meals and snacks, prioritizing low-fat* because fat has the most calories per gram. **Fasting** achieves a *deficit by skipping meals and snacks entirely,* keeping calorie intake at zero.

Think about how a square is a rectangle but a rectangle isn't a square. Similarly, fasting meets the requirements for creating a caloric deficit, but eating a diet based on *eating calories* is not the same as a protocol defined by *not eating calories at all.* Of course, that's an oversimplification—obviously, people who fast still need to eat food. They do that in their eating window.

The difference is that **low-calorie diets** provide *low satiety alongside high cravings* by avoiding fat and often being carbohydrate predominant. The continuous nutrient deficit *affects brain function, causing irritable "hangry" moods.* Compare this to people who practice **intermittent fasting** and report feeling *alert, sharp, and have increased focus.* Since fasting is *focused on gaining metabolic flexibility to maintain adenosine triphosphate* (ATP) s*upply, eating natural, unprocessed fats actually helps fuel the process.* As fat burn and ketosis start, *satiety is high, hunger is low and cravings are reduced.*

The **low-calorie diet** advises *eating small, frequent meals,* but these *don't allow insulin levels to drop.* The insulin secretion *prevents fat burn,* eventually forcing the body to *slow down metabolism* as it sees nutritional deficits but can't access any stored energy. This is how low-calorie diets reach a weight-loss plateau. Not only is there a *loss of lean muscle mass,* but as a result of these *metabolic adaptations,* only further calorie restriction will aid in maintaining weight.[2]

Since most people find that difficult to do, they struggle with sustainability. When they resume previous eating habits, they find themselves regaining more than they had initially lost, probably due to the slowing of their metabolic rate. **Intermittent fasting**, on the other hand, is made effective through *consuming sufficient nutrition in eating windows, getting sufficient recovery, and engaging in progressive workouts* that support muscle gain and fat loss. A four-day fast can boost your metabolism, *increasing your resting energy expenditure* by 12 percent.[3] Increased energy and engaging in workouts help to avoid plateaus, and *lean muscle is preserved when this is all done correctly.* The longer the fast, *the more body fat is burned,* and since *insulin levels stay low for longer, this contributes to reversing insulin resistance.*

When a healthcare professional tells you what you can and can't eat on a **low-calorie diet**, it creates a *locus of psychological control that is external*, meaning, from a location outside of you. By committing to following their rules, you experience *low flexibility* and can become rooted in a *mindset based on deprivation, restriction, limitation, and rigidity.*

When it comes to **fasting**, the *locus of psychological control is intrinsic*, or self-driven, or from within you—you get to decide whether, how long, how often, and when to fast. When you are in charge, you have *high flexibility*, and are more likely to operate from a *mindset of empowerment, autonomy, and choice.*

With that in mind: How would you prefer to achieve a caloric deficit?

6.3: What does the body do during the fast?

Understanding what fasting brings to the table isn't too hard, but understanding what the body *does* when you fast, is a little more complicated. Before understanding what your body does, **we first have to understand how it's fueling itself through the fast.**

While you may not be taking in any calories, your body generates constant energy through metabolism. Metabolism during a fast includes burning stored fuel for energy and recycling old tissues for raw material when insulin levels drop. In the previous chapter, we learned how your metabolism and energy expenditure improves from fasting, which shows that just because you consume zero calories doesn't mean your metabolism stops.

We haven't used the word "calorie" too often in this guide, and that's purposeful. Do you remember how I told you in Part 2 to think about nutrition in terms of hormones instead of calories?

That's because this difference comes into play when we compare fasting and dieting.

If you have been made to believe that you need to eat a certain amount of calories every day to sustain your energy levels, then it's only natural that you would worry about where your energy will come from during a fast, because fasting equals no food, and no food equals no calories.

Right?!

If that were true, then how does one maintain energy during a fast, and why do people report higher energy levels once their body gets used to fasting? Conversely, if the calories from food fuel us, then why do we use the phrase "food coma" when feeling stuffed after a delicious calorie-laden buffet?

I've said it before, and I'll say it again: The body counts energy in a different currency than scientists use in the lab. *The energy currency in a nutrition lab is calories, while the energy currency of the body is adenosine triphosphate* (ATP).

Adenosine diphosphate (ADP) is the raw material on site right before a third phosphate is added to make ATP (di means two and tri means three). The body is constantly changing metabolic gears based on the availability of ATP versus ADP, and has established multiple metabolic pathways to easily convert different types of fuel into a constant supply of ATP.

This metabolic machinery is set up in the energy powerhouse of the cell—the glorious mitochondria of Part 1.6. No matter what, your mitochondria are responsible for ensuring ATP is always readily available. Why?

Because you don't need constant food in your mouth for energy.

You don't need constant carb intake for energy.

You don't need constant glucose in your food for energy.

You need constant ATP for energy.

Sure, food and carbs can give you energy. The difference is that humans can go weeks without eating any calories but if someone's body stops making ATP—they'll die within minutes to hours.

It's that serious.

The mechanisms that constantly produce ADP and ATP for your body to use as energy are the foundation to intermittent fasting. The **energy source for producing ATP changes over time** as the fasting duration increases. Initially, glycogen (the storage form of glucose molecules) is used to create ATP; after glycogen stores run out, the mitochondria switch gears to burn stored body fat.

A special feature of pure water fasts is **the process of autophagy**, in which *the body is able to repair, recycle, and reuse old tissues during fasting.*

Autophagy literally means *"self-eating."*

Some members of the Jain and Hindu communities have been observing pure water fasts during times of spiritual significance for centuries. Still, the discovery that *autophagy provides the necessary protein* needed by the body while fasting is quite recent.

Yoshinori Ohsumi, who discovered that autophagy provides protein and described its relation to fasting, was awarded the Nobel Prize in Physiology or Medicine in 2016 for his contribution to medicine.[4]

He found that when we fast, even though we are not *consuming* any proteins, the body's recycling team goes around and breaks down any cells that are old, diseased, dying, dysfunctional, and damaged. It then reuses the spare parts, including amino acids, for new building and repair work. The body provides the energy for these catabolic (breaking-down) and anabolic (building) activities by initially burning stored carbohydrates (glycogen) and, as the fasting duration progresses, by burning fat. It's like reusing, recycling, and repurposing old useless plastic bottles to turn them into shopping bags.

Ohsumi describes the protein balance in the context of a sixty kilogram person. They would have an approximate daily protein turnover of 240 grams, of which seventy grams are eaten, seventy grams are excreted, and *170 grams of daily protein needs are obtained from recycling* body tissues. This is why some people interested in longevity opt for a seventy-two-hour water fast every six to twelve months; to recycle dysfunctional cells as a form of detoxification. Pure water fasting is a powerful stimulus that can be leveraged to help achieve the body's protein needs by increasing autophagy.

Can triggering autophagy help in any other ways?

Actually, it helps in quite a few different ways. When it comes to **cosmetic benefits**, autophagy has your back. When losing fat from below the skin, also known as subcutaneous fat, the clean-up crew will clear up any dead or dysfunctional fat and skin cells to *help prevent loose, hanging skin*. Autophagy is also **anti-inflammatory**! After a few fasts beyond thirty-six hours, we've seen people's knee pain, frozen shoulder, joint stiffness, and diabetic neuropathy *pain improve or disappear*. When this happens, they obviously don't miss the pain and don't always notice the specific moment when the pain left. The best is when we ask about the pain and they have to scratch their head to remember because the pain had not showed up for a while!

Since mitochondria are the energy powerhouse responsible for creating ADP and ATP, it's essential that autophagy **improves mitochondrial health**. Autophagy recycles the damaged, dysfunctional mitochondria in the body in order to preserve mitochondrial quality and quantity. The process of clearing damaged mitochondria, specifically, is called mitophagy.[5]

So now you know about the cosmetic, anti-inflammatory and mitochondria-upgrading potential of autophagy. Whether those perks appeal to you or not, you might be interested to know that dysfunctional autophagy might play a role in many major human diseases.[6]

If dysregulated, it's possible that missing out on its anti-inflammatory properties can directly affect things like *neuropathy* or *lung fibrosis*.

Diseases associated with aging, like *Alzheimer's, age-related macular degeneration* or *glaucoma, osteoarthritis,* and *osteoporosis* could be tied to the age and degeneration of cells that have yet to be cleaned up or recycled.

At any age, a build-up of old, dysfunctional cells can cause a wide array of ailments. Whether there's a stockpile of *bacteria and viruses* causing infections, backlogged uterine cells causing *endometriosis*, fat cells gathering causing *obesity*, bad cells replicating and creating *many cancers*, the accumulation of substances in artery walls causing *atherosclerosis*, or a development of scar tissues that leads to *cirrhosis* of the liver, there's a chance autophagy could be the key to treating–or even preventing–these maladies.

The list goes on. Rogue autophagy is implicated in diseases like *cardiomyopathies* and other *degenerative myopathies, inflammatory bowel disease, acute and chronic kidney disease, systemic lupus erythematosus, chronic obstructive pulmonary disease* (COPD), *nonalcoholic fatty liver disease* (NAFLD), and of course, our familiar character, *type 2 diabetes.*

While there is no peer-reviewed proof that autophagy is the solution to these issues, it just means that we need more research. We already know how autophagy and fasting can help with diabetes, and that's the focus of this section.

6.4: Addressing safety concerns before fasting

CAUTION: Regardless of whether or not you suffer from any of the previous diseases, we only allow our patients to proceed with fasting once they are getting at least 1.2 grams of protein per kilogram of body weight per day **and** are engaged in strength training, pushing each muscle group to failure twice a week.

Why?

So that they preserve and gain muscle and burn fat as they fast. I have seen so many people trying to fast **without ensuring those two essential safety precautions** who end up *facing plateaus* in fat loss, *slowing metabolism, hair loss, low energy, lack of muscle gains, drops in immunity, disappointment,* and *frustration.*

Consider fasting with diabetes as a form of medication. It needs the dose and frequency adjusted because of the powerful effects it has on insulin and overall metabolism. So please, only fast under the medical supervision of a professional who knows how to help you ensure correct (1) nutrition, (2) sleep habits, (3) stress management, and (4) exercise before using fasting as a treatment option.

When you begin fasting with diabetes, the **two main safety concerns are hyperglycemia and hypoglycemia.**

During the initial stages of fasting with uncontrolled severe diabetes, you may see a paradoxical rise in glucose levels. How? Why? If you aren't eating any food, where is this high glucose coming from?

From inside your body, of course! If you remember from the three musketeers analogy, the role of the liver is to be the glucose provider during a fast; **hyperglycemia**, or **high glucose levels** during a fast *is a sign that your diabetes is still uncontrolled* and is exactly why you need to partner with a healthcare provider who can support this process for you.

Think of this stage as the time when all the toxic excess fat from all the organs is being offloaded. For years, the *high insulin levels kept the body in fat-storage mode.* Fasting allows insulin levels to drop low enough to finally access and burn fat, and the first site that the body seems to burn fat from is the visceral compartment where fat is considered the most toxic.

Although your mind may want to see cosmetic improvements as soon as you start fasting, your body is prioritizing infrastructure and safety projects before beautification projects. Your body is focused on neutralizing the threat, building up the defenses, *and* then adding parks and gardens. To support your body's agenda, *consult with a professional to stay low-carb, get enough protein in the eating window, use strength training to build muscle,* and *then fast to burn the toxic fat* so you can turn diabetes around—your skin will glow and your aesthetic will improve later on.

Since hyperglycemia means glucose levels are high, I'm sure you can guess what hypoglycemia is!

Low glucose levels are also known as hypoglycemia. This may not seem like a safety concern when you consider that the point of fasting is to lower glucose, but this is why you have to work with your doctor to fast safely.

Glucose is expected to lower from fasting—but not to the point of danger. I have successfully used fasting as a treatment for thousands of people with either type 1 or type 2 diabetes under close supervision, and I know that it takes a team and one-on-one support to do this safely.

To minimize the risk of severe hypoglycemia you should only fast under your doctor's supervision so they can monitor and adjust your diabetes medication closely as needed, because fasting hypoglycemia is not normal in a person who isn't taking prescriptions to lower glucose. Your liver knows how to continuously maintain sufficient glucose levels to support the brain, so *if your blood glucose on a glucometer goes below 70 mg/dL* (3.8 mmol/L) *during a fast, you need to end the fast, treat the low glucose and discuss it with your doctor immediately.*

This is because **fasting hypoglycemia** is very different from **reactive hypoglycemia.**

Like I mentioned, **fasting hypoglycemia** is not normal. By definition, it strikes in the fasting state (more than four to six hours after the last meal) and feels better after eating carbs. This requires medical evaluation and treatment. The most common cause is the use of medication that causes hypoglycemia.[*] Some rare causes of fasting hypoglycemia include the presence of advanced liver disease or insulin-secreting tumors; the treatment is to identify the cause and remove any source of excessive insulin, either surgically or medically.

Reactive, or postprandial, hypoglycemia is simply an *exaggerated normal response to food* that happens in the postmeal state (within six hours after a meal) and feels better after eating carbs, too. This exaggerated response is likely caused by either an *excessive sensitivity to normal insulin* response, or by *excessive insulin secretion* in response to simple carbohydrates as a precursor to insulin resistance. You'll need to evaluate which foods are triggering the symptoms; the

---

[*] Insulinomas and surreptitious use of hypoglycemic agents or insulin are challenging rare conditions that I have seen and treated. Both are extremely rare and outside the scope of this book.

treatment is a low-carb lifestyle focused on reducing processed carb intake alongside getting enough good quality protein and fat.

Even if you are working with your care team to watch for hyperglycemia, fasting hypoglycemia, and reactive hypoglycemia, **there are still certain groups of people who should not fast.** The list includes *pregnant and lactating women* who need the nutrients for the growing baby and an adequate milk supply.

Similarly, *children* cannot fast—they need the nutrients to grow.

Additionally, *people who are underweight* shouldn't fast as they need the nutrients to avoid the risk of losing more muscle or lifesaving body fat.

People with an eating disorder or extreme love/hate relationship with food should not fast without addressing the underlying emotional needs first. Fasting might expose emotional triggers like we covered under yo-yo relationships with food, and can unearth deeper struggles that need attention.

6.5: Getting started with fasting

As I'm sure you're aware by now, fasting is the fifth lifestyle tool that can be added only after making sure your four wheels are in good condition and well-aligned. The same way that you can't expect to put luggage on top of your car, drive off, and expect to get somewhere if one or more of your tires is flat, you can't move onto fasting if you skip any of the four wheels.

Sure, you could try, but you're likely to end up stuck in the same ways others do when they try to skip steps. In most cases, this looks like headaches, weakness, hunger pangs and muscle loss. People experience acid reflux or acidity due to higher carb intake, processed and refined carbs, poor sleep or late night meals, protein malnutrition, lack of strength training and high stress levels.

Don't suffer like them. Remember that you are kicking off major metabolic changes when you expose the body to this shift, so *consider fasting as a medical intervention* that can come with side effects if not used or monitored properly like anything else.

Don't get caught up in words. I use the words *intermittent fasting*, fasting, and *time-restricted eating* to represent the same thing. Some people say "*IF*" or "*intermittent*" for shorter daily fasts and use "*extended fasting*" for fasts lasting longer than twenty-four hours.

I advise my patients to **start with a baseline overnight daily fast**, where we establish *a twelve-hour, overnight fast between the last meal of the day and the first meal the next day to track what happens*. If you feel like **you need a bedtime snack to fall asleep**, then before you fast, please go back to the nutrition chapters to be sure you're getting enough protein, and check to see if your sleep hygiene or stress management needs to improve. *Improving protein intake and recalibrating your stress management and sleep are reasonable ways to help you* get a baseline twelve-hour fast overnight and also give yourself a sufficient twelve-hour eating window the next day to achieve your protein intake. After you achieve your health goals through longer fasts, *you can come back to this overnight fasting schedule as a maintenance routine.*

Twice a week, advance the duration. Start small. It could be by thirty minutes, in which case you'd have your first meal twelve and a half hours after the last one. From there, once you are feeling confident, you can increase it by say, one and a half hours so that you have fourteen hours of time-restricted eating overnight twice a week. *Observe your hunger and fullness levels when the fourteenth hour comes to a close.* Research has shown that maintaining a self-selected ten-hour eating window with a fourteen-hour fasting window can improve insulin-resistance parameters out of proportion to weight loss. "Out of proportion" to weight loss means that even though the individuals in this study didn't lose much weight, their *insulin sensitivity, blood pressure, waist circumference, visceral fat, inflammation, and unhealthy lipid panels improved* after just twelve weeks of fasting fourteen hours each day.[7]

After you have optimized nutrition, sleep, stress management, and exercise as discussed in the previous chapters, **if fourteen-hour fasting is still not giving you normal glucose levels,** then a *longer fast* will probably help.

The issue is that getting to twenty-four hours is the hardest phase of extended fasting.

Why?

Because as the fast progresses, insulin levels drop, and the body starts burning stored glycogen–but you only have approximately one sedentary day's worth of glycogen (carbohydrate) stores. A trained athlete could burn through their glycogen stores within one hour of intense exercise. If you are untrained as an athlete, then as your body senses glycogen levels falling, it will kick in a **counter-regulatory hormonal response that creates real hunger pangs** to get you to hunt and gather by going to the kitchen or ordering a meal online. Those hormones want you to eat something before you run out of glycogen.

You can always eat to get relief from hunger because, thankfully, food is always available for people reading this book. As soon as you eat, however, insulin secretion will resume in people with type 2 diabetes and an insulin dose will be needed in people with type 1 diabetes. Your body will burn the fuel that came from the meal, which prevents you from burning stored body fat. This is where clarity helps. *You can take care of the short-term feeling of hunger pangs with the immediate gratification of eating, or you can address your long-term goal of burning the toxic fat stores by fasting.* That's the therapeutic ketosis you are aiming for to turn around insulin resistance.

When it comes to **things like exercise, cold exposure,** and **fasting**—*they're not supposed to be fun.* They're just good for you. It's called *hormesis.*[8] Having clarity about why you are bothering with it helps you pull through.

In addition to clarity on your "why," you should also have a toolkit of ways to overcome the hunger of the first twenty-four hours. But don't worry–when it comes to tips, I've got you covered!

First, **stay ahead of salt and water losses.** Excessive insulin levels cause fluid and sodium retention, so as you fast and your insulin levels drop, your body may start discarding excess water and salt (sodium) that was being retained. While this can make you feel shaky and low on energy, *a pinch of salt, a glass of water,* or *salted lemon water* may help preempt these symptoms. If you are on blood pressure medication, you'll need to monitor your blood pressure and keep your doctor posted because the dosage will probably need to be reduced as your blood pressure trends down toward normal. Eventually, you can move to pure water fasting as the body achieves a new homeostatic balance.

The second tip to have in your toolbox is to **take a walk**. The body is intelligent. If it realizes the hunter-gatherer is hungry but on the move, potentially searching for food, *it will mobilize energy from stored fat sites to power your expedition.* Your body knows that if you are successful at finding food, you and your tribe will survive, so the counter-regulatory hormones will coordinate with the liver for gluconeogenesis, and your glucose levels will rise even without you eating to support muscular activity. I have seen this on my own personal continuous glucose monitoring as well as in my patients with diabetes.

Sometimes, exercise can cause glucose levels to spike very high in people with uncontrolled diabetes, which is why you need to do this under medical supervision so that your doctor can support your lifestyle-change efforts with the right medication doses.

Another fun tip is that **soluble fiber can ease hunger pangs**. A teaspoon of chia seeds, fresh flaxseed powder, or psyllium husk in a glass of water will absorb water and expand to form a gel. *It can trick the stomach into feeling like a meal has arrived*, providing some short-term relief. Consider this a crutch while you are at the beginner levels of fasting. In order to get the highest returns from your fast, a pure water fast is the ultimate goal, but don't let that drive you crazy. **Perfection is not necessary on day one**. What matters is finding ways to *enjoy the fast or make it less painful so that you are willing to try it* again and build it as a habit.

Most of the world will not understand what you are trying to do, and one of the most underrated options you have is to **lean on a support system and accountability partner.** So many of my patients have been discouraged and scolded by well-wishers who tell them their condition cannot be turned around, and that they will need to be on progressive prescriptions forever; they almost gave up completely.

With that said—avoid ignorant advice and work with a supportive professional. People with type 1 diabetes get scared by those who don't understand the difference between ketosis from low-carb or fasting versus diabetic ketoacidosis (DKA). Even people with type 2 diabetes are often discouraged from fasting. Remember to work with a qualified healthcare professional who knows how to monitor therapeutic ketosis and differentiate it from DKA. You will need the professional input to manage your diabetes medication to prevent hypoglycemia, too, so find someone who provides the health care you deserve. *This provider needs to be someone who understands how lifestyle changes can turn around insulin resistance.*

Early in your fasting journey, before moving to pure water fasting, you may struggle **knowing which fasting fluids are best for hydration besides water.** What should you even look for in a fasting fluid?

I recommend that you *try to select one without nutrients that would activate mechanistic target of rapamycin (mTor).* We want mTor and insulin to be as low as possible during the fast to allow for recycling of old cells. *Black coffee* and *green tea* may be your best options for fasting fluids if pure water feels too difficult at first. The caffeine in these may reduce mTor activity, but be sure to limit caffeine after 2:00 p.m. to protect your sleep if you are caffeine sensitive.[9] There are also fluid options like *bone broth* that are not considered "pure" because while they help reverse insulin resistance and suppress hunger, they also have enough protein and fat to activate mTor, create minor insulin secretion, and stop autophagy.

The most urgent goal of fasting, however, is to reverse insulin resistance and uncontrolled diabetes, and you can achieve that even without autophagy by fasting long enough to let insulin levels fall low enough to enter ketosis and burn the excess body fat. Although you don't need to monitor insulin or ketone levels, the fact is that high insulin levels prevent fat burn and ketosis, so some people like to monitor their ketosis just for curiosity. While it's not necessary, it can be done by testing urine with urine ketone strips or testing blood on glucometers that double as ketone monitors. The Lumen device I mentioned in Part 5 will also indicate fat burn as the respiratory exchange ratio (RER) approaches 0.7 throughout a long fast.

Using tools like these can be a powerful stepping stone to help you get comfortable with the changes you'll go through as your body learns to burn body fat efficiently (fat adaptation). This happens because the mitochondria are being trained to switch gears from burning carbs for energy, to burning fat. This is metabolic flexibility.

The ideal stage is where **fat adaptation and metabolic flexibility** meet. *Once you are fat adapted, you won't need as many fasting fluid crutches.* Bulletproof coffee with lots of fat in the form of butter, cream, or cacao butter might help you start fasting, but the body senses nutrient abundance and will increase mTor; we want mTor to be as low as possible if you are aiming for autophagy. Being overenthusiastic about fats in fasting fluids can backfire long term, so if you must add something to your tea or coffee, a teaspoon of pure fat would cause less of an insulin spike than milk, because milk has carbs and protein. Fats, on the other hand, cause the lowest insulin response of the three macronutrient categories.

Indians also sometimes use diluted buttermilk as a fasting fluid, which is a beverage that's popular across the country. Made by blending homemade yogurt in water and adding a few seasonings, it has carbs and protein which stimulate insulin. I help my patients to wean off of this as soon as possible for better results; even when they use it, we modify the recipe to have them add yogurt very sparingly–no more than a teaspoon in a glass of water.

By fasting, you are trying to get insulin levels to be as low as possible. That means trying to avoid your brain telling the pancreas to release insulin as part of the *cephalic response* to food, when the mind is anticipating a meal. As buttermilk is associated with *meals* in Indian culture, thinking about it or other yummy foods during the fast can cause insulin secretion, causing trouble in two ways. On one hand, you will feel hungry and fasting will be difficult, and on the other, insulin secretion will instruct the body to store fat, even though the whole point of fasting is so that you can *burn* fat. Do you want the brain to prepare for eating, or for fasting?

That's why I don't recommend Indian beverages like chaas (buttermilk), jaljeera, or pani puri water because they remind you of mealtime and can then backfire by causing Pavlovian insulin secretion in people with type 2 diabetes.

Another data point is that **a fasted workout can increase the return on investment.** A vigorous, one-hour workout will deplete most of your glycogen stores and force the body to switch metabolic gear to burn fat. Our goal is to have better diabetes levels with less medication, so work with your doctor so they can review the medication and prevent hypoglycemia.

If the fast continues, your body will start burning fat for two reasons, to maintain a constant supply of ATP through ketosis and second, to keep blood glucose levels steady. Remember, active muscles are the glucose takers of the three musketeers, and they can bring glucose levels down into normal range. The liver is the glucose provider and will switch metabolic gear as glycogen gets depleted; it starts converting fat into glucose through gluconeogenesis to support the fasted workout. This way, you are getting two benefits at the same time; *a fasted workout can preserve muscle and burn excess stored fuel during a fast.*[10] Sometimes, fasted workouts will paradoxically make your glucose levels go higher before they come to normal. This is a sign that there is still insulin resistance, and is another reason to do this under medical supervision.

There is growing research to suggest that ketosis itself can be muscle-sparing, as achieving ketosis by being very low-carb sends a muscle-sparing message to the brain, encouraging ketones to be used as the primary energy fuel source.[11] For now, the research is in mice models and needs to be validated in humans, but from an evolutionary perspective, it makes sense to preserve hunter-gatherer muscles when they are fasting so that they can go find that next meal without becoming frail.

Finally, when you decide to start fasting, **decide if you want to fast on a mentally busy day or a slow day.** You might be the kind of person who can be so busy at work that you forget to eat, and that might make fasting easier. You might be someone who wants to fast on a day when you are relaxed at home, where you have access to your fasting fluids and family support. Find the strategy that works with your personality and the demands of your day by doing whatever helps you feel confident and safe. The key is to observe and learn how your body responds to the initial fasts.

I have worked with cardiac surgeons, chief executive officers, investment bankers, and homemakers, and all of them had different ideas about how to incorporate their initial fasts into their already busy schedules. While there are no set rules, you may still need some inspiration.

I have seen people align their fasting schedule with things they would rather avoid. They specifically choose to fast when traveling so that they don't have to rely on the airport meals, or when at a conference so they wouldn't have to deal with the provided buffet. They even fast before meeting friends and family to avoid unwanted questions, unwanted attention, and unnecessary concern.

Others fast when it comes with external structure, like the days when you have back-to-back meetings scheduled because it's easy to skip a meal. Other outside influences like having an accountability partner who wants to give you company or fasting on religious or spiritual days can make it easier to stick to a fast.

Some people don't really need a reason at all, and they fast on days that mean something to them personally, or just fast when they want to have a calm, quiet day to themselves.

If you consider fasting as a type of prescription for diabetes, it makes sense why some people call it therapeutic fasting (fasting as treatment). Done right, it can be very powerful and life changing. Done wrong, it could make your health worse, so hopefully, you've followed all the steps to ensure you're ready to fast correctly. **Once you have your toolbox packed with all these tips and you figure out your fasting patterns, then it's time to focus on the right fasting "dose."**

Fasting beyond thirty-six hours is when most people can expect to be in ketosis. This means that you have depleted all of your carbs stored as glycogen and are now using fat for energy. Glucose is provided through gluconeogenesis, and blood glucose levels may go up before they go down due to the excess fuel being dumped into the bloodstream when you have uncontrolled diabetes. The more insulin resistance, muscle losses, and fatty liver you start with, the longer this may take, and it's why you should work with a medical professional who can adjust your medication as the glucose levels fluctuate before settling down.

Learn how Annabelle customized a thirty-six-/forty-two-hour fasting schedule within her week

Annabelle had been living with diabetes for eighteen years, and as a senior school teacher in her upper fifties, she was planning to retire soon. She worked with us on stabilizing her four lifestyle wheels and I adjusted her medication to make sure she would not experience a low-glucose reaction. She was ready to start fasting.

As her first step, she picked her busy days to extend the overnight fast to sixteen hours by skipping breakfast.

She carried her protein to school and sipped on green tea from the teacher's lounge. She started with Tuesdays and Thursdays because those were full of morning classes, so she knew time would fly by, and it would be lunchtime before she knew it.

Slowly and steadily, she kept advancing the duration of the fast by an hour or two. Sometimes she even forgot and fasted for twenty-one hours when aiming for twenty!

We supervised her protein intake, and as expected, her appetite was shrinking. This was because her previously high insulin levels from insulin resistance had been keeping her hungry, but as the insulin levels dropped with fasting, so did her appetite. It became more difficult to achieve her protein target in the narrowing four-hour eating window, especially because she was vegetarian. She was physically ready to go for a thirty-six-hour fast, but she had to get mentally ready.

She chose a Tuesday when there was a school play being hosted for parents because she knew she would be running around backstage until the end of the day. After dinner on the Monday before the play, she knew that all she had to do was get through Tuesday.

On the big day, she made it a point to stay hydrated with salted lemon water and crossed the twenty-four-hour mark at dinnertime without even noticing. She got home on Tuesday night, exhausted, and fell asleep. On Wednesday morning, she woke up feeling like she had experienced a much deeper, better-quality sleep than she'd had in years. Oddly, she wasn't even hungry. She decided to carry her meal to school and instead of ending her fast on Wednesday morning at thirty-six hours, she stretched it to a late lunch, reaching forty-two hours.

Because it seemed easier than she had expected, she added two forty-two-hour fasts to her week, taking care to ensure strength training during the fasting window. If she had a public holiday on a day that was supposed to be a fasting day, she would just move the fast to the next day because she preferred fasting when busy at school.

She's not the only one to gradually turn diabetes around by integrating fasting into her lifestyle. Having coached people through this process hundreds of times now, I'm sure you probably still have some specific questions when it comes to intermittent fasting.

6.6: Frequently Asked Questions when Fasting

Including all the questions I've heard over the years would be too much, so I decided to boil them down to the top thirteen (I just couldn't take out more to make it 10!). We'll start at the top.

#1 How long do I need to fast?

It's a great question, but *the ultimate answer comes from your body.* You know you have achieved your diabetes goals when the overnight fasting glucose level is below 100 mg/dL (5.55 mmol/L) and the two-hour postmeal glucose is below 140 mg/dL (7.77 mmol/L) with the least amount of medication possible. When that goal is achieved, you can scale back from longer fasts to a maintenance routine of daily time-restricted eating windows. The variables that determine how much therapeutic fasting you need are:

- **Muscle mass:** Muscle is the glucose taker. Having more muscle increases insulin sensitivity, so *the more muscle you have, the better your glucose levels become,* especially the postmeal levels. Remember that fasting without strength training will backfire and cause muscle loss. If you want better metabolic health with less fasting, *intensify muscle-building workouts* to ensure gains in strength and performance.

- **Carb intake during the eating window:** Eating more than 100 grams of carbs per day in the eating window raises the insulin levels significantly, causing the initial part of each fast to be spent bringing those insulin levels back down again. If you want better metabolic health with less fasting, *stay low-carb in the eating window so that you can enter the fast at a lower insulin level,* allowing for more progress with each fast.

- **Protein deficiency.** As your appetite shrinks in the eating window, you may find yourself slipping behind on your daily protein targets. This becomes metabolically very expensive because you run the risk of a slowing metabolism, like what happens on a calorie-restricted diet. You cannot build muscle without enough nutrition. This is one of the biggest reasons for stagnation.

	Protein is below target in the eating window	Protein is at target in the eating window
Fasting without strength training	1. Muscle loss ✗ 2. Slowing metabolism ✗ 3. Weight-loss plateau ✗	1. Muscle loss ✗ 2. Slowing metabolism ✗ 3. Weight loss plateau ✗
Fasting with strength training	1. Muscle loss ✗ 2. Slowing metabolism ✗ 3. Weight-loss plateau ✗	1. Muscle gains ✓ 2. Increased metabolism ✓ 3. Fat loss ✓

My observation is that people on plant-based protein diets take much longer to find this balance than those who move to mostly animal-based protein. If you want to maximize the output of your strength-training workouts so that you need less fasting, *ensure enough high-quality protein in the eating window, and then, as your appetite reduces, increase the fasting window.* A fine balance between anabolism (growth) for muscle and catabolism (breaking down) of excess fat is required when using therapeutic fasting to reverse insulin resistance. Work with a health professional who understands these nuances of metabolism.

- **Sleep quality and quantity:** I have seen people reach plateaus because they are fasting on top of very poor sleep patterns. The bad sleep keeps worsening insulin resistance every night. If you want better outcomes with less need for fasting, *invest in better restorative sleep* like we covered in Part 3.

- **Chronic stress:** This raises cortisol and worsens insulin resistance. You might be doing everything right, and your body is just not giving you the expected results. Starting a fast from a place of emotional well-being and mental clarity has helped many of my patients not just experience rapid results, but also chart out a journey that they are happy to continue long term. These are things that cannot be published in medical journals because there are no clinical trials that study this. I reversed my own prediabetes in 2013 by doing an about-turn on my victim mindset years before I had optimized my low-carb, protein-sufficient nutrition; strength training; or fasting. If you want more return on investment from your efforts but long fasts are causing you even more stress, then you may want to *focus on deeper stress management techniques first.*

- **Fatty liver:** The more severe the fatty liver you have to start with, the longer it will take for fasting glucose levels to come to normal. Remember the liver is the glucose provider. Fatty liver is a sign that insulin resistance reversal is still a work in progress.

- **Number and length of fasts beyond thirty-six hours:** Many people stop at twenty-four hours and get frustrated. Remember that fat burn starts after the twenty-four-hour mark. If you want your fasts to result in meaningful fat loss, *the threshold to cross is the twenty-four-hour duration mark, and you'll know the work is done when your fasting glucose comes down to below 100 mg/dL* (5.55 mmol/L) with the least possible medication. That's a sign that your liver, the glucose provider, is no longer dumping excessive amounts of glucose into the blood.

- **Duration of diabetes:** *The longer you've had insulin resistance, the longer it will take to put it into remission.* When you struggle, it might be that you are feeling conflicted between the immediate need to be relieved of hunger pangs versus the long-term need to reverse insulin resistance. This is where you always have choice. Why do you want this? How badly do you want this? What will long-term success look like for the future version of you?

- **Personal fat threshold:** *Every body is different.* Some people have been carrying excess body fat for decades, so they'll need longer fasts. If you took years to develop insulin resistance, do you trust the process of lifestyle change enough to put in whatever it takes? Some people hate seeing others drop weight effortlessly while they struggle, but comparing yourself to others will always cause frustration. This is a personal journey of self-discovery. Long before you see fat loss, the body will start rewarding you with non-scale-related victories. Are you looking for those rewards with self-love and curiosity? Or does the self-sabotaging inner critic keep you constantly disappointed?

- **Consistency in self-care and mindfulness over perfectionistic yo-yos:** Some people get into on/off patterns with fasting, using it for a few months with a dieting mindset to "clean up" the effects of life events like weddings, vacations, or personal stress. This will often cause stagnation, guilt, frustration, and impatience at the lack of results. *Losing contact with the present moment of life on a regular basis is what adds up to a lack of results in the long term.* Remember, life is what happens to you, lifestyle is how you react or respond to it. It is extremely difficult to catch the mind when it uses stories to disconnect you from the present moment with mindless eating, lack of self-monitoring of glucose, and reasons why exercise and self-care should stop. That same monkey mind comes back online with fatigue, guilt, and self-blame when it asks, "How long will I have to do this for? My problem is consistency!"

#2 Why is the morning glucose level higher than the bedtime one, even without eating anything?

That's an excellent question and observation! Remember, your liver is the glucose provider, working all night to ensure your brain gets a constant supply of glucose during your overnight fast when you sleep. If you did a deep Diwali or spring cleaning and saw lots of dust come out when you pulled the furniture away from the wall, you would take that as a sign of a good deep clean, right?

If the morning level is rising higher than the bedtime one, it's a sign of all the toxic excess fuel that's being dumped out by the liver as the overnight insulin levels finally fall low enough to allow the overnight cleaning process. The higher reading obviously didn't come from food because you haven't eaten anything. That's exactly what we refer to as *uncontrolled diabetes*. If you have type 2 diabetes, it's a sign that you still have insulin resistance that has not yet fully reversed. If you have type 1 diabetes, you need to determine if the problem is insulin deficiency or insulin resistance. Your doctor needs to supervise and adjust medication during this stage, based on the glucose levels. Intensify the lifestyle options mentioned earlier, and you will see this level gradually come below 100 mg/dL (5.55 mmol/L) and stay there.

#3 How do I fast when I am traveling?

Actually, this is entirely up to you. Airport and hotel staff won't be offended if you don't eat. Still, you get to decide. Is it too complicated to search for low-carb foods when you travel? You might decide to fast instead.

Are you traveling to a new place where you want to enjoy new restaurants and dining experiences? *You get to decide how to balance that with your overall goals.* You are the master of your journey. You decide. There are plenty of ways to improve your glucose levels with less medication, and that's why fasting comes after those four major lifestyle wheels.

#4 On what days of the week and how often do I fast?

This is where you get to customize this to suit your life. Some people plan two fasts of thirty-six to forty-eight hours per week, ensuring enough protein in the eating window, and add exercise throughout the week. A fasted strength-training workout twice a week can increase your growth hormone response and empty out glycogen stores, so some people plan the fast on their strength-training day. See how your body responds. You might find it harder to do cardio on the fasting day, perhaps due to the increased salt and water loss through sweating and perhaps because your mitochondria have not aerobically adapted to burn fat yet. Some of my Indian patients plan fasts on vegetarian days that align with their spiritual beliefs; for example, wanting to avoid animal protein on Tuesdays or Saturdays is a common Hindu practice.

#5 Should I skip breakfast or dinner?

Let's say you want to start with sixteen hours of fasting. The word *breakfast* itself refers to the meal you eat at the end of a fasting period. For most of us, the most common fast is the overnight fast in our sleep. So, the first morning meal of the day was named *breakfast*.

But your first meal of the day might be at 2:00 p.m., which someone might call lunch, although technically, it's breakfast for you. So, *don't get caught up in the vocabulary.* Find a rhythm that works for your life in a way that you can sustain and enjoy.

For example, if you have a few nuts first thing in the morning, followed by a biscuit with your morning tea, and eat a full meal much later, the nuts break the fast because they result in insulin secretion and digestive system activation. The body switches into "store-fuel" mode. *Decide when you want to truly "break the fast" and start insulin secretion.* Are you even physically hungry when you are deciding to eat? If you're not hungry, why are you eating?

Maybe it's because you've been told to eat breakfast like a king and dinner like a pauper. Your stomach size and physical capacity to eat stay the same in the morning and evening. So, I don't see any logic in stuffing yourself first thing, except that you may buy more carb-predominant breakfast foods, need more medications, and keep someone's stock prices up.

Dr. Satchin Panda mentions in his book *The Circadian Diabetes Code* that a fourteen-hour overnight fasting window and a ten-hour eating window (for example, from 8:00 a.m. to 6:00 p.m.) works well, and additionally, a research trial looking at weight loss in overweight women showed more weight loss in the group that had dinner early (7:00–7:30 p.m.) versus late (10:00–10:30 p.m.).[12] The body does have a natural circadian rhythm to hunger and appetite, and eating late at night (10:00 p.m.) does have a worse metabolic effect than eating at 6:00 p.m.[13],* *Decide what works best for you by listening to your hunger and fullness patterns, seeing what fits in your life, and how it affects your glucose levels.*

I have seen twelve to fourteen hour hour overnight fasts to be helpful as a maintenance duration once the insulin resistance is reversed. Some "alternative therapy" folks may discourage you from skipping morning meals because they say morning cortisol is high and skipping breakfast increases stress levels, so you "don't want a double whammy" that results in increasing cortisol levels.

This is an inaccurate representation of how cortisol works. Acute rises in cortisol and noradrenaline in response to natural stressors like fasting, cold immersion, or exercise are normal. Cortisol is an essential hormone; we need it to survive and respond appropriately to stress. The healthy response to moderate, intermittent amounts of stress makes you stronger by the adaptive process called hormesis. The daily circadian rhythm of cortisol is normal, too. Hunter-gatherers historically would have woken up and gone about their hunting and gathering in the fasted state—they didn't need to be served a bowl of carbs so that they could champion the day. It's *chronically* high cortisol levels that make you sick, not brief intermittent ones. In general, I avoid advice that makes someone fearful of their own natural body physiology.

#6 Can't I just do one meal a day (OMAD)?

I strongly discourage my patients from long-term OMAD. We only use the twenty-four-hour fast as a brief *physiological* stepping stone (shifting from glycogen to fat burn) before making the *psychological* jump to a thirty-six-hour fast. Done long term, OMAD ends up becoming a half-hearted attempt at fasting without the fat-burn benefits, plus a half-hearted attempt at eating, with a feeding window that's inadequate to complete your protein requirements. This results in a failure to build muscle, slowing metabolism, failure to burn fat, and disappointing results. I compare long-term OMAD to camping in Frankfurt airport which was meant to be your transit city on the way from New York to Mumbai.

Remember, you are using *therapeutic fasting as medicine that needs a dosing strategy for long-term outcomes.* You need an anabolic (growing) phase to build muscle and a catabolism (breaking-down) phase to burn fat. It's a fine balance that needs to be monitored by working with a professional to ensure you are improving body composition, gaining lean muscle, and losing belly fat, not just briefly losing weight on the scale, only to slow your metabolism down in the long run.

---

* Some religious groups in India, such as the Jains, have a lifestyle of finishing dinner before sunset. The Jain community got the circadian part right. Considering that there are plenty of Jains with uncontrolled diabetes and obesity, it's a matter of working with them on the other wheels of the lifestyle car.

#7 Should a twenty-four-hour fast be from breakfast to breakfast, lunch to lunch, or dinner to dinner?

Much like my answer when it comes to skipping breakfast or dinner—*this one's up to you.* Depending on what fits in your life, you may want to have dinner with your family for social bonding, and plan accordingly. Since hunger tends to peak around 5:00 p.m. for many, per the body clock and circadian rhythm, you could plan around that and see how it feels.

On the other hand, you might plan a forty-eight-hour fast from lunch to lunch so that you get a bigger eating window on the first and last day. For example, if you fast from Tuesday lunch to Thursday lunch, it psychologically only feels like one full day (Wednesday) without food, leaving enough of an eating window on Tuesday and Thursday to complete your protein requirements. I personally planned my first seventy-two-hour fast on the last three days before relocating my office to a new address. I was so busy with the long days of patient appointments and packing that food was the last thing on my mind during the move. It felt right, so I did it. Experiment a bit, then decide.

#8 Can women fast? If yes, can they fast on their period?

Women were exposed to the same hunter-gatherer lifestyle as men. *The only time we don't want women to fast is when they are pregnant or breastfeeding* because the body has increased demands for the growing fetus and for making breast milk. Other than that, women can fast for their metabolic goals. It's totally up to you whether to fast during the menstrual or premenstrual period, based on how you feel. I have seen some functional medicine practitioners say women should match their fasting schedule to their menstrual cycle.

Frankly, we don't have clinical trials proving the "best" time of the month to fast, and for all we know, hunter-gatherer women had to fast at various times of the month regardless of their period. If you have insulin resistance or uncontrolled diabetes, the sooner we turn that around, the better. *So find what works for your menstrual cycle.*

#9 Can people with hypothyroidism fast?

Yes, as long as your thyroid-stimulating hormone (TSH) is normal, you can fast for insulin-resistance reversal. Always work with your doctor so that they can adjust thyroid medication as your body changes with fasting.

#10 Should I force myself to eat protein before the fast?

If you are struggling to get enough protein in the eating window, this can be good news, depending on how you interpret it. I think it's great news that *you're now aware of your body's satiety signals,* and your *hormonal signals are also telling you the body is ready for a longer fast.*

It's crucial to use fasting carefully here because protein malnutrition in the eating window can sabotage all your efforts at insulin-resistance reversal. I sometimes have to stop patients from fasting to create a larger eating window. We take another look at their nutrition to ensure sufficient protein and we recalibrate their exercise to intensify hypertrophy workouts for muscle gains. We focus on better sleep and stress management *without* fasting, and then reintroduce fasting based on how their glucose levels respond. Interestingly, many patients see their appetite coming back as they build muscle and get stronger in their workouts. That's those beautiful myokines saying the growing muscles want protein!

Again, it's all about that crucial balance where we want both anabolism (build more muscle to reduce insulin resistance) and catabolism (break down excess toxic fat to turn around insulin resistance). You may notice that I am saying this repeatedly. I am. Many people make this one mistake through different misunderstandings and reach the same negative outcome: "Fasting didn't work for me."

#11 Are there other side effects or benefits that I can expect when fasting, besides fat loss?

Recall from the previous chapter, when we said that if you consider therapeutic fasting as a type of prescription for diabetes, then it can come with side effects if not used or monitored properly. So, yes, fasting done correctly does come with fat loss and an improvement in insulin levels, but it also comes with possible side effects like:

- **Insomnia:** this usually settles after the first one or two fasts that cross 36 hours. The counterregulatory hormones settle down, and the body embraces the opportunity for rest, restoration and repair. Talk to your doctor about this to see if any lifestyle intervention can help.

- **Hair loss:** This is the most troublesome side effect of fasting for some. I see this happen especially when patients get enthusiastic about fasting for longer hours at the expense of achieving enough protein intake in the eating window because of their shrinking appetite. In these situations, I have to ask them to stop fasting, get enough protein, and intensify other ways of getting glucose levels down, such as lowering the carbs or intensifying the muscle-building workouts, walking after meals, and tweaking stress management and sleep. The hair loss can take up to six months to settle down as the stress of fasting (worsened by protein deficiency) pushes large numbers of hair follicles into a resting phase called telogen *effluvium*. It usually helps to coordinate your fasting plans with a dermatologist to help the hair loss settle down.

- **Cramps, headache:** As long as you get enough whole-food nutrition and hydration in the fasting window, you should not experience these. Talk to your doctor about a magnesium supplement if it persists. Salted lemon water or just a pinch of salt on the tongue helps, too. Always monitor your blood pressure and work with your doctor if you have high blood pressure or are taking medication for it.

- **Increased uric acid on your blood tests:** Uric acid levels may temporarily go up as a byproduct when the body breaks down old cells and tissues through autophagy. Work with your doctor to keep an eye on this, and stay hydrated till the level comes down. I cover uric acid in more detail in Parts Seven and Eight.

Don't worry; it's not just negative side effects—there are additional benefits to look for, too! We want to focus on non-scale victories that we might see on a daily basis, things like **increased energy, mental focus, alertness,** and **concentration.** Additionally, you may experience **better sleep, less pain, less fluid retention, less swelling, fewer inflammatory symptoms,** and **enhanced performance and strength** in workouts—just like a hungry hunter-gatherer in the wild.

#12 How often should I weigh myself during the fast?

I've stressed numerous times that the scale cannot differentiate between fat loss and muscle gain, and I caution clients away from using the scale as their primary metric to assess success. But that's not the only reason why. When you begin turning around your diabetes and fasting, your body goes through a lot of different changes.

Once you start fasting beyond thirty-six hours you will first lose water weight and then slowly lose fat, starting with visceral fat, because this is the most toxic and important site to clear first. As you get enough protein and push each muscle group to failure twice a week, you will build muscle and gain lean muscle weight. Not only are **the scale and BMI calculators unable to tell the difference between fat loss and muscle gain**—they **can't tell you whether you've dropped some water weight** either.

Unfortunately, many of your health professionals are just telling you to reduce the number on the scale without paying attention to how you do it or what changes are occurring in your muscle mass, fat-depot distribution, or body composition. The truth is, the number on **the scale will be the *last* place to reflect improvements** in body composition and metabolism. Even if your health provider doesn't understand the limitations of the weighing scale in the early stages of your journey, I am going to teach you about non-scale victories with a visual analogy.

Vegetarians: Visualize a bowl of miso soup with tofu chunks. The tofu is mostly protein and sinks to the bottom. The fat in the soup floats at the top.

Meat eaters: Visualize a bowl of chicken soup. The chicken sinks, and the fat droplets float on top.

Basically, protein, or muscle, is heavier than fat. So, as you gain muscle and lose fat, **it's possible that you will gain weight on the scale.** Does that mean you're doing bad? Don't let the weighing scale fool you.

Please don't step on the weighing scale for at least six weeks. Even the "smart scales" that give you fat and muscle estimates are prone to errors and inaccuracy. Instead, focus on the principles outlined in the book so far. When you follow the steps to get the four wheels of the lifestyle car aligned before fasting, *you will notice a leaner, trimmer look with inch loss before you start seeing weight loss on the scale.*

#13 Are all fat-storage sites the same?

When it comes down to it, **some fat is more harmful than others.** In Part 1, we discussed how brown fat, or BAT, is rich and mitochondria and is only trying to help your body. Then, in Part 6.4, we described how visceral fat is burned first, as the body considers it to be the most toxic. There is clearly a range of roles played by body fat starting from helpful all the way to toxic, but like many other changes, the weighing scale cannot illuminate the changes in the amount of fat in these different depots or the effects.

There are four main fat storage sites to be aware of when fasting and even though they are all fat stores, they're still all different.

- **Subcutaneous (SC) fat** is *located below the skin*. You can identify if it's subcutaneous by pinching the skin away from muscle. To see how much you are carrying, you want to *measure the skin-fold thickness at multiple sites,* or how much skin you can pinch away from the muscle. What's typically *seen as a dimply look under the skin, or cellulite,* is a mix of brown adipose tissue (BAT) and white adipose tissue (WAT). Of course, the more BAT, the better. The *approximate storage capacity of subcutaneous fat is ten kilograms* (twenty-two pounds).[14] The role of SC fat in health is that it serves as a *prelimi-*

nary "metabolic sink" to store excess energy while preserving metabolic balance.[15] ***Moderate amounts of superficial subcutaneous fat are associated with better survival rates from severe illness.***[16] If we accumulate SC fat beyond that, the metabolic effects are not great. This fat becomes *metabolically toxic* after around ten kilograms of weight gain, releasing inflammatory fats and cytokines into the blood.

- **Visceral fat** is *located deep inside the abdomen around the organs.* As belly skin cannot be pinched away, this is harder to measure right away. However, you can measure waist circumference and look at a dual-energy X-ray absorption (DEXA) scan to get some basic information. *Advanced imaging techniques like computed tomography (CT) and magnetic resonance imaging (MRI) give direct visualization and can give you a more accurate measurement but these are used more for research purposes.* This type of fat accumulation is usually *noticed as inch gain around the belly,* and its approximate *storage capacity sits at three kilograms* (six pounds). As visceral fat is made of mostly WAT, it drains inflammatory fats and cytokines directly into the liver, causing insulin resistance. This is a negative metabolic effect and *is considered to be metabolically toxic.* Not only does it get involved in a vicious cycle of insulin resistance, but it is also associated with ***poorer cardiometabolic outcomes and cancer survival rates.***

- **Hepatic fat** is *located in the liver,* and is associated with nonalcoholic fatty liver disease [NAFLD] or hepatosteatosis, and fatty pancreas. Unfortunately, levels of hepatic fat can *only be measured by ultrasound or MRI.* It *is externally invisible* due to being mostly toxic triglycerides inside the liver cells. While the *approximate storage capacity is less than 0.25 kilograms* (half of a pound), *the metabolic effects are immediately harmful, inflammatory,* and directly *drive insulin resistance and metabolic syndrome.* Hepatic fat plays a role in disease by being a *leading cause of liver scarring, fibrosis, cirrhosis,* and *liver failure,* ***even overtaking alcoholic liver disease.***

- **Muscle fat** is located in the muscle, specifically between and inside muscle cells, and is also called *myosteatosis.* To measure it, *you'll need a CT scan, MRI, or ultrasound* because it's *externally invisible* when it precedes muscle wasting. The *approximate storage capacity is up to 0.3 kilograms* (just over half a pound).[17] As this is fat inside or in between the muscle cells, the *metabolic effect is negative in sedentary people and positive for those who are active.*[18] Sedentary individuals will see the negative side of muscle fat by having unhealthy mitochondria, while trained endurance athletes enjoy muscle fat as a helpful energy source.[19] Muscle fat can *play a role in insulin resistance, altered mechanics, muscle loss (sarcopenia),* and *can trigger a harmful phenomena called "inflammaging,"* or inflammation plus accelerated aging.[20,21]

So to answer the question, *all fat-storage sites were not created equal,* but the good news is that fasting allows your body's intelligent self-repair mechanisms to go through and clear away toxic fat that can cause negative health outcomes.

If you have other questions before you begin fasting that I have not covered, feel free to reach out to me and my team at www.reisaanhealth.com. We are eager to answer any additional questions you may have and get you all the clarity you need.

6.7: So, what happened to Mr. Shanti?

If you recall, Mr. Shanti was on the waiting list to receive a lung transplant. He continued his physical therapy six days a week, determined to increase his muscle mass and improve his diabetes. He started fasting to see if it would reduce the inflammation while waiting for the donor lung, and also to reduce excess body fat to improve his chances of surviving the transplant surgery.

But then, he noticed something I could've never predicted from any textbook, training, or experience.

On his eating days, his oxygen saturation would fall below 90 percent within six minutes of walking with the therapist, because his inflamed lungs struggled to support his oxygen needs. On his forty-eight-hour fasting days, he could walk uninterrupted for fifteen to twenty minutes without the oxygen saturation dropping. Within three months of working with us, he had lost inches from the waist, gained strength and was down by a net of fifteen kilograms on his scale. His lungs were still inflamed, and still needed the transplant, and yet, his aerobic walking capacity was drastically better during the long fasts. On one of his latest fasts, he even managed to walk uninterrupted for thirty minutes!

It seemed that **his lung function was better when he was burning stored fat for fuel,** and once he ended the fast and resumed eating, his walking capacity dropped back to less than ten minutes. This was visible proof that *his mitochondria and aerobic capacity were more efficient when he was in ketosis* (using stored body fat as the fuel during the fast) and less efficient when food was the fuel source.

Over the years, my team and I have used therapeutic fasting with hundreds of people with diabetes or people on steroids, and despite being on these medications, they've been able to stabilize their weight by focusing on protein intake and muscle mass as best they can. They have been able to counteract the side effects of steroid-induced myopathy and steroid-induced diabetes by focusing on carefully monitored lifestyle changes. So, if you learn anything from Mr. Shanti, it's that fasting is not just for biohackers. It's for anyone who wants to enhance their metabolic flexibility and metabolic resilience.

Part 6 summary

- Fasting is an additional tool to reduce insulin resistance and needs to be handled like medication, with careful monitoring and adjustment under professional supervision when used with diabetes.

- Watch your mindset about fasting so that you are fasting by choice towards your long term goals.

- Fasting can cause harm if done without ensuring your four lifestyle wheels are in good shape first.

- Fasting is flexible and can be tailored to your reality of both the response from your body and the daily situations in your life.

For Bonus Materials, Visit the Website Here:

PART 7

UNDERSTANDING INVESTIGATIONS AND PRESCRIPTIONS

7.1: Gathering the facts

The underlying driver of insulin resistance is the same across the continuum of progressive diabetes and it just gets worse as you go from prediabetes to type 2 diabetes, or from needing low doses of insulin in type 1 diabetes to needing more and more insulin to get the same glucose-lowering effect. This part of the book is dedicated to giving you what you need to know *before* you go to the nutritionist, doctor, or hospital. I will get into prescription medication (and their side effects) and even bariatric surgery. I will walk you through the basics of understanding labs, leveraging screening tests, and recording your own data. **That way you can be prepared to advocate for your health with *confidence* at the next visit with your healthcare provider.**

The most powerful study of lifestyle change for insulin resistance done by the US government was called the Diabetes Prevention Program, and was published in 2002 in the prestigious *New England Journal of Medicine*.[1] The results were impressive: *lifestyle change in people with **prediabetes** was more powerful at preventing diabetes than taking metformin or doing nothing at all.* While we have this compelling data for prediabetes, we don't have it for established type 2 diabetes, even though the disease process of insulin resistance is exactly the same along that continuum; it's only getting worse. Once you exceed the magic threshold of 6.5 percent from prediabetes into diabetes, we don't have any large-scale study comparing the power of lifestyle change alone to diabetes prescriptions alone.

Perhaps study regulators consider it unethical to design a trial where no medication is used in established type 2 diabetes, because doing *nothing* for uncontrolled diabetes would be harmful—and I agree. But lifestyle change would be far from doing nothing.

Such a study would have to be done long-term and would be prohibitively expensive to do correctly. Though the research could do a lot of good, it just might reduce pharmaceutical revenue. Who then, besides a government who would be motivated and able to fund it?

Our only option is to talk about the data we do have.

Three studies came out during my endocrine fellowship training that took the diabetes world by storm. The ACCORD, ADVANCE, and VADT trials looked at the impact of pushing the HbA1c below the standard goal of 7 percent.[2] They made patients reach an HbA1c of 6 percent and 6.5 percent by using **sulfonylureas** (gliclazide/glimepiride) **and insulin**, *which make insulin resistance worse*, and the **thiazolidinedione rosiglitazone**, which *causes weight gain and fluid retention and has been implicated in increased rates of heart attack* (myocardial infarction).[3]

The results of these brute-force studies were not encouraging.

The intensive treatment group in **ACCORD** and **VADT** *experienced more hypoglycemia and weight gain*, thanks to the types of prescriptions used to push the HbA1c lower. The **ACCORD** study was halted prematurely because it *demonstrated more cardiovascular events and deaths in the intensive (lower HbA1c) group* compared to the group that had standard (higher) HbA1c targets.

None of the three trials showed meaningful cardiovascular protection by pushing the HbA1c lower with more aggressive prescriptions. **This led many to conclude that it's preferred to target a higher HbA1c goal if the person** with diabetes is *older, has other coexisting health conditions, has a tendency for hypoglycemia,* or *has limited life expectancy.* These studies left people thinking that a lower HbA1c was harmful, and as an endocrinology fellow in training, I too, was caught up with this conclusion.

Looking back now, I suspect that the more precise conclusion was that a lower HbA1c achieved in type 2 diabetes by aggressive use of *sulfonylureas, insulin,* and *rosiglitazone* was making people sick. Now I know we have safer ways of helping people to achieve a normal HbA1c (below 5.7 percent). Studies aside, here's what I can tell you. If you have type 2 diabetes, with a C-peptide level that confirms your pancreas is still making insulin (discussed in Part 1), *I know you can safely achieve a normal HbA1c without medication, provided you change the lifestyle that gave you insulin resistance in the first place.*

If you have type 1 diabetes, I know you can achieve a near-normal HbA1c – with minimal glucose variability and with the lowest possible insulin dose – if you work with your doctor and embrace the lifestyle concepts covered earlier in this book plus the points in the dedicated section for type 1 diabetes in Part 10. But before we go deeper into whether HbA1c is a concern you need to address, let's go over what we can figure out ourselves. Then we can get the lab involved.

Using glucometers to do your own investigations

Ever since Lakshmi had been diagnosed with diabetes in her late twenties, she'd been taking insulin. She would take the morning injection and be out the door to work. She could tell when her glucose levels were above 250 mg/dL (13.8

mmol/L) because she would feel a particular tingling around her lips. As long as she wasn't feeling that symptom, she wasn't checking her levels.

She would take her evening insulin dose and keep some candy close to her bed in case she felt like her blood glucose was going low in the middle of the night. Sometimes she would wake up and eat something to be safe. She replaced rice with quinoa because it was supposed to be healthier. She had sacrificed eating mangoes for years, although they were one of her favorite fruits.

Despite this effort, frustratingly, her hemoglobin A1c (HbA1c) was never below 7 percent, so every visit to the doctor just meant higher insulin doses. It's not what she wanted, but she didn't know what else to do.

Having blood samples collected and getting bloodwork done is great, but it's not a consistent solution to knowing and managing what's happening in your body. I had to tell her what I am telling you: *data is your friend.* Data gives insight that provides a better understanding of your body, and seeing your body responding to your efforts boosts your confidence. So don't forget about Lakshmi, because by the end, it will all make sense.

In Part 2.14, I told you how using your own glucometer can give you insight into how your nutrition changes are directly affecting your glucose levels. This knowledge gives you power here, because now the doctor isn't the only one determining how your diabetes journey will unfold. You get to drive.

As exciting as it may be to take control of your diabetes journey, unfortunately, **it won't happen if you don't have your own data and only rely on the lab.**

Maybe you're fine with showing a lab report to your doctor once every three months and letting them adjust (possibly increase) medication based on that single report. That's absolutely your choice. Most people with diabetes do exactly that because neither they nor their doctor has any idea how the day-to-day lifestyle choices are directly affecting their glucose levels. And because uncontrolled diabetes is chronic and progressive, unless you make lifestyle changes, the cycle predictably continues.

The glucometer measures glucose in capillary blood in your fingertips, and the lab measures glucose in a bigger vein, so some difference is expected. Some highly curious, data-oriented patients of mine carry their glucometer to the lab, take a drop of the sample collected by the lab technician from the vein, and place it on their glucometer strip. That way, they can cross-check their meter with the lab. Usually, a good meter will have a margin of error of approximately 20 mg/dL (1.1 mmol/L) compared to the lab, and that's quite acceptable, so don't take it personally.

Cross-checking the precision of your glucometer with the lab is not necessary for most respected brands. You are using the meter to measure the effects of your habit changes, not to win the glucometer accuracy award.

Let's say your glucometer always reads twenty points higher than the lab. Fine. This means that when you eat two rotis or two slices of bread, if your glucometer reads 160 mg/dL (8.8 mmol/L), then maybe the lab would've reported 140 mg/dL (7.7 mmol/L). Similarly, if you cut the bread to 50 percent, the glucometer may show 130 mg/dL (7.2 mmol/L) where the lab might have said 110 mg/dL (6.1 mmol/L).

The expected difference between the lab and meter is due to technical differences and cancels out, because what matters is that you saw a drop of 30 mg/dL (1.6 mmol/L) by reducing your carbs by 50 percent.

I'm not saying to never get labs again. I'm just saying that *the glucometer readings provide day-to-day feedback between your doctor appointments.* The only reason to use your own glucometer at home is to help decide which habit changes you want to apply from this guide in order to reduce your glucose levels. As you make positive lifestyle changes, your doctor's job switches to *reducing* medication to support your *efforts* at achieving better diabetes outcomes. Seeing the drop in glucose helps you decide what direction you want to go in so that *you* are driving your diabetes care plan at your next doctor's appointment.

But doesn't it hurt to prick my finger? This is another common fear that prevents people from getting started with a glucometer. It does hurt, but did you know that *it could hurt much less if you use the lancet on the side borders of your finger* instead of right in the fleshy middle pulp of the finger? Why does it hurt more if you poke the middle pulp of your fingertip? You interpret much of your environment through the sense of touch, pain and temperature in those fingertips. This is possible because the pulp is sensitive; it's enriched with a very high density of nerve receptors that accurately pick up important cues from the world around you.

This nerve density is meant to protect the hunter-gatherer from picking up something that's too sharp or too hot—so why would we knowingly go and stab a needle right into that most sensitive protective tissue?

How do you find a less painful spot to apply the lancet? Place your *hands in the namaste position,* pressing your fingertips together. *The side borders of your fingers that you can see* are the edges that have enough blood for your glucometer strip and hurt much less than the central sensitive part. If you squeeze your fingertips together (the way you make hand mudras or finger shadows), the side edge becomes firm enough to easily apply the lancet with less pain. Sometimes my patients tell me they're concerned because they only have ten fingers and there isn't enough space to keep checking, but if you use the side edges, you have double the real estate. Two edges per finger gives you twenty edges to rotate between. Even if you check your glucose reading four times a day, you won't come back to the same edge until five days later. Along each edge, you have plenty of spots to choose from while letting the old sites heal so there's no need to keep poking at the exact same spot. Chances are, you won't even remember where you poked last because your finger has already healed.

Often, patients will tell me that **it's scary to see the high readings**, and I agree. If you see a high number and have no idea what to do with it, it could create a sense of powerlessness and doom. Better not to know and stick your head in the sand!

But you wouldn't do this if you realized you had termites in your home. You'd find out how they got into the house and stop them from destroying your place of residence. *Your body is the only permanent home you'll get in this lifetime, and seeing a high reading could become a learning experience if you knew what to do with the data.* From reading the earlier chapters in this book, you have five lifestyle categories to introspect on.

- Nutrition: What did I eat to cause this? How can I help my pancreas? For type 1: How can I change my food to lower my insulin dose?

- Sleep: Did I sleep poorly last night? How can I help my body?

- Stress management: Was there more stress than usual? How can I help my mind?

- Exercise: Did I move less through the day? How can I help my muscles?

- Fasting: Have I been snacking all day or late into the night? How can I help my liver?

If you reflect on those categories, I'm confident you can come up with plenty of ideas on how to make your glucometer data less scary.

Outside of those common fears, the most popular question I hear is, **"What numbers am I looking for on my glucometer?"**

When it comes to fasting glucose targets, you're aiming for *a fasting glucose reading below 100 mg/dL* (5.5 mmol/L) in type 2 diabetes (without medication) or with the lowest slow-acting insulin requirement in type 1 diabetes (without hypoglycemia).

After food, you're looking for a *two-hour postmeal reading below 140 mg/dL* (7.7 mmol/L) in type 2 diabetes (without medication) or with the lowest quick-acting insulin requirement in type 1 diabetes (without hypoglycemia).

That's it! Just prick your finger on the side when you need to, and aim for lifestyle choices that will help you meet the glucose targets. This may be difficult, however, if your next question is **"How can I get enough blood on the strip?"**

Some people tell me they don't get enough on the strip because they don't have enough blood in their bodies. Wrong. You have around five liters of blood, and the glucometer strip only needs one drop.

If your lancet has been reused multiple times, it's probably blunt and not piercing the skin. That's when you won't get enough of a sample without switching to a new lancet. This struggle is worse if you have thick, hard, dry skin, so even with a new one, *you may need to dial up the lancet so that it goes deep enough* past any dry callus.

For those scared of pain and hesitating while using the lancet, you may be unconsciously pulling away from the lancet so that it's not going deep enough; *placing your hand on a table or firm surface* can prevent any unwanted movement. On the other hand, if you have untreated *anemia*, you might need to *get your doctor to fix that.*

The one complaint that I can't help too much with, is when clients are upset that **the testing strips are expensive**, and I agree. Checking glucometer readings indefinitely with no plan would be frustrating, and it's completely natural that you would question the whole point and wastefulness of it all.

Hopefully, the readings will help you work with a competent professional to make strategic changes and achieve better glucose levels within a few months. That way you don't need as many useless pokes for the rest of your life, and you get to reduce your long-term health expenses. Uncontrolled diabetes gets much more expensive (financially, emotionally, and physically) down the road. You get to decide if the short-term investment is worth the long-term rewards.

Unless the glucometer readings are faulty. This can happen for many reasons, and you may see inaccurate readings. Some of my patients keep a backup glucometer, especially if they have type 1 diabetes and every reading has an impact on the next insulin dose. In any case, check if the old batteries in the meter need to be replaced or if there's a need for recalibration of the glucometer. Inspect whether the test strips have expired or been contaminated, and even look for chemicals on your fingertips that could be interfering. If nothing helps, you might just have a faulty glucometer.

If you're already comfortable using a glucometer and want other options to monitor glucose trends, **you can always wear a continuous glucose monitoring (CGM) device.**

Wearable technology has really changed the landscape of diabetes self-management. I have always believed that knowledge is power when used correctly.

If your neighbor tells you about some miracle food for diabetes, why blindly believe them? Your body doesn't gossip or lie. If you see your own glucose spiking after a particular event, you might not need a health professional to tell you what to do. Your body is already telling you. Your body offers more accurate feedback than social media influencers or your own doctor can about how specific foods or experiences do or don't work for you at that stage in your journey.

The difference between a CGM and a glucometer is worth understanding. The sensor of the **CGM** *is a filament that sits under your skin.* Because it *checks* *the glucose level of the interstitial fluid* (the space between the cells under the skin) instead of measuring glucose in an actual capillary blood vessel, *it's an indirect and delayed marker* for what is happening in the blood. When the glucose levels are steady, I've seen a difference of up to 40 mg/dL (2.22 mmol/L) between a glucometer and CGM compared to times of rapid glucose fluctuation when I've seen differences from 80 up to 100 mg/dL (4.44–5.55 mmol/L).

The fact that the CGM is *less accurate than a glucometer* is one thing, but the fact that *it becomes very inaccurate and delayed during large, rapid glucose shifts* (high-carb, high-sugar meal; high insulin dose; intense workouts) is one of its biggest **disadvantages**.

That's why CGM is also *insufficient to make changes in diabetes medication doses. Being on vitamin C or aspirin can also interfere* with CGM readings. Not only can it *get kinked when sleeping on the same side and give falsely low readings that you might think are hypoglycemic events,* it's also susceptible to inaccuracy after being exposed to high temperatures. According to the different manufacturers, these devices are designed to be stored at 36°F–80°F (2°C–27°C) because *they can give inaccurate readings when exposed to high heat.* Many distributors don't store the sensors in the fridge. Room temperatures across India and other warm countries are much hotter than this, which means that wearing these sensors outdoors or in high temperature rooms might come with inherent inaccuracies.

Finally, a CGM can be expensive out of pocket, especially if worn continuously and still requiring a glucometer to double-check. It might feel like an unjustified expense if no action is taken based on the insights from the data.

On the other hand, **there are quite a few advantages of wearing a CGM**, primarily when it comes to managing your data. You can r*eceive twenty-four-hour insights for seven days* with new measurements every five minutes; other models offer *fourteen days' readings taken every fifteen minutes.*[4,5] This continues even in your sleep! The reports *display trends over a daily and weekly time frame* so that you can zoom out and get a bigger picture. A CGM can provide *data on how a meal or a workout affects you, even up to four to six hours later.*

But wait, there's more!

Not only is the *information relayed to the reader or your phone*, but you also have the *ability to export data as a .csv or .pdf file* to your computer. You can even share your *data dashboard* view with your clinical care team to generate more insights.

Continuous glucose monitors are also *able to translate a theoretical glycemic index or glycemic load into real time data so you can understand how a particular carbohydrate affects your glucose* at that particular phase of your diabetes turnaround journey.

This is a *powerful visual way to show you the impact* of lifestyle changes, especially by changing the amount of carbohydrates and protein in meals. The ability to manipulate and analyze the data can *help you correlate periods of low energy in the day with glucose levels and give you confidence* that the glucose level is not dropping dangerously low during a fast, an office meeting, or a workout. I often *plan a two-week insight-generating activity with my patients on CGM,* where they observe patterns for the first seven days, make changes based on customized feedback, and then observe the impact over the subsequent seven days. Even though I don't have diabetes, I have personally used a CGM as have many of my health conscious friends, family and preventive health minded patients. The CGM has shown me how my body responds to favorite Gujrati comfort foods like mango pulp (aam ras) and sweet stuffed flatbreads (puran puri). I have noticed how the glucose remains steady in a 60 hour fast and rises up in a fasted workout. The most unexpected finding was seeing the lowest level in two weeks coincide with the three hours when I was teaching meditation to a physician colleague.

And depending on who you ask, **the biggest advantage to a CGM is that it's painless.**

We know that a glucometer or a CGM can give us more information and control, but we should also know that there are some things you can't monitor yourself. Things like blood tests and lipid panels are things your doctor will and should look at periodically.

7.2: Why we use lab work to assess diabetes

There is one caveat when thinking about blood tests. A blood test is a one-time, static photograph of constantly flowing blood. It's like a closed-circuit television (CCTV) photograph of a vehicle at a busy junction. Imagine a truck full of fresh produce is captured on the CCTV camera while crossing an intersection. After the photo was taken, the truck driver got in and out of the vehicle, loaded and unloaded the produce, and went back on the road multiple times. The truck probably also transported other goods on the return journey.

What would traffic police understand if they only looked at a still image from the CCTV footage? They wouldn't assume the truck has been parked at that intersection with those same fresh goods ever since that photograph was taken, right?

Like the truck, our blood never stops moving.

For the average person with a resting heart rate, or pulse, of seventy beats per minute, the contracting heart pumps around five tablespoons (75 mL) of blood forward with each squeeze. This means that your entire approximate blood volume of five liters gets pumped all the way around the body about once per minute, at rest. So on average, your heart pumps your entire blood volume around the resting body at least 1,440 times per day without any breaks.

Blood tests are a snapshot of something that is constantly in motion for as long as we are alive. After providing a blood sample, the contents of your entire blood volume would have circulated tens of thousands of times over by the time you are looking at the test results.* To take the example of cholesterol, constant blood flow normally prevents clotting and buildup of material by carrying and

---

* There is some data to suggest that you don't really need to provide a fasting sample for lipid assessment and that nonfasting lipids may actually provide more information about cardiovascular risk. See: Børge G. Nordestgaard, Anne Langsted, Samia Mora, Genovefa Kolovou, Hannsjörg Baum, Eric Bruckert, Gerald F. Watts, et al., "Fasting Is Not Routinely Required for Determination of a Lipid Profile: Clinical and Laboratory Implications Including Flagging at Desirable CONCENTRATION Cut-Points—A Joint Consensus Statement from the European Atherosclerosis Society and European Federation of Clinical Chemistry and Laboratory Medicine," European Heart Journal 37, no. 25 (2016): 1944–1958, https://www.ncbi.nlm.nih.gov/pmc/articles/PMC4929379/.

transporting fats to various locations in the body via the help of lipoprotein carriers. The information we get from a blood sample is helpful, but is only a snapshot of what is constantly happening.

The blood carries and delivers thousands of materials that are constantly needed by the body. Some of those are solid, some are attached to the solid, some are liquid, and others are dissolved in liquid.

Your red blood cells (RBCs) have a protein called *hemoglobin* that delivers oxygen to all the cells in the body. You also have glucose traveling in the blood to deliver energy to each cell in the body. Glucose and RBCs interact with each other on their daily commute along the bloodstream highway, and the friendly RBCs give a lift to some of the glucose molecules on the journey because they are headed to the same destination—that's how HbA1c is formed.

HbA1c stands for glycosylated hemoglobin, which is the percentage of RBCs that have glucose attached to their hemoglobin. The average lifespan of a RBC is ninety days, so the HbA1c gives you a ninety-day average of how your blood glucose has been for the last three months, twenty-four hours a day. To describe this, I like to use the waterpark analogy.

Have you ever seen a lazy river in a waterpark? It's a popular water ride with donut-shaped tubes that float in a pool that's shaped like a winding river. When people enter the lazy river, some people climb inside the ring tube and lazily float along the river until they decide to get out.

Now imagine that the *person sitting in the float is* **glucose***, the ring is the RBC with* **hemoglobin***, and the flowing water is your* **bloodstream***.** If you were to measure the *average percentage of ring floats that have people, versus the rings that don't have people in the river over a ninety-day period, that's the* **HbA1c** *in this analogy.*

In insulin resistance, the liver is holding excess glucose from the meals as fatty liver for years before the HbA1c starts to climb. Imagine the liver works like a security guard at the entrance of the lazy river ride, holding excess guests behind the gate to ensure the right number of people inside the ride at a time. The liver has to make sure too many people don't enter the lazy river all at once so that the ride flows smoothly and everyone can have a good time. When a huge crowd accumulates and exceeds the capacity of the liver, the security gates get breached, a stampede happens, and too many people start jumping into the water.

Now, with a chaotic mob crowding in the water (elevated blood glucose), the water gets dirty and turbulent (inflammation), multiple people are bumping into the walls and the tiles are getting chipped off (damaging the blood vessel lining or endothelium), and too many people are climbing into each ring and refusing to leave the park for ninety days (elevated HbA1c). This is not good, and if this goes on for years the ride and the whole park will be a mess.

---

* Geeky fact: adults have an average of 4–6 million RBCs in one cubic milliliter of blood!

Now, let's consider the role of HbA1c in diabetes management. **Blood work can tell us our HbA1c levels,** and it's considered the standard of care to use the quarterly HbA1c to determine how you are doing and to inform treatment decisions. *The goal is for HbA1c to be below 5.7 percent without medication in type 2 diabetes and to be as close to normal as possible with the lowest insulin doses in type 1 diabetes.* Research has shown that higher HbA1c levels directly translate to more complications of diabetes, so your doctor is programmed to prescribe medication to get your HbA1c below 7 percent.[*]

A word of advice here: if you want to use lifestyle change to reduce your risk of diabetes complications while still needing less medication, you may have to *specifically inform* your doctor.

I know that sounds crazy, but doctors are being bombarded with research data on how drugs are better than the placebo (of doing nothing) to reduce the risk of complications. The doctor doesn't have the luxury of a trial that proves how many more complications or deaths are avoided by making the aggressive lifestyle changes mentioned in this book, versus taking medication without any lifestyle changes. That type of trial is unlikely to ever be published, so their solution to save your life and reduce suffering is by giving you something they are trained to prescribe. But why let your doctor increase prescriptions based on medication research alone?

I tell everyone to start with getting lab work done so that you can get an idea of where you stand instead of relying only on medication research. In cases like Harry's, the results of his blood work changed his life.

For reference, when we first met, Harry was used to the old-fashioned way of seeing his doctor for diabetes checkups. Once a quarter, he would go to the lab and get a fasting glucose and a two-hour postmeal glucose sample drawn. He didn't trust the glucometer and could not be bothered with pricking his own finger. His wife did it for him sometimes, but mostly he would resist.

The night before the blood test, he would finish dinner early by 8:00 p.m. and avoid his daily dessert or extra helping of rice, which always made his 8:00 a.m. fasting glucose reading look slightly better. The lab in Bengaluru would feed him a carb-heavy meal, then measure the two-hour postmeal reading. The extent of his diabetes appointment included the doctor frowning at the quarterly reports and adjusting medications up or down by a few milligrams based on those two numbers. The next three months of treatment were determined by reviewing data from fourteen hours of Harry's life.

When Harry came to see me, I told him that we were going to measure his HbA1c for the first time in the twenty years that he'd been living with diabetes.

---

[*] Based on the UKPDS and DCCT trials showing reduced microvascular complications of diabetes when the HbA1c is below 7 percent.

While I'll be sure to tell you what we learned about Harry's diabetes later, read on to understand the power of the HbA1c first.

When getting bloodwork done to measure HbA1c levels, it's important that you understand the results. This table can help you translating the HbA1c into estimated average glucose levels for the last ninety days in type 1 and type 2 diabetes.[6,7]

Hemoglobin A1c (HbA1c) *as a percentage*	5	6	7	8	9	10	11	12
Estimated 90-day glucose average *as mg/dL*	97	126	154	183	212	240	269	298
Estimated 90-day glucose average *as mmol/L*	5.4	7	8.6	10.2	11.8	13.4	14.9	16.5

Using lab work to monitor HbA1c, has many advantages.[8] For starters, we are given a retrospective *look at the last ninety days of twenty-four-hour averages* of fasting and postmeal glucose levels. Lab work *lends more information* than isolated glucose readings because you may consciously or unconsciously "eat clean" for a few days to prepare for a fasting glucose or postmeal glucose reading to show the doctors. Sound familiar? The best part is that fasting is not required to measure HbA1c, so if you're anything like Harry, the HbA1c results might influence you to change your diet for more than fourteen hours.

On the other hand, there are a few **disadvantages of HbA1c testing.**

Since the test is measuring hemoglobin inside RBCs that are chemically changed by exposure to glucose, HbA1c is *not directly measuring glucose* or counting all the people in the lazy river or the water park. It's counting the percentage of rings that have people inside relative to how many total rings are in the river.

Because of the ninety-day RBC life span, HbA1c testing *will take three months to reflect the impact* of any intervention. Being a lag indicator, it *cannot predict what is going to happen with your future glucose levels.* It only tells you about the past. So, if you changed your diet or medication and your glucose levels drastically improved within the last four weeks, that means it will take two more months to reflect in the next HbA1c.

Nowadays portable HbA1c kits are available that give you an instant reading from a finger prick. These results are less accurate compared to the HbA1c from a lab sample taken from your vein.

There are also reasons that a *lab HbA1c* can be inaccurate, or *falsely low.* Imagine dumping out a chunk of water and its contents from the lazy river—that's what blood loss is like to the body, and it can skew HbA1c due to a different blood concentration. Conversely, a recent blood transfusion is like adding water from a different pool into the lazy river. That means you have donor RBCs circulating amid yours, so the HbA1c cannot be used until ninety days after a blood transfusion.

Pregnancy changes almost everything in the body, and can falsely lower the HbA1c. The results can also be thrown off due to genetic variants of hemoglobin, like having uncomfortable ring floats in the pool. Imagine damaged ring floats that get removed by the safety check and quality control team faster than new rings can be replaced. That illustrates any conditions that reduce the lifespan of RBCs, which can also taint your HbA1c numbers. Anemia, or low hemoglobin, is like not having enough rings in the pool, so your doctor would evaluate the complete blood count, ferritin and iron status to address the cause of anemia. Regardless of what caused inaccurate results, in many cases your doctor may track fructosamine instead of HbA1c.

Lab work can track your glucose levels, fructosamine, and HbA1c, but it also can shed light on other important diabetes tests, like **fasting C-peptide levels**.

In Part 1, we discussed how C-peptide *helps confirm whether your pancreas is still making enough insulin or not.* The good thing about this test is that it can help even if you are on insulin prescriptions.

Blood work can tell us if you have low, normal, or high C-peptide levels. *If C-peptide levels are normal or high, you have type 2 diabetes* that can be put into remission through the lifestyle changes discussed in this book. *If your C-peptide levels are low, it shows that the pancreas is not making enough insulin*, so depending on how low it is, you might need insulin therapy. Your doctor may also check anti-GAD and anti-islet cell antibodies to check for autoimmune causes of pancreatic damage, like latent autoimmune diabetes of adulthood (LADA). As some types of autoimmune diabetes can run in families,, this may guide you to **visit the lab for genetic screening** in case you are planning a family of your own.[910] Even if your pancreas is not making enough insulin, the lifestyle changes in this book will help you work with your doctor to achieve the most stable glucose levels possible with the lowest insulin dose.

On the journey to achieve those stable glucose levels, your doctor may want to look at the Homeostatic Model Assessment for Insulin Resistance (HOMA-IR) index.

The HOMA-IR index is a measure of insulin resistance. The test can be expensive and is not really going to change the treatment plan, because any good clinician can pick up clues to confirm insulin resistance from your history, examination, and the results of basic lab tests. Some people opt to monitor it to document progress and improvement in insulin sensitivity over time.

7.3: Using blood tests to understand the relationship among cardiac risk, lipids, and cholesterol

In regards to cardiovascular risk, there are many names for the same thing, but they are all talking about narrowing of the coronary arteries. Whether it's called *coronary artery disease* (CAD), *atherosclerosis, atherosclerotic cardiovascular disease* (ASCVD), myocardial infarction, or ischemic heart disease (IHD), **it's caused by plaques that block the coronary arteries** and become dangerous when they rupture, causing a heart attack or death. When this happens in the brain, we call it a *stroke or cerebrovascular disease.*

Before diving in, I want to make something clear: *I am not an atherosclerosis researcher.* I'm a clinician who sees patients every day to navigate test results and manage medications to reduce side effects while working on the lifestyle changes that help.

The work of internist Eric Westman, MD MHS; insulin researcher Ben Bikman, PhD; cardiologist Allan Sniderman, MD; internist and data scientist Adrian Soto-Mota, MD, PhD; and engineer Dave Feldman are excellent resources to get more technical about cardiovascular risk.[11,12,13,14,15,*]

As an endocrinologist, it's my job to help you understand metabolism, so instead of repeating what they have already written and spoken extensively about, I'll tell you the minimum you need to know about your blood tests to improve your cardiometabolic health in the context of insulin resistance.

---

* See the Cholesterol Code website https://cholesterolcode.com/.

This section is a bit technical but explains what to look for on your lipid panel so that you can assess your cardiac risk and discuss your medication and lifestyle changes with your doctor. But before we look at the lipid panel, let's discuss how it even relates to the plaque buildup that puts you at cardiac risk, because the world agrees on one thing—nobody wants a heart attack.

While the world *also* agrees that uncontrolled diabetes is a major contributor to the risk of heart attack and stroke, they are still debating whether or not all LDL cholesterol is purely evil.

Even though the controversy regarding diet as it relates to the heart, cholesterol, and statins is beyond the scope of this book, cholesterol is one of those areas that needs to be understood in the context of metabolism and energy transportation.*

The first thing to understand about cholesterol, is that **there are two main types called HDL and LDL**, and we referenced HDL specifically in Part 1.3 in regards to metabolic syndrome. LDL stands for *"low-density lipoprotein,"* while HDL stands for *"high-density lipoprotein."* They're both composed of fats and proteins; the word "lipoprotein" simply combines lipid (fat) and protein. These lipoproteins carry cholesterol and blood fats (lipids), so it makes sense why cholesterol is part of a lipid panel.

If you recall from our soup analogy in the FAQs of Part 6.6, protein sinks and fat floats, so it makes sense then that *high-density lipoprotein* is the one that has more protein than fat. The letter "H" really should stand for "the higher, the healthier," **as higher HDL levels seem to correlate with better cardiac outcomes**.[16]

There seems to be an inherited basis to HDL, but unfortunately, there is no medication that effectively raises HDL. No need to worry—research shows that lifestyle change can make a difference.[17,18]

I have seen patients' HDL improve when they eat whole eggs, build muscle, and practice intermittent fasting correctly, but I've also done my own experiments. As an endocrinologist who was diagnosed with prediabetes, I've tested my HDL levels before, but I wanted to experiment and see what happened when I tested in the middle of a sixty-hour fast where I was also building muscle and staying low-carb in the eating window.

The results?

When comparing my previous numbers to my levels at the sixtieth hour of the fast, *I saw an increase in HDL by almost 50 percent* (from 57 to 85 mg/dL). This is an "n of one" experiment I did on myself and is not something I am suggesting anyone do, because we don't have standardized ways of interpreting lipid profiles during extended fasting. The drastic difference tells me that lipoproteins seem to

---

* The two major opposing camps are those who support the lipid energy model versus the diet–heart hypothesis.

be carrier molecules that move lipids around the body depending on the hormonal and metabolic signal, and I look forward to seeing more studies on lipoprotein metabolism.

Until then, there is growing research suggesting it's the *lipoproteins, more than the cholesterol* carried inside them, that correlate with the amount of athero-sclerotic damage to the blood vessels. As insulin resistance intensifies, the LDL particle type shifts from large, buoyant, and benign; to a smaller, denser particle that is considered more dangerous because it seems "atherogenic" which means capable of starting atherosclerosis.[19] A more advanced and expensive lipid test called *nuclear magnetic resonance* (NMR) can show you the distribution (size and particle count) of large, buoyant, benign LDL versus their small, dense ath-erogenic LDL counterpart.

Because **apolipoprotein B** (ApoB) captures the various forms of the main atherogenic particle, it's considered by many to be a superior cardiovascular risk marker than LDL or triglyceride levels.[20] So, **instead of thinking of cholesterol as good or bad**, we should *focus on reducing the presence of atherogenic lipopro-teins.* These atherogenic particles are directly implicated in atherosclerotic dis-ease, as it's the stuff that blocks the arteries. The good news is that ApoB is very responsive to lifestyle changes that reduce insulin resistance, so you have already learned through this book how to get ApoB levels below 100 mg/dL. An indirect estimate of ApoB particles is provided by the ratio of triglycerides to HDL, but first–what are triglycerides?

The body stores excess fuel as fat in the form of triglycerides.

If you consume sugar, fructose, simple carbohydrates, or alcohol, your liver converts them into *triple* fatty acid molecules called triglycerides (TG). These fats are then carried around the body by VLDL (*very*-low-density lipoproteins) for storage.*

When the storage sites can no longer handle the excess fuel, "the grease spills into your vessels," as Dr. Robert Lustig puts it. As your blood TG and remnant cholesterol levels increase—so does insulin resistance and cardiac risk.[21]

Triglycerides and remnant cholesterol levels (but not LDL) have been **cor-related with higher rates of a first episode of a major cardiac** event in a life-style intervention study on people with insulin resistance.[22] Reducing your intake of sugar, refined processed carbohydrates, and alcohol are powerful ways to rap-

---

* I get this question a lot at dinner parties. There really is no "healthy" dose for alcohol in diabetes. Alcohol puts you at risk for low blood glucose if you are on certain medications. Cumulative alcohol intake has the same effect as sugar on the liver; it worsens insulin resistance. I tell my patients that the definition of a "safe" alcohol limit is lower for women than men, because women are built smaller. Smaller body: smaller liver: less alcohol tolerance. Well, those standards were assigned for Caucasians with larger body frames than Indians and South Asians. So by that logic, Indians would be able to tolerate even less than the recommended daily limit. Considering that one in three Indians are estimated to already have fatty liver from their carbs alone, I wonder how much alcohol they can safely manage.

idly reduce triglycerides. Although most labs say a TG below 150 mg/dl is normal, I want my patients to aim for a TG below 80 mg/dL. Once you are aware of your triglyceride and HDL levels, you can calculate their ratio to get an estimate of ApoB particles in the bloodstream.

The **TG/HDL** ratio is a reliable marker of insulin resistance and is available on standard lipid panels. The ratio is made of two numbers: dividing TG by HDL and from this ratio alone, you can identify two of the possible five criteria for a metabolic syndrome diagnosis, which correlates with cardiac risk (Part 1.3). The ratio between them should be less than two, which means that the TG should be less than double your HDL. I try to get my patients to a ratio below one through lifestyle change alone. In that case, their TG is less than their HDL.

An elevated TG/HDL ratio marks the presence of those dangerous small, dense ApoB particles and can help you get an idea if it needs deeper assessment.[23,24,25] The European Society of Cardiology has published that this ratio has been able to predict first coronary events regardless of body mass index (BMI), providing evidence that an elevated TG/HDL ratio could be a principal marker for assessing cardiac risks like coronary disease and atherosclerosis.[26]

It also means that, despite taking statins, an elevated TG/HDL ratio could help identify extreme high-risks in people with diabetes, and maybe even work to predict heart attack or cardiovascular death.[27] While I always want to see more research, we currently know that a high TG/HDL ratio is at least as powerful as high LDL levels when it comes to predicting ischemic heart disease over eight years of follow-up.[28] The TG/HDL ratio is not affected much by statins but responds very well to lifestyle change.

Despite the evidence, this ratio gets less mainstream attention than it should, and certainly gets less attention than LDL or total cholesterol.

There's another lipoprotein called **Lp(a)** that is associated with early cardiac events but gets less attention because the risk is genetic. You can still ask to have your levels checked. While knowing if it's high may give you more reason to invest in a healthy lifestyle, you should be sure to discuss the risk or benefit of statins with your doctor—especially if there's a family history of early cardiac events—as this lipoprotein is considered less amenable to lifestyle changes.

Regardless of whether you have the genetic lipoprotein, family history can influence how you approach cholesterol.

Take Omar, for example. His father and paternal uncle both had diabetes, both had stents placed after mild heart attacks, and both were taking insulin by the end. They had both died of sudden heart attacks in their seventies; he wanted to prevent this.

Omar had a lot to live for and wanted to reduce his cardiac risk as much as possible, and in addition to working with us on his uncontrolled diabetes, he wanted to know if there was anything actionable on his lipid panel. He had never had a heart attack and wanted to know if taking a statin to keep his low-density lipoprotein (LDL) normal was all he could do.

He was forty when we met, and he had already been on a statin for his cholesterol for nine years. Available data strongly suggest that heart attacks do occur even in people on statins with normal LDL, and that persistent cardiac risk can be picked up by the TG/HDL ratio.[29] By now you know why the team and I helped him reduce his TG/HDL ratio as his best next step.

Bottom line, don't shiver just because someone in the room said the word *cholesterol*. Most forms of cholesterol are made by the liver and are necessary for health.

The physician researchers who asked the question, "Why is cholesterol present in plasma?" received the 1985 Nobel Prize in Medicine for their discovery of the LDL receptor and its role in atherosclerosis. Their research brought them to state the "most logical conclusion. . . is that the receptor mediated LDL pathway functions in man *to protect* against atherosclerosis."[30] Cholesterol makes the backbone of important hormones (testosterone, progesterone, estrogen, and cortisol) and is part of every healthy cell membrane, playing a role in immunity and normal cellular repair processes.

The body doesn't put cholesterol into every cell just to block your arteries and kill you, so when a patient asks me whether they should be concerned about their cholesterol profile, I know what they're really asking is what they should do to improve their cardiac health outcomes.

7.4: Screening for complications[*]

The main reason people with uncontrolled diabetes experience progressively debilitating and devastating complications is due to the unchecked inflammation inside the blood vessels.[31,32] This **inflammation is caused by insulin resistance, often worsened by coexisting high blood pressure.**

Buildup of inflammation worsens atherosclerotic plaques *inside large blood vessel walls causing macrovascular* complications like heart attacks, strokes and peripheral vascular disease. The inflammation and damage *in smaller blood vessel walls causes microvascular* complications.

Smoking tobacco has been linked with new cases of type 2 diabetes along with increased macrovascular and microvascular complications. A particularly troublesome complication that demonstrates the additive effect of macrovascular and microvascular complications is diabetic foot. Thankfully, quitting smoking starts accumulating risk reversal over time as the body starts its healing process, but **taking preventive measures before complications occur has been proven to be cost effective.[**]**

Obviously, the way to prevent these events is by achieving normal glucose and blood pressure levels with the least amount of medication through the lifestyle steps outlined in this book, but you should still work with your doctor to discuss your options when it comes to screening for complications beyond a routine physical examination. Like Sid.

Sid was fifty-six when he came to my office with diabetes that had been uncontrolled for the past twelve years. He had recently been diagnosed with moderate sleep apnea and low total testosterone levels. He loved his wife, but they both were dissatisfied in the bedroom. It would be straightforward to say, "Yeah, your testosterone is low, so let's replace some." But to do justice to someone's symptoms, a more thorough evaluation is necessary.

Upon detailed questioning, we realized that he had not yet started continuous positive airway pressure (CPAP) treatment for sleep apnea, which is a known

---

[*] The American Diabetes Association Standards of Care document published every January specifies the screening frequency for these, and they should be individualized with your doctor.

[**] 2024 ADA Standards of Care in Diabetes

cause of erectile dysfunction (ED) and low testosterone levels. Besides controlling his glucose levels, starting CPAP, and considering couples therapy, we gradually reduced unnecessary medications because his medication list (that I'll share in this part) included many that have ED as a side effect. Within eleven months of working consistently on his lifestyle changes, he reported more mutually satisfying sexual experiences for himself and his partner.

You may not have considered it, but **macrovascular and microvascular damage** is a *real cause of sexual dysfunction in men and women* and can be aggravated by the side effects from many medications that people with diabetes often take, besides the direct hormonal and psychological impacts of uncontrolled diabetes.[33]

The good news is that even though further research is needed on things like the effect of pelvic floor exercise on sexual dysfunction in men and women with diabetes, people like Sid have experienced improvement in their sexual health by following the steps we have already covered in the earlier chapters.[34] Many of my patients have been pleasantly surprised to notice improvements after having given up on any hope of a healthier sex life with their partner.

Sadly, since there tends to be some shame surrounding sexual dysfunction, people often continue on without seeking help. When it comes to other parts of the body, people sometimes seek help when it's too late.

Sadly, there are thousands of Indians who discover the importance of glucose control for the first time after they rush to the eye doctor with sudden loss of vision out of one eye. Diabetic retinopathy and diabetes-related macular edema can progress undetected for many years before getting diagnosed in drastic ways, so I strongly urge patients to seek **retinopathy screening**. All you have to do is get a dilated fundus exam once a year in order to catch retinopathy early before diabetes causes any visual symptoms. I have seen patients halt progression of mild to moderate cases of retinopathy once they turned around diabetes through lifestyle changes. Although artificial intelligence (AI) is increasingly being used in retinopathy screening, nothing replaces an old-fashioned dilated exam with a good ophthalmologist. You don't want to wait till your vision is being threatened and needs expensive injections in the eye, and this goes for everything else in the body.

If you don't want to be blindsided by ailments after it's too late to reverse them or stop the progression, I **recommend that you talk to your doctor about the screening tests you feel are right for you.** While we will dive into how to communicate with your care team later, for now, take a look at the table below to get an idea of the different options available.

Organ system	Screening options	To prevent or detect
Circulatory system Cardiovascular Cerebrovascular Peripheral arteries	Electrocardiogram (ECG), ECG treadmill stress test (TMT), chemical stress test, two-dimensional echocardiography (2D ECHO), coronary artery calcium (CAC)* score, carotid intima media thickness (CIMT), foot pulse, ankle brachial index (ABI), toe blood pressure Screen for tobacco use Monitor blood pressure to keep below 130/80 mm Hg	Heart attack (a.k.a. atherosclerotic cardiovascular disease [ASCVD], coronary artery disease [CAD], or coronary heart disease [CHD]), congestive heart failure (CHF), ischemic cardiomyopathy, strokes, peripheral vascular disease (PVD) or peripheral arterial disease (PAD)
Brain Cognitive function[35] Psychosocial	Ask about cognitive function Mini–Mental State Exam (MMSE) Screen for diabetes distress using Diabetes Distress Scale for type 2 diabetes (T2-DDAS) or type 1 diabetes (T1-DDAS)	Mild cognitive impairment (MCI), dementia (now also referred to as type 3 diabetes), Diabetes distress
Eyes	Ophthalmological testing Retinal examination by an ophthalmologist	Glaucoma, cataract, diabetic retinopathy, and diabetic macular edema (leading causes of blindness)
Kidneys	Urine routine Estimated glomerular filtration rate (eGFR) Urinary microalbumin/creatinine ratio (more sensitive than albumin/creatinine ratio)	Urinary infection or bladder cancer associated with diabetic medication Diabetic nephropathy (a leading cause of kidney failure)

---

* Anyone worried about radiation exposure from the DEXA or CAC score can compare the radiation dose from these tests with the background cosmic radiation exposure from living on Earth at sea level (0.01 mSv per day) and exposure from sitting on a six-hour flight (0.015 mSv). See: RadiologyInfo.org, "Radiation Dose," November 1, 2022, https://www.radiologyinfo.org/en/info/safety-xray.

Organ system	Screening options	To prevent or detect
Nerves	Testing for balance, stability, position (proprioception), coordination Monofilament sensation testing of the feet (ability to detect 10-gram force) Nerve-conduction studies	Diabetic neuropathy (a leading cause of diabetic foot, amputations, and falls)
Feet Footwear Foot care	Examine skin for callus or ulcer Check for deformity or flat foot Review protective footwear and foot-care habits	Diabetic foot (a leading cause of amputations)
Liver	Liver enzymes aspartate aminotransferase (AST or SGOT) and alanine aminotransferase (ALT or SGPT) Calculate Fibrosis-4 (FIB-4) index Ultrasound to look for fatty liver Elastography Screen for alcohol use	Nonalcoholic steatohepatitis (NASH), nonalcoholic fatty liver disease (NAFLD), fibrosis or cirrhosis
Bones	DEXA scan with body composition analysis (BCA) Gait assessment	Fall and fracture risk

While we'll only go in depth about a few later, they all are important. Regular screenings help you stay updated on the health of your body systems and catch health risks early. Even if your glucose levels are normal, lab work and screenings can provide clues that point to insulin resistance. This can help you take preventive measures to turn around insulin resistance before it affects your glucose.

Clinical, lab, and radiology clues that you have may have insulin resistance include **elevated** *blood pressure, HOMA-IR, TGs, TG/HDL ratio,* and *liver enzymes* (ALT and AST), **increased** *uric acid, echogenicity* (brightness) and *hepatomegaly* (enlargement) *of the liver* on ultrasound, suggesting fatty liver; and low *HDL*. These clues come from all different places, so discuss which screenings would be the best for your situation with your doctor, like Lakshmi, Harry, and Omar.

7.5: Whatever happened with Lakshmi, Omar, and Harry?

I shared stories throughout this part of the book and said I would revisit them once we have covered enough information to really assess their situations. Now that we've made it to this point, it's time to update their journeys.

Let's start with Lakshmi–

Once we started working together, she wanted to know what her quinoa was doing to her glucose levels. She'd read about glycemic index and glycemic load but didn't really know the impact of these on her body until she started using her own glucometer.

It turned out that reducing her quinoa and replacing it with protein gave her better postmeal readings, so I was able to quickly reduce her insulin dose. After her glucose stabilized, she wanted to test what happened with the forbidden mango—she was pleasantly surprised to see how a few bites of mango did not cause the level to go as high as other foods did, especially when she had the mango as dessert, after her protein and vegetables. She was no longer blindly wondering what to eat and was able to self-adjust her carb intake while also achieving more stable glucose levels with lower insulin doses.

Back to Harry

By tweaking dinner on the night before his lab test, Harry was usually able to show his doctor a fasting reading of around 140 mg/dL (7.77 mmol/L). Since the postmeal usually hovered around 170 mg/dL (9.44 mmol/L), that came to an average glucose of 155 mg/dL (8.6 mmol/L). When he tested his HbA1c, however, it came back at a startling 8.8 percent. At 8.8 percent, it meant that on average, his blood glucose levels were around 207 mg/dL (11.5 mmol/L) all day, for the past ninety days.

Imagine driving on a long road trip on the highway, and your engine is in trouble, and your dashboard light fails to alarm you that something is wrong.

Both he and his doctor were working under the false impression that his diabetes was relatively well-managed because his glucose numbers looked "reasonable" during the doctor visits. The data science buffs may have noticed that since his fasting levels were always lower than his postmeal readings, it's likely his readings were actually exceeding 207 mg/dL (11.5 mmol/L) after food. Even though he thought he was mostly fine, these levels had been silently causing harm in his body for years undetected. The results of the HbA1c changed Harry's outlook, especially once he realized he could turn things around.

Remember Omar?

Omar's HbA1c was 9 percent, indicating uncontrolled diabetes. That itself was a major cardiac risk factor, so we decided to continue his statin. But a statin alone does not reduce anyone's risk of heart attack or cardiovascular death to zero; he was clearly still at high risk.

His LDL was thirty and his HDL was twenty-six, but his TGs were *sky-high at 2,791* mg/dL, putting him at risk for acute pancreatitis.

That put his TG/HDL ratio among the highest I've seen in years. If you recall, the ratio should be less than two, and doctors tend to get nervous if the ratio is above three.

His TG/HDL ratio was thirty times higher than that, clocking in at a whopping 107.

He looked like he was at high risk for a heart attack just based on his blood work. His cardiologist insisted on an angiography, and one of his major coronary arteries had a 90 percent blockage of calcified plaque. He was only thirty-nine, and he had aggressive atherosclerosis already.

This is the sad part of the cardiometabolic epidemic we face, with people being affected from their thirties.

We began working on his nutrition and intensified his prescriptions. He is still a work in progress, struggling with stress management, emotional eating, binge eating, and addiction to processed food, but he's working with a therapist and doing the best he can.

Seeing patients like Omar is a sad testament to why this is the first time in history that the current generation has lower life-expectancy projections than their parents, but this is the epidemic doctors fight every day, especially when it comes to the role of medication.[36]

7.6: How doctors give you hypoglycemia

I have not told you too many negative stories about diabetes because the focus of this book is on what to do to *prevent* bad outcomes. Self-love is a stronger long-term motivator for sustained habit change than fear. Most people don't quit smoking because "tobacco kills." They quit because they decide their life is worth it. Still, it's important to show you the full picture that you have probably seen around you in life, too. All diabetes outcomes are not as rosy as the inspiring stories you have read about in this book. The suffering from diabetes and its complications or side effects from its treatment are real. Millions face it every day.

Take Marco, for example. His mother was eighty-seven and had just been found unconscious as a result of a low-blood-sugar hypoglycemic reaction. She had been on insulin for years, so her family recognized the pattern and knew it was an emergency.

But it took fifteen minutes for her to be revived by her family.

Marco was a friend of mine and called me in a panic, "Is Ma having a small heart attack every time her sugar fluctuates?"

Usually, making her eat a packet of biscuits and drink a small box of juice was enough, and they always left home with her bag of rescue foods. Things had gotten worse in the past year. She had lost some weight, and this was her fourth severe hypoglycemic reaction in six months.

The family had heard that diabetes could cause silent heart attacks, and because each hypoglycemic event caused Ma to end up sweating and unconscious on the floor, they worried that each episode was a mini-heart attack. They also worried about how frail she had become; each fall was a risk for her breaking a hip. These episodes made everyone very nervous.

His mom was *not* my patient and was on a 70/30 premixed insulin twice a day, five different blood pressure medications, isosorbide mononitrate and aspirin "for her heart," a multivitamin, calcium supplementation, and three different tablets for diabetes.

The interesting part about the diabetes medication was that she was on **gliclazide**, which works by *getting the beta cells of a working pancreas to release more insulin.*

But this patient was also on forty-four units of injectable insulin a day, which meant the treating team had assumed her pancreas was no longer making enough insulin (burned-out pancreas or failing beta cells). Giving gliclazide with insulin made no clinical sense, so make up your mind, Doc. *Is Ma's pancreas working?*

Or is Ma's pancreas burned out? Is our clinical logic burning out?

I asked about Ma's last few blood reports to assess the health of her kidneys and inquired about her last meal and insulin dose. Ma had eaten very little that day. Her appetite was low, but the family pointed out that she always loves her little sweet at the end of each meal. She figured that if she must endure insulin injections twice a day, she might as well enjoy some chocolate in the bargain. Naturally, the family summarized that Ma's level would touch a maximum of 320–340 mg/dL (17.7–18.8 mmol/L), average around 150–210 mg/dL (8.3–11.6 mmol/L), and hit a dangerous low about four times a year.

Despite the regular chocolate, the family knew they had to keep sweet things handy for when a low blood glucose episode threatened to strike. Do you see the paradox? Diabetes itself is diagnosed by a high blood glucose, not a low one. The **low blood glucose in diabetes** comes from *specific prescription tablets and insulin injections.* So if the doctor prescribes a certain type of medication whose job is to *lower glucose by brute force no matter what the glucose level is, only then* will the patient potentially be at risk of having low sugar.

Remember the ACCORD, ADVANCE, and VADT trials from Part 7.1?

The effect of sulfonylureas like gliclazide is to keep pushing the glucose level down for as long as the medicine remains bound to its receptor. The drug effect can last for six to twenty-four hours—or even longer in the elderly or those with reduced kidney function. Again, sulfonylureas do this regardless of whether the glucose has reached normal or not. This doesn't sound safe at any level, does it? A working pancreas would intelligently reduce natural insulin release as it sees glucose levels approach normal (remember it's the glucose regulator among the musketeers). The normal range would be a fasting level below 100 mg/dL (5.55 mmol/L), and the two-hour postmeal glucose levels below 140 mg/dL (7.77 mmol/L). Ma's glucose was going below that thanks to gliclazide and prescription insulin on board, raising the risk of knocking her unconscious.

It never fails to grab me, the insanity and futility of it all.

We were treating Ma's high blood glucose by giving her a risk of low blood glucose, which we treated with sweets, sugar, chocolate, juice and biscuits, which rebounded her back into the high blood glucose range. What exactly were we treating?

We were chasing our own tail and keeping her sick, so it seemed like my friend's question about small or silent heart attacks was not far from reality. Indeed, it was a very important one. Were we, in fact, keeping Ma's heart safe with all the prescriptions?

Or were we somehow silently aware and passively accepting that one day, despite all the effort, suffering, prescriptions and expense over the years, diabetes would eventually get to her heart?

7.7: The web of polypharmacy

Every January, the American Diabetes Association (ADA) releases its *Standards of Care in Diabetes* publication to guide health professionals, policymakers, and individuals about diabetes care. You might hope that the prescription algorithm guides doctors to help people with diabetes to achieve better glucose levels with less medication, but frankly, that's not the way a busy doctor ends up using the guidelines.

The 2024 *Standards of Care in Diabetes* publication is 328 pages long. I don't know about you, but reading that many pages of technical text can get exhausting. It's natural to want to skip to the colorful charts and pages that are easier on the eyes and brain, so most physicians don't read the whole thing cover to cover. Your doctor probably refers to the colorful ADA **pharmacotherapy algorithm for glucose-lowering medication** to decide which drug to prescribe you next, and I know I relied on it for years as well. In recent years, I have spoken out extensively online about how that algorithm *effectively serves to inform doctors on how to increase medication as diabetes progresses along but does not show people how to achieve better diabetes with less medication.* Don't just take my word for it, check out the 2015 TEDx talk by the brilliant late Dr. Sarah Hallberg. Titled "Reversing Type 2 Diabetes Starts by Ignoring the Guidelines"; it's perfect for those who want to know whether the diabetes treatment algorithms sufficiently guide doctors to engage deeper with lifestyle change *before* organs start falling apart.

That's not to say that the entire publication is bad, incomplete or wrong—all of the right words can be found on page S166 where a colorful algorithm helps doctors navigate through options for glucose-lowering drugs. Key terms like *motivational interviewing* and *person-centered management* appear elsewhere in the fine print, but the mere presence of these words in writing doesn't really tell busy doctors how to do any of these things with their patients.

The ADA guide may be 328 pages long, but it is taking me even longer to explain the "*how*" of lifestyle change to you after over a decade of experience with it. By going out of my way to learn, refine, enhance and expand on what was often mentioned in passing, I was able to bring life to my patient's care plans by working with them on all the points highlighted by the ADA:

- Healthy lifestyle behaviors
- Diabetes self-management education and support
- Social determinants of health
- Achievement and maintenance of glycemic and weight-management goals
- Avoiding therapeutic inertia
- Identify barriers
- Individualized weight-management goals
- General lifestyle advice
- Medical nutrition therapy
- Support self-efficacy
- Tailor therapy
- Eating patterns
- Physical activity
- Intensive, evidence-based, structured weight-management program

Saying all the right words and *explaining how to do* them are two different things. To me however, *medication guidelines* seem like a way to **react** to the problem, whereas taking the time to get into the *how and why of lifestyle changes* is the way to **prevent** issues. While it's great that the ADA documented important things like motivational interviewing and person-centered management, **the rest of page S166** visually, and hopefully unintentionally, *nudges doctors to expect diabetes to keep progressing.* It colorfully implies that they will have to keep adding more medication when HbA1c is not at goal levels.

It almost looks like the document suggests *that doctors should expect that organ damage from diabetes is inevitable*. If doctors are reading about what to do *after* we lose the battle without strategizing how to win—we've lost before the fight's even started. By reading the page from left to right, doctors are *almost conditioned to wait for organ damage* and then add value by identifying "high risk" patients; the algorithm then suggests what medication to prescribe. *Wait, what? When did the patient become high risk? What did we do for them when they were low risk?*

Because different drugs have different risk-reduction benefits under different dire circumstances, page S166 helps doctors think through different drugs *after* the patient has atherosclerotic disease (or its risk factors), heart failure, or kidney damage.

It's great that drugs have "protective" benefits, but to me, it's only giving the illusion of choice—it's too little, too late. A doctor is not of much use in prevention if they don't know how to help their patients with any of the fourteen points mentioned previously, but again, the visual algorithm in itself is ineffective at getting doctors to use lifestyle change more aggressively as a prevention or treatment option in diabetes. The medical education system will have to change if we truly want more doctors to be competent and confident in a lifestyle-first approach. Right now, most physicians' only skill is a medication-based approach.

I know. I was there, too.

7.8: Diabetes prescriptions

In the United States, patients get a tiny handout along with the prescription; it's in fine print that's almost impossible to read. In India, most medication comes in aluminum foil packs with no accompanying safety information at all. For more details on each medication, you can visit the manufacturer's website or online resources like Epocrates.com, drugs.com, medlineplus.gov, mayoclinic.org drugs, and supplement information pages.

Epocrates.com lets you check for drug interactions; you'd be surprised how many of the medications you are taking might cross-react with each other and start accumulating side effects like bone loss, brain fog, sexual dysfunction, constipation, and sleep or mood disturbance, causing you to get caught up in the web of polypharmacy and never-ending doctor visits.

It happened to Rita.

I will never forget my first consultation with her in August of 2020.

She looked like a zombie on that first day, when she saw me for severely uncontrolled diabetes at the age of sixty-two. The family told me that she was first told about "borderline" glucose levels in 2014. Their general physician had said it was nothing to worry about, so life went on as usual. *Nobody checked glucose levels for another few years.*

In January of 2020, she was started on an antiseizure medication, divalproex, by a psychiatrist for her complaints of low mood. The family reported that after starting this medication, Rita became more withdrawn and quiet, taking almost no initiative in her daily activities of life. She needed a continuous caretaker to bring her things.

In July of 2020, Rita started experiencing urinary incontinence. She would feel an intense urge to pass urine and could not control herself until she reached the washroom. The family took her to a urologist, who prescribed some tests and started her on solifenacin for the "bladder symptoms." While waiting for the test results, she started the solifenacin, and three days later, she had a fall in the bathroom that resulted in a vertebral fracture.

Then the test results came in.

With results showing glucose levels of 333 mg/dL (18.5 mmol/L), the family was shocked—they had no idea that she had developed severe diabetes.

Her story has a happy ending, but you may want to become aware of the different medication options that can affect your diabetes journey, like they did Rita's. We've spent so much time understanding the effects of the food we put in the body; it's only fair to also cover the medications that we might swallow or inject.

Doctors like me may prescribe a multitude of medications, including **metformin, DPP-4 inhibitors, SGLT-2 inhibitors, GLP-1 agonists, sulfonylureas and glinides, alpha-glucosidase inhibitors,** and **insulin,** so we want to be sure we understand the effects of the common diabetes medications.

Some of these medications have many different variations, and new drugs are released every year. My logic is not to use cheap drugs just because they are cheap, and I say this at every invited lecture on diabetes. If the sponsor of a conference is not willing to have me speak about reducing medication once diabetes gets under control through lifestyle change; I don't speak at that conference.

Drugs that are cheap in the short term can cause harm in the long term if they don't allow the person to safely invest in lifestyle changes to turn around diabetes. Doctors sometimes use cheap drugs because they think it will help patient "compliance". I weigh short term medication costs against long term value addition. If a person with diabetes invests in lifestyle change, it makes sense to use safer drugs that support the process. Once the lifestyle changes kick in and the glucose levels approach normal, long-term costs come *down*. Patients save money through needing less medication and avoiding expensive organ damage. People value that.

Trying to save a few pennies on pills is a poor long-term strategy; being penny-wise but pound-foolish is what keeps too many people stuck in the vicious cycle of insulin resistance, marching toward progressively increasing glucose levels, medication burden, and devastating complications.

As we talk about common medications for diabetes and their side effects, I'll be sure to touch on cost, but again, I like to focus on the long-term benefits. Let's jump in.

Biguanides: Metformin

Metformin is *the most common drug I use* for people with type 2 diabetes in my practice. It *also helps the insulin resistance seen in polycystic ovarian syndrome (PCOS) and people with type 1* diabetes on very high insulin doses.

Mechanism of action: Metformin improves insulin sensitivity by helping insulin do its job more efficiently. Scientists are still not exactly sure what metformin does inside the cell to achieve this and are also looking into any longevity benefits it may offer. We do know that metformin improves insulin sensitivity inside the liver and reduces the liver's tendency, as the friendly glucose-provider, to make excessive amounts of glucose. *This is the first drug of choice in diabetes* and insulin resistance from a safety, efficacy, and cost profile, with a long safety track record of use in millions of people.

Possible common side effects: You may experience an upset stomach, reduced appetite, nausea, diarrhea, or vitamin B12 deficiency. The stomach side effects usually settle in a few weeks and can be prevented by a slow, gradual increase in dose, and taking it with food may reduce stomach upset. It is safe to take this during a fast, and a teaspoon of chia seeds or freshly ground flaxseed powder in a glass of water will expand to a jelly that can reduce any stomach upset with the dose. *A minority of people in my practice, particularly the elderly, have had to stop metformin because of unacceptable diarrhea or weight loss.*

Effect on weight: Neutral or weight loss. Fascinatingly, new research suggests that metformin may have protective effects on loss of muscle (the friendly glucose-taker) in older adults.[37]

Safety: Metformin does not cause hypoglycemia when taken as a single prescription. It may be used in pregnancy and breastfeeding, and may restore ovulation in a woman with insulin resistance, causing restoration of fertility and unexpected pregnancy if sexually active and not using contraception.

Dosing: 500–1,000 mg twice a day

Cost: Low

Precautions: The risk of lactic acidosis seems extremely rare and I have not seen a single instance in my practice yet, but in cases of reduced kidney function, you need to adjust the dose.

DPP-4 inhibitors: Sitagliptin, linagliptin, vildagliptin, teneligliptin, saxagliptin, alogliptin

I could keep listing more, as cousins keep entering the pipeline, but I prefer using medications with a longer track record and don't feel obliged to rush to start prescribing every new drug on the market just because it gets newly approved. Long-term safety data helps build confidence in a molecule, and like I said—don't take cheap drugs just because they're cheap.

I use dipeptidyl peptidase 4 (DPP-4) inhibitors as a step-two drug if the person with type 2 diabetes *needs more than metformin while working on lifestyle change,* as it makes sense to use medication to support the process. The goal should be to reduce long-term medication costs by tapering down the dose once the lifestyle changes kick in, eventually stopping the medication when glucose levels approach normal levels.

Mechanism of action: DPP-4 inhibitors work on the incretin pathway and help incretins stay in the system for longer. Incretins are gut hormones that help insulin do its job more effectively; they lower glucagon levels, and glucagon is a hormone that counterbalances insulin.

Effect on weight: Neutral

Safety: DPP-4 does not typically cause hypoglycemia when taken as a single prescription or with metformin. We don't have enough human pregnancy data.

Dosing: Different for different gliptins, and needs adjustment for liver and kidney disease

Cost: High

Possible common side effects: Headache, joint pain, runny nose, cold-like symptoms, rash

Rare but important possible severe side effects: Pancreatitis, kidney damage, severe rash, heart failure, and rarely, muscle damage (rhabdomyolysis)

- While rare, *severe pancreatic damage on DPP-4 inhibitors is possible.* I have one patient who had been taking a gliptin for type 2 diabetes for many years, did not drink alcohol, and led a very disciplined lifestyle. He developed pancreatitis that was severe enough that his pancreas (the friendly glucose regulator) lost the ability to make enough insulin, and he became dependent on insulin to manage his glucose levels. Although these incidents are rare, I try to get people off gliptins as soon as the lifestyle changes kick in to reduce any possibility of medication side effects. This is the reason why I only prescribe medication in the context of a longer association with ongoing coaching, to help my patients work on lifestyle change, so that I can help them move toward better health with less medication.

- *Mild pancreatic damage on DPP-4 inhibitors is also possible.* I had one patient who came to me with uncontrolled type 2 diabetes with a low-normal C-peptide. She was sure she did not want to start insulin and insisted on getting off her gliptin because she wanted to see if her C-peptide would improve. We worked on lifestyle change, and I stopped her gliptin.

I cannot explain how or why, but her C-peptide actually came up from 0.99 to 1.99 ng/mL—not the trend I expected from a "failing" pancreas. Since DPP-4 inhibitors are known to rarely cause severe pancreatic inflammation (pancreatitis) and the C-peptide test tells you about the pancreatic reserve of beta cells, I began to wonder. Is it possible that DPP-4 inhibitors are causing some low-level pancreatic inflammation in people that is not getting picked up on in routine monitoring? The prevalent observation in the world of diabetes treatment is that eventually, uncontrolled diabetes results in pancreatic beta-cell failure—are drugs playing any role?

SGLT-2 inhibitors: Canagliflozin, dapagliflozin, empagliflozin

Similar to DPP-4 inhibitors, more cousins keep entering the market. **Sodium-glucose cotransporter 2 (SGLT-2) inhibitors** have become popular thanks to their additional effects on kidney health, heart health, weight and blood pressure.

I use these drugs as a **step-three drug** *when metformin plus a DPP-4 inhibitor or glucagon-like peptide 1 (GLP-1) agonist is not enough* while the person is working on lifestyle change, but I am uncomfortable continuing these drugs indefinitely. My focus remains on helping people get off these drugs as soon as possible by coaching them on safer lifestyle changes that naturally lower glucose levels, body fat, and blood pressure as described throughout this book.

Mechanism of action: These medications work by blocking the SGLT-2 transporter in the kidney so that more sodium and glucose are excreted and removed from the body as waste through the urine. Some of these drugs have gotten the nod for providing cardiac and kidney protection in people with type 2 diabetes and renal or cardiac disease, but you know how I feel about waiting till organs get damaged before reconsidering treatment plans.

Effect on weight: Can cause initial weight loss and lowering of blood pressure, presumably as a result of salt losses. There is growing concern that some of the weight loss on SGLT-2 inhibitors may be due to loss of lean muscle mass, which is a metabolically expensive approach.[38] I cannot justify indefinitely prescribing something that costs muscle. The long term value equation doesn't add up for me when I think about the person's need to preserve muscle for healthy aging and glucose metabolism.

Safety: Does not typically cause hypoglycemia when taken as a single prescription or with metformin. Not enough human pregnancy data.

Dosing: Different for different SGLT-2 inhibitors

Cost: High

Possible common side effects: Urinary tract infection or fungal infection of the skin around the groin and genital areas in men and women, slight weight loss that includes muscle loss, low blood pressure, digestive complaints[39,40]

Rare but important possible severe side effects: Severe urinary tract infection, diabetic ketoacidosis (DKA), severe infection of genitals, loss of bone density, fracture, risk of lower-limb amputation, pancreatitis, kidney damage, kidney cancer

- Everyone loves a pill that causes weight loss. But I am not okay with close to half of that being muscle loss. I don't like prescribing drugs that can potentially harm the kidney or pancreas or cause bone loss, and I don't like prescribing things that cause infection in around 10 percent of people. With India's hot, humid, and sweaty climate, the infection rates already seem to be higher than 10 percent.

GLP-1 agonists: Liraglutide, exenatide, dulaglutide, semaglutide

I used to prescribe cousins of these drugs more often over a decade ago, especially when I was working in the United States; still more are entering the market. Back then, my training had taught me that these are a great option when someone with type 2 diabetes also needs to lose weight. They told us you could get two effects with one drug and back then, I didn't really focus on whether that weight loss was truly fat loss—we just looked at the scale.

In regards to **glucagon-like peptide-1 (GLP-1) agonists,** I still *occasionally use dulaglutide and liraglutide*, with the constant nudge for my patients to intensify lifestyle changes so that I can deprescribe them. When I prescribed these medications earlier in my practice for Indian people with type 2 diabetes and obesity, they experienced more gastric side effects like intolerable nausea and vomiting. Once I discovered the power and safety of lifestyle change, my need to prescribe the entire class of GLP-1 agonists went down drastically and I use them much less frequently now. People love this drug class for its effect on appetite and cravings; my patients all report reduced appetite after getting enough protein in their meals. Most of their "food noise" has settled by addressing our lifestyle wheels. I have a basic question for you here: Would you want your appetite to be reduced by medication, or by food?

Mechanism of action: These work on the incretin pathway by acting like (or mimicking) the incretin GLP-1. That's what agonists or analogs do. They mimic and support normal processes. Incretins are gut hormones that collaborate with the pancreas (our friendly glucose regulator). They help insulin do its job more effectively and they lower glucagon levels; glucagon is a pancreatic hormone that has effects opposite to insulin. GLP-1 agonists slow down the emptying of the stomach, reduce appetite, and keep people feeling full for a longer time. Some of these drugs have gotten the nod for providing cardiac and kidney protection in people with type 2 diabetes who have established renal or cardiac disease, or cardiac risk.

Effect on weight: Can cause weight loss as a result of initial nausea and loss of appetite. Most of the weight is regained when the dose is stopped. The drug manufacturers suggest people should *take this as long as they want to maintain weight loss.* I'm pretty sure nobody wants the fat to come back, and we have no long-term safety data on what it means to take these drugs indefinitely. Unfortunately, a significant portion of the weight loss is from lean muscle mass, which can be metabolically harmful long term.

Safety: Does not typically cause hypoglycemia when taken as a single prescription or with metformin. Human pregnancy data not available.

Dosing: Most of these are injections, daily or weekly. Researchers are working on once-a-month options. Semaglutide comes in injection and tablet form and recently became extremely popular for off-label use as a weight-loss drug.

Cost: High

Possible side effects: Nausea, vomiting, gastritis, loss of appetite, constipation. People experience less nausea when a low initial dose is gradually increased over a few weeks.

Rare but important possible severe side effects: Pancreatitis, thyroid cancer, kidney damage, muscle loss, paralysis of the stomach (gastroparesis), paralysis of the small intestine (ileus), reflux of stomach contents into the lungs during anesthesia (aspiration)[41,42]

Take caution with the GLP-1 craze, as semaglutide is very popular right now as a "magic" weight-loss drug. Most people want to lose weight, and many are willing to try it, so it's important you decide with your doctor whether this is an option for you after you get all the facts. If you are one of the people whose life has been changed for the better by taking these medications, I am glad you have found what works for you. Celebrities talking about it in the news, healthcare professionals willing to prescribe it off-label, and sales of the drug in the gray market have resulted in shortages of the drug, to the extent that people with diabetes could not get it for their glucose needs. Desperate consumers have even been sold counterfeit versions. It's intense.

When people at a party ask me if I will prescribe a GLP-1 analog for weight loss, my answer is a flat-out no. It would be against my ethics to prescribe something without an endpoint in sight, without a detailed conversation with the person so that they can introspect on their lifestyle in the way we have covered in this book. I won't prescribe a drug that exposes people to possible serious side effects when I have safer, effective lifestyle options available that can be continued indefinitely as a way of life. It's possible that getting on a weight loss drug misses healing the person's relationship with their food and their body. If that conversation needs to happen in the distant future when they want to get off the drug without regaining weight, what stops us from working on it now? If that means the person needs to work with a doctor other than me who feels right about prescribing the medication, that's between that patient and their doctor, and I truly wish them well.

I am thankful that science is continuously advancing and providing more options for people to find what works for them, and I have found a way that allows me to do no harm, uphold my oath, and work with people in a way that is deeply rewarding and fulfilling for us all. I see no point in judging or having an ego clash with someone who is feeling better in a way that works for them. You do you. We've had the opportunity to work with people who benefited from GLP-1 therapy but wanted to find a way off of the medication without having the weight all come back, because remember, the manufacturer says *this medication has to be continued if you want continued weight loss benefits.* People who stop the drug have seen that the weight comes back. GLP-1 agonist supporters argue that if you stop your healthy habits, the weight and diabetes will come back. Yes. Correct, and throughout this book, we have discussed how to get out of yo-yo habits. We have worked with people who want to transition off the GLP-1 agonist to reduce side effects, while maintaining fat loss and muscle gains. Deprescription and off-ramping of GLP-1 analogs is possible when you find a sustainable lifestyle that works for you.

Sulfonylureas and glinides: Glimepiride, gliclazide, glyburide, gilbenclamide, glipizide, repaglinide

I've barely used **sulfonylureas** *and* **glinides** *since my training days.*

Mechanism of action: These drugs stimulate the pancreas to secrete (release) more insulin independently of the blood glucose level.

Effect on weight: Weight gain

Safety: Can cause hypoglycemia between meals or fasting. Inadequate human pregnancy data available. May cause hypoglycemia in the newborn.

Dosing: Different for different molecules

Cost: Low (repaglinide is the most expensive in this group)

Possible common side effects: Hypoglycemia, weight gain

Rare but important possible severe side effects: Severe hypoglycemia, reduced bone marrow function. *Long-term use seems linked to pancreatic beta-cell failure.*

I stopped prescribing these drugs over a decade ago when I realized how they were keeping my patients on lifelong medications, with no diabetes remission in sight. They work initially to get the pancreas (our friendly glucose regulator) to release more insulin, so everyone is happy with the improvement in glucose levels, and the doctor's prescription looks powerful and impressive. But these drugs seem to be directly linked with long-term failure of the pancreatic beta cells that secrete insulin causing some people to eventually become insulin dependent. Does that count as diabetes treatment?[43]

I saw how the medication was causing people's glucose levels to quickly move toward normal, but the levels would not stabilize there. During the initial years of the medication working, the glucose would crash below normal, causing terrible symptoms of hypoglycemia. If a person experienced it even once, they learned that they should eat more carbohydrate-rich foods to prevent low glucose levels, like Marco's mom. This meant they were eating more food or midmeal snacks than planned, just to avoid the side effects of medication. The sulfonylurea had turned type 2 diabetes from a high-glucose problem into an "avoid low-glucose" problem.

What was worse, eating the extra food and snacks caused more weight gain, and if their baseline habits stayed exactly the same over the years, the disease progressed, and they kept needing more prescriptions! It felt insane that a prescription was forcing someone who has excess body fat to eat more foods which just worsened the problem. I rapidly de-prescribed these drugs, cleared a path for patients that did not include hypoglycemia, and started reassuring my patients that it was safe to reduce carbohydrates and snacks.

This opened up the entire range of possibilities for reducing medication and supporting them with behavior change. A common argument I hear from doctors is that these drugs can be used long term because they are not expensive. I don't make budgeting decisions on behalf of the patient without a conversation with them. If your doctor offered you two choices: a cheaper drug that might cause hypoglycemia, weight gain or long term pancreatic failure; versus possible short-term use of slightly more expensive drugs that don't cause hypoglycemia or weight gain, while you make lifestyle changes to improve glucose levels so that you can hopefully stop long-term medication—which would you choose? What do you value?

I have never seen a patient request a cheaper drug just for the sake of saving money on tablets. People value getting better with less medication. When informed about side-effect profiles and chances of turning diabetes around, most people opt for increasing the dose of lifestyle change. Everyone knows how devastating diabetes complications can be. They want help deciding the right approach for their situation.

Alpha-glucosidase inhibitors: voglibose, acarbose, miglitol

Like sulfonylureas and glinides, *I don't use the **alpha-glucosidase inhibitor** drug class at all anymore.* Put carbs in your mouth only to malabsorb them after you swallow them? Sounds like a prescription for mind-body disconnect and a disordered relationship with food.

Mechanism of action: These work by delaying digestion and absorption of carbohydrates that have been eaten.

Effect on weight: Neutral

Safety: Do not typically cause hypoglycemia when taken as a single prescription or with metformin. Human pregnancy data not available.

Dosing: Different for different molecules

Cost: Low

Possible common side effects: Gas, diarrhea, and bloating as a result of fermentation of undigested carbohydrates. The drug stops you from digesting them, so the gut bacteria do.

One retrospective study showed an association of acarbose use with decreased muscle mass, handgrip strength, and gait speed.[44] Acarbose has also been associated with liver injury and paralysis of the small intestine.[45] Seems like a risky option to put the carbs in your mouth and then block your digestive tract from doing its thing. Oops.

Thiazolidinediones: Pioglitazone, rosiglitazone

Thiazolidinediones and I don't mix. Something that causes weight gain, bone loss, fluid retention, and possibly cancer and heart attacks? I know that lifestyle change is stronger and safer, so *I don't touch this drug class at all anymore.*

Mechanism of action: Works by increasing insulin sensitivity

Effect on weight: Can cause weight gain and fluid retention

Safety: Does not cause hypoglycemia when taken alone or with metformin. May help fatty liver. Pregnancy safety data not clear. May restore ovulation in a woman with insulin resistance, causing restoration of fertility and unexpected pregnancy if sexually active and not using contraception.

Dosing: Pioglitazone comes in seven-and-a-half, fifteen, and thirty milligram preparations; lower doses can cause less fluid retention.

Cost: Moderate

Possible common side effects: Bone loss and increased fracture risk. Can trigger heart failure. Pioglitazone has been linked with bladder cancer. Rosiglitazone has been linked with increased rates of heart attacks (myocardial infarction) and has been withdrawn from many markets.

Last but not least: Insulin

I rarely use **insulin** if a person with type 2 diabetes has a C-peptide level that confirms a working pancreas. *The rare times I prescribe it, it's for a specific short-term reason* with a clear-cut plan to taper it off as soon as possible. We will also cover insulin in more detail later when we get to type 1 diabetes, where it becomes a lifesaving prescription. In type 2 diabetes, however, the brief insulin dosing is to reduce the effects of glucose toxicity while the person is investing in habit changes.[46]

Mechanism of action: Pharmaceutical insulin acts like natural active insulin to increase glucose uptake into cells, reduce glucose production by the liver, block the breakdown of body fat, and regulate glucose metabolism. Pharmaceutical insulin is active when it's injected; it does not have C-peptide attached.*

Effect on weight: Can cause weight gain, particularly accumulation of toxic visceral fat with increasing inches around the belly when used in

---

* The Nobel prize in 1977 was awarded to Yalow, Guillemin and Schally for developing the radioimmunoassay that allowed testing of levels of protein based hormones. Combined with the separate Nobel prizes for the discovery of insulin and sequencing its molecular protein structure, multiple Nobel laureates paved the way for making life-saving synthetic insulin as we know it today.

high doses.

Safety: Can cause hypoglycemia. The dose needs to be adjusted by the doctor to prevent hypoglycemia. Can be used in pregnancy under supervision.

Dosing: Differs for different insulins and from person to person. Need to reduce dose in case of hypoglycemia or kidney disease.

Cost: Older insulins=low; newer insulins=high

Possible common side effects: Hypoglycemia, weight gain, lipodystrophy (inflammation of the fat tissue under the skin at the injection site that causes erratic absorption).

Rare but important possible severe side effects: Severe allergic reactions

If using insulin to treat insulin resistance, the problem only gets worse, requiring higher doses to keep the glucose levels in the blood "normal."[47] Where is all the glucose going? Inside the cells, where it is toxic! Diabetes causes complications in the entire body largely due to cells across the entire body being exposed to the toxic effects of high glucose and high insulin. To take the water park analogy from Part 7.2 even further, after the lazy river is being swamped by a stampede of people chaotically swarming into the water, the management asks their "lifeguard and engineering service (aka insulin)" to send reinforcements. Instead of the few happy lifeguards who easily keep the lazy river moving smoothly, now you have an *army* of lifeguards, who keep scooping up the extra people and stuffing them with brute force into *other* water rides and attractions across the entire amusement park. Those visitors are not allowed to leave the other rides, because the corporate headquarters are satisfied with the optics, adding more lifeguards when needed as long as the river doesn't look crowded. Is anyone actually having fun anymore?

7.9: Other medications every person with diabetes is likely to be prescribed at some point

As we just discussed, one of the main reasons that diabetes causes complications in the entire body is because over time, the cells across the entire body are being exposed to the toxic effects of high glucose and high insulin. In addition to muscular, hepatic (liver), and pancreatic complications as they relate to glucose taking, providing, and regulating, diabetes can also affect the heart, kidneys, and nervous system.

When this happens, there's an array of medications doctors can prescribe. As with everything else, we want to make sure we are aware of how each works, and what possible side effects there might be.

Medications for heart health

When it comes to heart health, medications may not be prescribed just for the heart itself, but also for the blood the heart pumps around. If you recall, there are cardiac events associated with changes in the blood, and here, we're specifically talking about blood pressure and lipids (blood fats). Many prescriptions for the heart are targeting cholesterol and other molecules in the blood.

Angiotensin-converting enzyme (ACE) inhibitors: Enalapril, ramipril, lisinopril, benazepril

Angiotensin-converting enzyme inhibitors still have more cousins entering the market. These drugs are focused on angiotensin, which is a hormone that regulates blood pressure, and therefore has an impact on cardiac health.

Mechanism of action: As the name implies, these block the *conversion* of angiotensin I into angiotensin II, thereby lowering blood pressure. They also help reduce protein spillage into the urine, which slows the progression of diabetic kidney disease, and they offer additional cardiac protection.

Effect on weight: Neutral

Safety: Can cause dry cough. Need to monitor blood pressure, potassium, and renal (kidney) function when starting. Additive effect if taken with angiotensin receptor blocker (ARB). Avoid in pregnancy.

Dosing: Different for different molecules

Cost: Low

Possible side effects: Can cause elevated potassium levels and worsening creatinine in specific conditions. Need to be taken under supervision of a qualified physician.

Angiotensin receptor blockers for blood pressure and nephropathy: Losartan, olmesartan, valsartan

We also keep seeing new iterations of **angiotensin receptor blockers** entering the pharmaceutical market.

Mechanism of action: As the name implies, these block angiotensin II *receptors*, thereby lowering blood pressure. They also help reduce protein spillage into the urine, which slows the progression of diabetic kidney disease, and offer additional cardiac protection.

Effect on weight: Neutral

Safety: Can cause joint/musculoskeletal pain, gastrointestinal symptoms. Need to monitor blood pressure, potassium, and renal function when starting. Additive effect if taken with ACE inhibitor. Avoid in pregnancy.

Dosing: Different for different molecules

Cost: Low to moderate

Possible side effects: Can cause elevated potassium levels and worsening creatinine in specific conditions. Need to be taken under supervision of a qualified physician.

I work aggressively with my patients on reversing insulin resistance, a key driver of heart attacks. I discuss with each of my patients the data behind statins, and we review their goals and priorities. Some of them opt to take the statin, and some of them opt out. It's my job to give them the available information so that we can make a decision together. Whichever way they decide, I support their efforts to improve their lifestyle. I always work with their cardiologist and don't claim to know everything about atherosclerosis. I do not consider low-density lipoprotein (LDL) and total cholesterol to be nature's most reliable and primary murder weapons, and I am convinced we need a better understanding of what drives cardiovascular risk. A statin reduces your chance of a heart attack if your diabetes is not okay. Since you're reading this book, I know you want to get your diabetes to be well-managed so that you can reduce your cardiac risk.

Statins for cholesterol: Rosuvastatin, atorvastatin, lovastatin, simvastatin, pravastatin

We agree that uncontrolled diabetes is a definite cardiovascular risk factor. Most people with uncontrolled diabetes are prescribed a statin indefinitely, encouraging even more variations to enter the market.

The guidelines say everyone with diabetes should be given a statin to prevent the first heart attack because having diabetes is equivalent to having cardiac risk. The data says taking a statin after your first heart attack or stroke improves clinical outcomes and reduces your risk of a second heart attack. These guidelines and data make convincing a doctor to stop an existing statin prescription quite difficult, because no doctor wants to be the last person who touched a patient's prescription before something bad happened to their heart. So, many feel it's safer to do nothing—which means keeping you on the prescription once you're on it.

There is currently no data to clarify what happens to cardiac risk if you turn around diabetes to achieve a hemoglobin A1C (HbA1c) of below 5.7 percent through lifestyle change and then stop the statin.

That said, even with my bias, I believe that *if someone is doing their best and lifestyle changes are taking time to reverse insulin resistance, then they might benefit from staying on a statin.* I do prescribe statins on an individual case by case basis after an in-depth conversation with my patient.

Common **side effects of statins** include *muscle damage* (one musketeer), *liver damage* (another musketeer), *pancreatitis* (the third musketeer!), *brain fog,* *confusion, insomnia, cognitive impairment, headache, dizziness, abdominal pain, joint pain, constipation, kidney damage* or *changes in urine*.

Additionally, another side effect could be new-onset diabetes.

Considering that statins are now considered to cause diabetes in a handful of people who didn't have diabetes in the first place, it feels conflicting to plan to keep someone on a statin forever. The justification seems to be circular: if a statin prevents a heart attack, it's fine to give the patient diabetes as a side effect. Even though diabetes is considered equivalent to cardiac risk, we have you covered because you are on the statin!

After evaluating your individual risks and benefits with your doctor, these will still remain individual decisions. You can try discussing cardiac risk calculators like QRISK3 with your doctor when deciding whether to start a statin to prevent the first heart attack or stroke, while also, hopefully turning around diabetes.

Fenofibrate

This is a medication that *reduces triglyceride levels*. I have not had to prescribe it in over ten years because reducing carbs, sugar, processed food, and alcohol brings triglycerides down naturally, rapidly, and safely. **Fenofibrate** comes with *possible side effects like abdominal pain, headache, nausea, constipation, a drop in high-density lipoprotein* (HDL)*, and inflammation of the liver, muscle, and pancreas* (all three musketeers!).

I can't justify using a drug that can inflame all of the three musketeers and also cause a drop in helpful HDL; remember from Part 7.3 that we want HDL to be higher. Also, being on both a statin and fenofibrate together can worsen muscle inflammation.

Medications for kidney health

Allopurinol is a medication that **reduces uric acid levels**. Uric acid is implicated in gout attacks. I have not had to prescribe it in over ten years because reducing carbs, sugar, processed food, and alcohol brings uric acid down naturally, rapidly, and safely.

This drug comes with possible side effects of reducing bone marrow function, drop in blood cell counts, kidney damage, rash, diarrhea and elevated liver enzymes (one of our musketeers in trouble again). Strangely, Epocrates and PubMed mention a *worsening of gout* as a common side effect, for which an anti-inflammatory should be prescribed in advance.[48]

Febuxostat is also a medication that *reduces uric acid levels*. I also haven't had to prescribe it in over ten years, because reducing carbs, sugar, processed food and alcohol brings uric acid down naturally, rapidly, and safely.

This drug comes with possible side effects of elevated liver enzymes and liver toxicity (again), muscle damage (a second musketeer), reducing bone marrow function, drop in blood cell counts, rash, and kidney damage. I am amazed at the number of people with protein deficient diets and insulin resistance who faithfully take febuxostat for their uric acid, while holding onto misplaced fear about protein supplements. There has never been any proof that fixing protein malnutrition harms the kidney or raises uric acid! Febuxostat, on the other hand, has kidney damage listed as a possible side effect. Do they know that their fear of protein might be imagined, while the risk of febuxostat is real?

Worsening of gout is a common side effect; remember it's being given as treatment for elevated uric acid levels to reduce gout risks! Rarely, this drug is associated with an increased risk of heart attack and stroke. In patients with existing cardiac disease, there is increased risk of cardiovascular death.

Umm, what?

The drug comes with an FDA black box warning mentioning that **people receiving febuxostat had higher rates of "heart-related death or death from all causes."**[9] We already agreed in the statin section that having diabetes is equivalent to having cardiac disease, so I really don't understand how this drug exists on the market or why people with uncontrolled diabetes are given this drug so freely.

Medications for neurological health

Here, we are mainly concerned with prescriptions for neuropathy but unfortunately, none of the available options give great results. The types of drug categories used are so varied that it seems like doctors don't really know exactly what they are targeting. They seem forced to try whatever works, even if it's not FDA approved.

The range includes seizure medications like pregabalin or gabapentin, or antidepressants *like selective serotonin reuptake inhibitors (SSRIs) or tricyclics*, and anesthetic medications like *lidocaine*. I have not met a single person who swears that taking these medications made their symptoms disappear or changed their life drastically for the better. The intensity of symptoms may have reduced, but they never felt normal. The side-effect profile has always made them an inferior choice for me, especially when my patients' neuropathy has consistently gotten better through lifestyle change without prescribing anything specific for the nerves.

The wide range of medications is because there are different ways in which diabetic neuropathy can manifest, depending on which part of the nervous system is most affected.

Different nerves perform different functions for us; some control the sensations from the feet, the sensations and responses of sexual organs, the movement of food forward along the gut, blood pressure, heart-rate variability and stress responses. Your sense of position in a three-dimensional space, along with your hearing, vision and eye movements, are all steered by separate nerves as well.

If no specific type of nerve damage is the villain then no singular medication can be the hero, and I see a sad paradox when people with decades of uncontrolled diabetes need various specialists. These different doctors prescribe various drugs to block or manage the symptoms of neuropathy in different regions of the body. Patients end up taking over eight tablets a day and still feeling like they have been hit by a truck. The intensity of nerve pain or tingling and numbness may have reduced, but they are anything but cured. I haven't needed to prescribe a single drug for neuropathy, and I think it's because the aggressive lifestyle change approach our patients embrace prevents the organ involvement and the related debilitating symptoms from happening in the first place.

I've seen drastic transformations in people who were told they had supposed end-organ damage. It takes many months of stabilizing glucose levels, but I see it happen. Across the board, patients have seen more stable blood pressure and fewer dizzy spells, suggesting possible improvements in autonomic neuropathy. Additionally, they experience less nausea and vomiting caused by a stagnation of food in the stomach, without being prescribed any motility agents. Along with the lifestyle changes in this book, we also leveraged the fact that *progressive muscle relaxation and mindfulness meditation have been shown to improve the fatigue severity and pain intensity of patients with diabetic neuropathy.*[50]

Time and time again, people have proved to me that improving diabetic neuropathy without medication is possible. In the case of a senior citizen I worked with, she started strength training and reported quicker reflexes, a steadier gait, and a reduced tendency to fall while washing her face.

Another lady was able to enjoy the sensation returning back in the soles of her feet. Originally experiencing numbness in eight of ten sites on her feet, upon examination with the monofilament again, she was now numb at only three of the sites! She reexperienced feeling the location of her footwear and sensing the floor beneath her feet again, instead of feeling like she was walking on clouds.

One case in particular was so validating. Over the course of working together, I worked with a man who was told he was gradually going deaf as a result of diabetes. As he improved his lifestyle, I noticed the improvement in his ability to hear without a hearing aid! At first, he needed to shout during our consultation, but within a year, his indoor talking voice came down to normal decibel levels because he could hear us better.

It made it a little less surprising when the ability to hear was restored in a twenty-six-year-old man with uncontrolled type 1 diabetes. After waking up suddenly with a loss of hearing from one of his AirPods, he needed a course of high-dose steroids. During that time, he embarked on an extended fast of fifty-four hours.

We managed to keep his insulin requirements low, despite the steroids; he stabilized his glucose levels by focusing on the changes outlined in Part 10 and earlier parts of this book. He started listening to inspirational health-related podcasts and worked on healing his relationship with food and his body. His morning journaling sessions helped him dig deep into his own resources and strengths.

Not every situation needs a complicated prescription. I've seen many patients get relief from the knife-like, burning pain that would jerk them awake at night; they were getting more restful sleep without any painkillers or sedatives—because the burning foot pain had reduced by 60 percent.

You might not need a million medications to address the pain and discomfort of neuropathy if you focus on treating the root causes. The body is always trying to heal and repair. My patients are living proof, but all I can do is share their stories with you in hopes that they inspire you as much as they amazed me.

7.10: Other common medications and their side effects

As life goes on, it's normal to get sick from time to time. From insomnia to heartburn, bloating to bone loss–some things are inevitable. When you take an over-the-counter (OTC) or prescription medication to ease your discomfort, you typically don't think too much about the side effects. While you may take medication to recover from a headache or upset stomach, sometimes that same medication can *cause the symptom you were trying to treat!*

Just look at how many times our trusted antacids show up on the list below (yes, you read that right, antacids)!

While this is not a complete list, it includes other medications you might come across. This list is to get you curious about how they compare and interact with your diabetes-related medications.

Abdominal pain, nausea, and vomiting are side effects of *antacids, painkillers, antidiarrhea medication, laxatives, antibiotics, cholesterol medication* (statins), *iron supplements, metformin, and allopurinol.*

Acid reflux or acidity is a side effect of *antibiotics, painkillers, osteoporosis medication, iron supplements, steroids,* and *metformin.*

Bloating is a side effect of *voglibose, acarbose, fiber supplements, aspirin, antacids, multivitamins,* and *iron supplements.*

Bone loss is a side effect of *pioglitazone, SGLT-2 inhibitors, acid-blocking drugs, high-dose steroids,* and *high-dose thyroid hormone.*

Constipation is a side effect of *antacids, antidepressants, blood pressure medication, pain killers, antihistamines, iron supplements, calcium supplements, diuretics, zolpidem,* and neuropathy medication like *pregabalin.*

Diarrhea is a side effect of *metformin, antacids, antibiotics, painkillers,* and *melatonin.*

Headaches are a side effect of *sedatives, zolpidem, melatonin, rebound* *headache from painkillers, antihistamines,* and neuropathy medication like *pregabalin* (yes, something given for nerve pain can cause a headache).

Insomnia (including poor sleep, daytime sleepiness, brain fog, and fatigue) **and cognitive or mood impairment** (including confusion, anxiety, lethargy, drugged feeling, and abnormal thinking) are side effects of *zolpidem and sedatives* (yes, sleeping medications can cause insomnia), *anxiety medication* and *antidepressants* (yes, medications for anxiety and depression can cause anxiety, depression, and suicidal ideation), *melatonin* (yes, the jetlag hormone can cause rebound insomnia), *antihistamines, statins,* and *pregabalin (yes something given for nerve pain can affect your brain).*

Liver damage is a side effect of *statins, contraceptives, antibiotics, uric acid medication, seizure medication,* and *acetaminophen/paracetamol.*

Muscle pain and joint pains are side effects of *statins, antibiotics, osteoporosis medication, isotretinoin,* and *pregabalin* (yes, even though it's often prescribed for pain).

Sexual dysfunction is a side effect of *antihistamines, antidepressants, sedatives, blood pressure medication, spironolactone, antacids, prostate medication,* and *diuretics.*

Unsteady gait, imbalance, and impaired coordination are all side effects of *zolpidem, antihistamines, melatonin, sedatives, anxiety medication, and* neuropathy medication like *pregabalin.*

Weight gain is a side effect of s*ulfonylureas, insulin, blood pressure medications, steroids, migraine medications, antipsychotics, antidepressants, antihistamines, mood stabilizers, neuropathy medications, seizure medications, pioglitazone, rosiglitazone,* and neuropathy medication like *pregabalin.*

Sometimes, despite taking multiple medications and trying various diets to lose weight, it all just becomes unmanageable. When it seems like there is no way to turn around the relentless weight gain, bariatric surgery becomes a last resort for some.

7.11: Prescribing metabolic and bariatric surgery

L et me start by saying: If weight-loss surgery was lifesaving for you, I am thankful.

I, however, have never had to refer someone to bariatric surgery, even as the world is prescribing more and more surgical treatments for weight loss and type 2 diabetes—even to adolescents who have their whole lives ahead of them.

Bariatric surgery has a role in medicine similar to the way an appendectomy does. If your weight has reached a level where your heart, lungs, or other vital organs are struggling to keep up, then it might be a lifesaving procedure for you because you don't have the time or capacity to spend another year trying to lose weight. It is an acute form of treatment that gives rapid results. If the primary problem is a burst appendix, then an appendectomy is curative. One major difference between the two surgeries is that for the appendix, we don't know exactly what lifestyle changes can prevent the appendix from getting inflamed in the first place.

If the primary problem is a chronically imbalanced relationship with food, imbalanced hormones, or impaired awareness of your body, surgery will give you weight loss on the scale but might cause you to lose many other things, too.

I have seen people develop mood disorders, depression, and anxiety, and there have even been case reports of debilitating hypoglycemia, dumping syndrome, bone loss, muscle loss, and malnutrition. In these situations, it doesn't feel like the metabolic surgery fixed the person's metabolism.[51] Sadly, people are at increased risk of reduced quality of life and the development of substance abuse disorders and suicidal ideation postoperatively.[52]

Like they say, bariatric surgery staples your stomach but not your brain. Did we cause bariatric surgery patients harm by replacing addiction to food with something else?

If you are considering bariatric surgery, talk to your doctor and request psychological support to address strategies for obtaining emotional relief, comfort, and pleasure so that you have tools when you won't be able to self-soothe with food. This looks like investigating what your psychosocial support system is; assessing your confidence around foods that trigger overeating; examining how you feel when you see yourself in the mirror; and deciding how will you handle cravings when you know that overeating the cherished food may cause guilt, severe digestive symptoms, or urgent trips to the bathroom.

The **people who decide to work with me on their weight loss** *have either already undergone bariatric surgery and gained all the weight back* (and sometimes more), or *were advised to undergo it*, but decided to work on lifestyle changes instead. I have witnessed people with severe obesity turn around their health one day, one meal, one good night's rest, one walk, and one act of self-care at a time. They have lost anywhere from fifteen to fifty kilograms over eight to twenty-eight months.

The best part is, they don't feel like they are on a diet, they enjoy their new way of life, and they can visualize themselves continuing on that path in a sustainable way going forward. They are done with the yo-yo diets because they changed their relationship with their food and their bodies. They feel in charge of their future and radiate a newfound spark in their lives. It has been nothing short of miraculous for me to witness.

7.12: So what happened to Marco's mom and Rita?

We were able to help Rita after key elements in her story were pieced together. Rita used to be very active and even exercised in the gym when she was in her forties. A few years of stress resulted in depression, and she had stopped exercising. The divalproex she started taking in January for depression had possible side effects of drowsiness, dizziness, blurred vision, constipation, somnolence, depression (!), amnesia, and an abnormal gait.

Sure enough, she had become expressionless and stiff in the first half of 2020. She was like this for months when the solifenacin was started for her "overactive bladder."

The side effects of solifenacin include confusion, drowsiness, blurred vision, constipation, fatigue, and urinary tract infection.

When I zoomed out to review this story, I realized Rita was probably experiencing overlapping side effects of the divalproex and solifenacin, with both causing her to be confused, drowsy, tired, lethargic, and forgetful, along with an abnormal gait and blurred vision.

This must have made her more prone to falling in the bathroom and fracturing her spine.

The urinary urgency may have been a result of the undiagnosed uncontrolled diabetes (her HbA1c was 9.9 percent), causing excess glucose to be excreted in the urine and causing the need to rush to the bathroom.

Her divalproex was probably reducing her agility and ability to reach the toilet on time, and the undiagnosed high blood glucose was adding to her blurred vision.

The perfect recipe for a fall at night in the bathroom.

As I explored her symptoms some more, we discovered that she had been sleeping alone in a separate bedroom, so nobody knew how severely she snored. She looked drowsy to me at one of our visits, and we did a sleep study that revealed undiagnosed sleep apnea—one more reason for her daytime somnolence, drowsiness, low mood, high glucose and impaired decision making. The untreated sleep apnea and high glucose levels gave her two reasons to need to urinate at night. Multiple doctors who had built up a pile of medications that made her worse, not better, had missed so many signs. It felt like a discordant orchestra, where the prescribers for mood, bladder, and diabetes were not talking to each other and treating individual organ systems without looking at what was happening with the patient.

It took us a few months to work with the psychiatrist to taper off the divalproex, but the solifenacin was stopped immediately after we updated the urologist about the high glucose levels. We started her on continuous positive airway pressure (CPAP), her mind was able to focus on lifestyle changes, and her glucose levels came down to 140 mg/dL (7.7 mmol/L) in two weeks with minimal medication.

Rita became a different woman over the coming months. The lethargic, sedentary zoned out person was gone, and she was working with her physiotherapist to rehabilitate herself after the vertebral fracture so that she could resume her workouts. Her mood improved, and her facial expressions were more animated. She was more awake and alert throughout the day as the drowsiness and confusion disappeared.

The family had their Rita back, and Rita had her life back. She started writing poetry again, a hobby she had abandoned years ago. Three years later, she remains off diabetes medication and is now the life of the party, as she always should've been.

It angers me to think how many people are still out there, popping pills daily and turning into placeholders of who they used to be, unaware of the cumulative side effects and drug interactions. The saddest part is that most of them are not even feeling like they are in the best of health despite so many medications. They are taking more than ten pills a day and feeling worse.

That brings us back to Marco's mom.

The family asked me if it was too late to start treatment with me and make lifestyle changes. They were willing to do anything to prevent these scary episodes.

So we checked the C-peptide level, and I was able to tell her *she was insulin resistant, not insulin deficient.* Lifestyle changes helped us reduce her insulin dose and glucose fluctuations.

At eighty-seven years old, she was able to reduce her insulin and improve her health. She didn't feel crazy anymore, and her family didn't feel so frightened leaving her at home and going to work. She was able to go for walks and meet her friends in the local garden.

She's no anomaly. I've seen lifestyle changes help reduce diabetes prescriptions (even insulin) at any age, thereby reducing the frequency of scary, dangerous hypoglycemic episodes and improving the overall quality of life. By working with professionals to assess your lifestyle car and making sure you are calibrated to your goals, nothing is impossible.

Part 7 summary

- Knowing your own glucose levels is the quickest way to evaluate how your habits are silently affecting your diabetes, so that you can decide what you want to change.

- The C-peptide level tells you whether your diabetes can be managed without insulin or not.

- Uric acid, liver enzymes and the triglyceride/HDL ratio are additional clues that can point towards insulin resistance.

- Some medications support your efforts to reduce insulin resistance and some don't.

- Consuming a medication for every symptom runs the risk of missing the root cause, polypharmacy and overlapping side effects.

- If considering an appetite suppressing drug or weight loss surgery, check whether you are doing it from a place of powerlessness or choice, since it's a long-term commitment.

For Bonus Materials, Visit the Website Here:

PART 8

HOW TO WORK
WITH DOCTORS AND
HOSPITALS

8.1: Working with doctors to protect your body

When it comes to the heart, kidneys, liver, bones, and muscles, you can't do it on your own. In order to protect your body and prevent further damage, you'll have to work with doctors to integrate different health screenings into your plan. While the table in Part 7.4 gives a big picture of the options available, I want to expand on some options.

That said, this book does not replace working with a cardiologist or physician who understands metabolic health and can discuss your individual needs and goals when it comes to managing cholesterol, lipids, and statins to reduce cardiovascular risk.

That said, the **noncontroversial way to improve your cardiac health** is to *reduce your insulin resistance, inflammation,* and *blood pressure* through the lifestyle changes you have learned about in this book.

Outside of this guide, there are whole books describing the link between **uric acid**, low energy levels, increased hunger, high blood pressure, weight gain, diabetes, and obesity. *High uric acid inside the cells may actually trigger these problems* by turning on a "fat switch" inside the mitochondria, and though most people only think of uric acid when they experience painful episodes of gout, it turns out that *uric acid is relevant for much more life-threatening reasons.*[1]

Most of the patients I assess have high uric acid levels despite being severely protein deficient. Someone told them to "reduce protein," so they severely minimize their already limited protein intake, leading to further malnutrition, but you can't blame dietary protein for elevated uric acid when you aren't even getting enough protein. It's the same shortcut-thinking as blaming dietary cholesterol for atherosclerosis even though a person is on a very low-fat diet. You are missing the actual driver of your high uric acid levels.

Dr. Richard Johnson, a physician, uric acid researcher, and board member of the Gout Education Society says that being dehydrated, drinking alcohol (especially beer), eating sugar, fructose, high-fructose corn syrup (HFCS), glucose, and starch, drinking liquid sugar in juices and sodas, and eating processed carbs combined with salt are all lifestyle choices that increase uric acid. So when you see high uric acid, first count what your daily protein intake is, and then reduce the foods that are actually known to raise uric acid before you randomly reduce your protein intake.

It works!

The only time I have seen uric acid increase with our lifestyle-change approach was in an 84-year-old Jain monk who worked with us to put his diabetes into remission. He had chronic kidney disease, relied on legumes and dairy as his only protein sources, and was fasting for thirty-six-hours on alternate days. The fasting protocol appealed to him because there is a Jain religious fasting schedule that looks very similar.

The catch was that he was not exercising to increase his muscle mass.

He kept meticulous notes of his progress and always came to our meetings with intelligent questions. He was able to get off insulin and reduce his blood pressure and diabetes medications. He even managed to fight off a bout of COVID before the vaccine was available, which was noteworthy considering that the people at highest mortality risk from COVID were elderly people with metabolic disease. Still, his uric acid kept climbing to concerning levels.

His dedication to his health was obvious. He knew what he wanted and made sure to document everything, which gave me everything I needed to see the big picture. It's patients like these that remind me that a well-informed patient committed to health can be an incredible partner when treating complex metabolic imbalances.

Ultimately, my explanation for his rising uric acid was that he had multiple forces working together. In addition to his advanced age, reduced renal function, and years of poor mitochondrial health, fasting itself can transiently raise uric acid levels as the body recycles old cells and breaks down the DNA into purines and their by-products. Then, take the combination of low muscle mass (severe sarcopenia) from persistent lack of strength training and muscle losses aggravated by fasting without exercise, and mix it in. The final contributor was that his top protein sources were legumes, beans, and milk which were more carbs than protein. This led me to suspect the uric acid was being driven by the carbs, not the protein in his diet.

I finally had to put him on allopurinol to get his uric acid levels down to a safe range. He has been the sole recipient of an allopurinol prescription from me in over a decade. And since I've said it before, I'll say it again—it's important to attempt lifestyle changes under medical supervision so someone can monitor how your body responds and keep you safe.

If you've addressed uric acid, the next thing you should talk to your doctor about when it comes to protecting your cardiovascular health is **c-reactive protein.** Atherosclerosis is a form of chronic inflammation of the vessel wall and since highly sensitive c-reactive protein (hs-CRP) is a marker of inflammation, especially in the vessel walls, an elevated hs-CRP mediated by inflammatory cytokines correlates with cardiac risk.[2,3] It may become elevated after a major illness or infection, so it's best checked when you are feeling well. When CRP levels are high it always helps to make lifestyle changes to reduce insulin resistance, so discuss further evaluation with your doctor and work with them on a lifestyle-change approach to get it down.

My patient Shirin was nervous about her kidney and CRP reports. She had been working with us on increasing her protein intake, and her latest urine reports showed the presence of protein on the computer-generated printout with the number marked in red. These reports suggested high levels of inflammation and a worrisome effect of diabetes on her kidney health. She wanted to double-check if she should stop eating all protein, like some of her well-wishers were insisting; so of course, we started working through the lifestyle changes discussed in this book.

To illustrate how stopping all protein wasn't necessarily the solution, I asked her to consider that if someone is injured in a car accident and is brought to the hospital with severe blood loss, would you offer them a blood transfusion, or would you say giving blood is bad for them because they are spilling blood? Similarly, uncontrolled diabetes harmed the mitochondria in the kidney filter, but the protein spilling into the urine does not mean dietary protein has harmed the kidney.[4]

Because diabetes can cause silent kidney damage, the best way to protect your kidneys is for a doctor to screen for it so you can catch it early. Doctors will likely recommend an analysis of the *estimated glomerular filtration rate (eGFR), serum creatinine, and urinary microalbumin-creatinine ratio* (MAC), so let's get an understanding of what these say about kidney health.

The **estimated glomerular filtration rate** (eGFR) formula factors in the effect of age, gender, creatinine, and body weight, and you don't want to wait till the eGFR starts to decline.

In fact, the first stage of diabetic kidney damage involves an *increase* in eGFR as the kidneys work hard to filter and throw glucose into the urine. Gaining muscle mass can increase serum creatinine, but does not mean there is kidney damage, so the eGFR is a better estimate of your kidney function than **serum creatinine** alone.

In fact, people with sarcopenia have low creatinine levels because creatinine levels are proportional to muscle mass. If the serum creatinine has gone up in the elderly in spite of age-related muscle loss, that means the kidney filtration rate has probably dropped quite a bit. Work with your physician or nephrologist on this.

In order to assess the **urinary microalbumin-creatinine ratio**, the urine sample provided needs to be a clean-catch midstream one. The result can be inaccurate if there is contamination, a delay in processing the sample, menstrual periods, urinary infection, or kidney stones.

Regardless, if any of these tests show protein in the urine it *doesn't automatically mean you have to reduce protein* in your diet. Always count your protein intake to make sure you are getting enough, and reduce your dietary carbs and sugar to improve your kidney function.[5]

You will need to work with your **physician** and possibly a **nephrologist** to manage glucose and blood pressure if you have diabetic nephropathy, and the medications for this were discussed in Part 7.9. I have a handful of anecdotes of working with people with very advanced kidney damage who did what they could to slow the progression toward dialysis. Ideally, we want to prevent this kind of permanent damage from happening in the first place by applying the lifestyle changes mentioned in this book; the good news is that these same changes can be applied to help protect the liver.

More people are developing fatty liver worldwide which may be the reason why, over the years, the "normal range" upper-limit cutoff for the liver enzymes **alanine aminotransferase** (ALT) and **aspartate aminotransferase** (AST) has steadily crept up from twenty-five to forty.[6]

Insulin resistance is a primary risk factor for fatty liver, also called nonalcoholic fatty liver disease (NAFLD); this name was coined because findings of fat infiltration in the liver were first noticed in people with alcoholism. As case numbers grew, physicians and hepatologists (liver specialists) suspected their patients were just secretly drinking and not telling the truth; it turned out people weren't drinking, and had a fatty liver anyway.

More than 70 percent of people with type 2 diabetes have NAFLD, which is becoming a leading cause of liver fibrosis, liver failure, and liver cancer. Children are getting it, too, with NAFLD rates going up by 20 percent in the last decade, correlating to the rapid influx of processed grains and sugars in mainstream food guidelines.[7]

This is why people with diabetes are overrepresented on liver transplant waiting lists.[8] Everyone with diabetes should have their **Fibrosis-4 score** (FIB-4) calculated (using age, AST, ALT, and platelets) by their doctor as a screening test for liver fibrosis.

Although NAFLD is classically associated with type 2 diabetes (insulin resistance), a recent study found NAFLD in 20 percent of people with type 1 diabetes—a rate of one in five.[9] This is startling, considering that type 1 diabetes starts as a result of insulin deficiency and insulin sensitivity.

Why does this happen? How? It's simple, people with type 1 diabetes are just as vulnerable to lifestyle diseases that cause insulin resistance, and that's why we want doctors to screen everyone, because the effects of diabetes don't discriminate.

We've talked about protein so much, it shouldn't surprise you that I also recommend having your doctor screen you for muscle loss and osteoporosis. Your primary doctor or orthopedic specialist usually does this.

The test is done on a dual-energy X-ray absorption (DEXA) machine designed to scan for osteoporosis, but for a little extra time, money, and radiation exposure (less than three additional hours of daily life at sea level), **you can ask the doctor to add a body composition analysis (BCA) to your DEXA scan.** The BCA gives you an estimate of the percentage of lean muscle tissue versus fat mass you have at various regions of the body. While it can't exactly differentiate between subcutaneous and visceral fat, it can give a general sense of how much of your body is made of fat and whether it's more of an android distribution (belly fat/apple-shaped) or a gynoid distribution (butt fat/pear-shaped).

We want to monitor these number trends over time, looking for an increase in lean muscle mass and a drop in fat mass, especially from the android region. This test is very operator dependent and provides more information when it is repeated after at least a year to check for interval changes, so it's best to do it *on the same machine* and, ideally, *with the same technician*. This is more useful than just looking at the number on your weighing scale, because as we discussed earlier, weight loss that comes from muscle loss is not good!

Doctors are here to help, so take advantage of any tools and tests they have to help protect your health.

8.2: Awkward: Recovering from fun

Elora came for their follow-up visit with a sheepish, apologetic look on their face.

"Doc, lots happened. I messed up. It was a wedding, an anniversary, and basically partying all week. Can you increase my prescriptions for a while? I will get back on track next week when the guests leave town and . . ."

Elora went on to explain how life had happened and made their diabetes worse; their request was putting me in a bind. I felt very conflicted. The request was to increase medication on the basis of a sudden elevated glucose level. I wanted to assess what life events and decisions *caused the glucose to go up in the first place.*

Prescribing a pill would take thirty seconds but was not going to solve the root problem. I wanted to help Elora look inward and introspect to treat the issue at its source. Sometimes this hesitation to give more medication has been interpreted as an unethical, cold-blooded, and outright "refusal to treat."

Who defines the word *treatment?* Who defines what is ethical?

You have every right to seek the treatment you believe is best for you. It's my job to explain what I think will treat the root cause of your problem. There are plenty of doctors out there who can prescribe more medication for "symptoms" of high glucose after a party. Maybe that's the right fit for you at a certain point in your journey, and that's totally okay. You do you.

If you've sought help after having a little too much fun, but only because you didn't know there were other options, you came to the right doctor!

If you want to avoid medicating the aftereffects of a good time, you can find the root cause and address it. I always tell my patients that the easiest way to get to the root cause of this is by playing a little question-and-answer game with yourself. Your answers may look different, but just to give you an example, here's a magical little hypothetical internal dialogue.

1. *Do I want my doctor to increase medication and write the following in my file?* "Diagnosis: Having fun. Prefers to deal with glucose later. Increase meds till . . . who knows." Or label you as "Noncompliant. Increase meds?" **No. That's not who I am. I want better**

diabetes with less medication.

2. *When I take a break from diabetes self-care, who is getting the break?* **My mind.**

3. *What happens to my organs and body during this mental break?* **They get exposed to high glucose levels.**

4. *Do my organs take weekends or public holidays off?* **No, they are working 24/7.**

5. *Do friends/relatives/loved ones that I celebrate with really want my diabetes to get worse?* **Nope.**

6. *Do they understand the level of diabetes I am dealing with?* **Probably not. I haven't explained it to them.**

7. *Would they get offended if I explained what I am working on (better health with less medication)?* **No, they might just be proud of me.**

8. *How would the bride, groom, or house guests feel if they found out their celebration caused my diabetes to get worse?* **Umm, they would feel bad. Maybe they would feel like they should not invite me next time? Or that I can't take care of myself.**

9. *Is there a way for me to manage my diabetes without even burdening them with any of this?* **Maybe. I could actually party with them and pay attention to my nutrition as well. Or just keep it all a secret.**

10. *Why would I take the trouble to do that?* **Well, I could keep it a secret, like I have, and take more medication. But I don't like being on more meds.**

11. *Sure. And won't these fun events happen again in the future?* **Yes, I hope so! I want to enjoy my life.**

12. *And right now, I feel like I can either have fun in life or I can control my diabetes, but I can't have both.* **Yeah, but I actually want both.**

13. *That's right– don't I have valid needs on both sides of these preferences?* **Yes, I want to have fun times with my loved ones and also have a life free from the burdens of diabetes.**

14. *So, being able to celebrate with loved ones and also not have uncontrolled diabetes are both important to me?* **Yes, 100 percent.**

15. *Do I feel like I have to do it perfectly or not do anything at all?* **No, I get it that there is a learning curve.**

16. *Do I feel like I have to get it right the first time I try to balance life's ups and downs alongside managing diabetes?* **I guess that's too much pressure, and it's unrealistic. Edison invented 99 ways not to make a light bulb before he invented the light bulb. I can give myself some space to learn.**

17. *I could just find a different doctor to write a prescription for more medication when future celebrations happen; that might be less work.* **No, I don't want that.**

18. *Does more medication even do anything for my diabetes?* **No, it's just pushing things out into some imaginary future, and I am kidding myself.**

19. *Okay, but I am saying that now, when the party music has faded. What goes through my mind when I make those choices in the middle of all the fun and games?* **I tell myself to enjoy now and get back on track later.**

20. *And that takes care of my mind's immediate need to "have fun." Deal with consequences later.* Yeah.

21. *And where is this track or this wagon?* **Hah! In my head.**

22. *How did my body feel during those party moments?* **I didn't even pay attention to my body that night. But the next morning, I felt tired and exhausted. My body was definitely complaining.**

23. *Right, so what needs to change so that my mind can enjoy the fun times in my life while I also learn to manage my glucose levels with less medication and feel healthier in my body, through the good times and beyond?* **Well, there are things I can do differently. Let's see . . .**

Maybe you want to get your glucose levels down after a life event with less medication. I offer these twenty-three questions to help you introspect and shed some light on how you think and feel before, during and after having fun; hopefully, you can use what you've learned from the past experience to prevent glucose from going up in the first place.

Even if you are able to prevent your glucose from increasing when exciting and fun events take place in your life, most people will visit the hospital at least once in their lives, diabetes-related or not.

8.3: Diabetes and the hospital

Diabetes sending you to the hospital is very different from going to the hospital as a person with diabetes.

Take Mustafa, for example.

Mustafa was admitted to the hospital **for a much-needed knee replacement,** but he had diabetes. He and his surgeon knew that uncontrolled diabetes would make the postoperative recovery more complicated. So he came to us.

He had been working with us for four months on turning around his diabetes. He was eating low-carb at home, with postmeal readings of around 130 mg/dL (7.22 mmol/L) before surgery. He had gotten his hemoglobin A1c (HbA1c) into a safe range and was approved for surgery.

He texted our support team from the hospital room on postop day one.

His message read, "The food here is crazy! The hospital dietitian realized I had diabetes and prescribed the 1,800-calorie diabetic tray. It's such crap! **More than half of the tray is carbohydrates, and** *there was barely any protein or vegetables in the last twenty-four hours.* The doctor just looked at the glucose of 190 mg/dL (10.5 mmol/L), and now the nurse came to poke me with insulin! Do they even talk to each other about this? I worked so hard to get the numbers down, and now this is totally backward! They have given me bread, biscuits, rice, and potatoes and two snacks. Are they insane? How can this many carbs be good for a person with diabetes? And then they are insisting on using insulin to clean up the mess that tray caused inside my body? Help!"

As part of his care team, of course I was concerned for him, but I was even more concerned for the people who didn't have a care team to text! Higher fluctuations in glucose levels (glycemic variability) on CGM seem to play a role in abnormal *immune cell behavior* in hospitalized patients with type 2 diabetes.[10] Even though Mustafa was able to stay in touch with us during his hospital visit, like so many other people with diabetes, he had no idea what to expect when it came to dealing with hospitals when diabetes was not the primary concern being addressed.

While Mustafa was smart enough to ask for help, his text message taught me that I need to be sure more patients knew **what to expect from their diabetes care team when admitted to the hospital.**

When it comes to tracking glucose levels in the hospital, there are both patient factors and logistical hospital factors that can cause unforeseen fluctuations. When it comes to **patient factors**, things as simple as *poor sleep in the hospital, fluctuating appetite, a change in taste buds or ability to eat,* and even *not liking hospital food options* enough to complete the tray can impact your glucose levels. On the other hand, there can be more serious patient circumstances like *fluctuating blood pressure and circulation, being given medications that raise glucose* (such as steroids and diuretics), or even *coexisting conditions* from the stress of infection, injury, or illness.

Comparatively, glucose levels can be influenced by **hospital logistics factors** like being met with *cold, unappetizing food trays* when you come back to the room. Even if it was perfectly warm, the hospital may have some *uncertainty about insulin dosing* for a meal that may or may not be eaten on time. This happens due to both a delay between checking the glucose level, administering insulin, and actually eating; and the unpredictable times you're wheeled off for tests and procedures, thereby missing meals. These things can affect glucose, sure, but the *quality of communication between the nurse and the primary doctor and between various medical consulting teams* **can greatly improve or worsen the experience and overall effect on glucose levels.**

Since you never know what the communication is like at the hospital, it's on you to advocate for yourself, so here's **what you should know about managing glucose levels in the hospital.**

For starters, *the target range in the hospital is a bit higher* than at home. An intensive care unit (ICU) team will probably aim for 140–180 mg/dL (7.8–10 mmol/L), while a ward team (non-ICU) may aim for 100–180 mg/dL (5.6–10 mmol/L). Some teams may aim for 110–140 mg/dL (6.1–7.8 mmol/L) if they can manage the risk of hypoglycemia (low glucose).

If you are wearing a continuous glucose monitor (CGM), you can continue to monitor trends, but *you will need a glucometer confirmation* to make treatment or dose decisions. However, if your circulation or blood pressure is affected, *the bedside glucometer readings may be less accurate* than an actual lab sample from the vein.

Medication side effects bring an increased risk to a hospital setting, so many oral diabetes agents need to be stopped on admission. You may end up *relying mostly on insulin* during your hospital stay because alongside the ease of dosing, insulin tends to have the least interaction with other medications.

To make things easier on the hospital logistics, the option for diabetic food trays is often designed *so each tray gives you a consistent amount of carbs*. This makes it easy for the doctor's insulin dose to match that carb load.

One study looked at what happened when hospitalized patients were allowed to control their own meals from an unrestricted menu.

Guess what?

The patients who were allowed to eat whatever they wanted experienced more hypoglycemia and their mean lowest-glucose was lower, compared to being given a consistent carb plan given by the hospital. Half of the patients who had a low glucose in the self-selecting group selected fewer than three carbohydrate servings per meal, or less than forty-five grams. The study concluded that the patients that were allowed to eat what they wanted had selected "inadequate carbohydrates."

The paper suggests that the patient-controlled menu group might have had less hypoglycemia if they had more nutrition "education" and monitoring by nutrition staff.[11] Results like this may be why patients are given "diabetic trays" with processed carbs at each meal.

But does any of that feel backward to you, having read this book, and especially after reading about Marco's mother in Part 7.6?

People were more satisfied when they chose their own food. If they were getting hypoglycemia by eating less carbs, perhaps the solution could have been for the doctors to reduce the prescription that was causing the hypoglycemia? Surely, the solution doesn't have to be that a nutritionist will come around and make sure the person with diabetes *eats more carbs?*

That can't be what the world needs, can it?

I'm just wondering where all these backward plans and money trails go, because you deserve to have a say in what you eat in the hospital, especially if the hospital food is raising your glucose levels and requiring more medication. Talk to your doctor. Most open-minded physicians will change the meal prescription; that way, the hospital dietary team will provide what's been ordered. Just remember, you might be going against the current here, so the medical team may reflexively judge you as being "difficult."

It's fine to be a little difficult if you're doing what's best for your health.

8.4: Why I stopped working in the hospital environment

Doctors are created from training grounds that are set up in hospitals. This was helpful for me because I was able to realize quite early in my career that my calling was to keep people out of the hospital.

I loved the powerful learning experiences I had throughout my medical school, residency, and fellowship, and I am thankful for all the hands-on training I received through caring for people in the inpatient hospital environment. Those internal medicine wards are what taught me all about the inner workings of the human body and how all systems coordinate with each other. But I was interested in more than just the body. I was deeply interested in the mind, and once I became an endocrinologist, I soon started *hating* inpatient rounds.

Why?

Because a large part of an endocrinologist's hospital job is to ensure tight glucose control for people with diabetes who have been admitted for various other illnesses. Keeping glucose levels stable in the hospital improves patient outcomes, and someone has to do it.[12] We did a pretty good job of it, too.

But it just didn't feel rewarding. Tweaking the insulin doses to stabilize glucose levels felt like putting on oxygen masks in a plane that's making an emergency landing. It might help, but you really wish you didn't need it in the first place. You wish the event could have been prevented.

The experience felt like a failure of outpatient health care to me. I saw every fluctuating glucose chart in people with elevated HbA1c levels as a sign that we had failed to help this person on the outpatient side to turn their diabetes around.

The other thing that always bothered me was the financial incentives.

The more doctors generated revenue value units (RVUs), the higher their compensation. The sicker the patient was, the more complex their case was. That meant more thinking and mental effort on the part of the doctor.

So? That's what we trained all our lives for. We are knowledge workers. I'm not an economics expert, and I know there are pros and cons of a capitalist and socialist approach to health care.

What felt backward to me was how level five medical billing for the sickest patients meant the highest possible income per minute. There was a financial reward attached to looking after the sickest patients.

Don't get me wrong; my ICU and super specialized surgical colleagues have dedicated decades of their lives acquiring the expertise to care for the critically ill and are saving lives in hospitals every day. We need highly skilled hospital teams to be compensated for their valuable hard work, and we need them when we get terribly sick. The doctor will treat whoever is in the bed to the best of their ability, but the doctor-patient relationship can become more sterile when the patient is highly vulnerable.

Often, the sickest person is the one you can't really talk to because they are hooked up to all kinds of monitors, tubes, and often life support. Sometimes they are sleeping, resting, or sedated when you stop by. For most hospital endocrinologists, rounds mean reviewing care plans, tweaking of insulin doses (most hospitals have protocols in place), quick notes in the system, a chat with a colleague about the patient, and an entry on the billing page. Brisk, efficient cerebral work.

I found it to be a soul-sucking endeavor after a while. I was good at it, and I designed protocols to synchronize my insulin orders to match people's food trays and glucometer checks so that the patient was disturbed only once per meal and the glucose levels were most stable. I also had a pretty solid understanding of internal medicine and endocrinology and could help patients navigate through rocky glucose control.

Excellent hospital nursing, pharmacy, and support staff helped them land safely with a more stable discharge plan. As soon as the patient was stable and didn't need daily level 5 endocrinology consults, I would put the diabetes orders on cruise control with sufficient safety checks in place. I'd then sign off on the case, noting to the primary medical or surgical team that they could reconsult our department if any new question arose.

This approach was not good for inpatient billing, my friend. Luckily, nobody chased me at the hospitals I worked at in Chicago or Mumbai to achieve specific "targets" from my hospital rounds.

Right now, *the twisted incentives of the financial compensation system cannot differentiate between someone who is critically ill because of a failed healthcare system and someone who is critically ill because of bad luck*. No single person is bad, but our systems are broken, and there's insufficient accountability for the failures of outpatient healthcare systems. One step in the right direction is that readmissions within one month of discharge are looked at negatively by some insurance companies. They are trying to reduce the "revolving door" costs of repeated admissions for the same problem. It takes lots of good people rallying together to fix broken systems.

Finally, in 2016, after twenty-one years, I stopped commuting to a hospital. **I left hospital practice to provide health care the way I wanted.** And that's what I've been doing ever since.

8.5: Shirin, Elora, and Mustafa: Where are they now?

Shirin, Mustafa, and Elora are a few of the people I've been able to help turn diabetes around since leaving the guidelines behind in favor of doing things my own way. But how did that turn out for them?

Back to Shirin

Shirin took two years to get her mind around all the lifestyle changes we had been discussing. She had first met me while coming for her mum's appointments for diabetes and had been considering some changes for herself, too. She wanted to remain healthy and enjoy more years of good life with her mother. They are a great mother-daughter team who motivate each other to keep upgrading their healthy habits. Trying the balloon for weight loss had not worked years ago, and now the wake-up call was coming from her own lab reports.

Shirin's CRP was forty-eight, indicating high levels of inflammation and cardiac risk. It should have been below three—the lower, the better. Her urine MAC ratio came back at 300 when it should have been below thirty. This was a sign that diabetes and high blood pressure were harming her kidneys.

Her cardiologist and I coordinated to adjust her medication, and she started a low-carb, sufficient-protein approach. Exercise came much later, once she felt enough energy to start building muscle. Finally came intermittent fasting. She ended up losing fifty kilos (over 100 pounds) by gradually increasing the duration of her long fasts to forty-eight hours, fasting twice a week.

Over a span of three years, she has normalized her blood pressure, and her cardiologist is delighted. We were able to reduce her medications, and more importantly, her CRP and urine MAC both came down to undetectable levels, and her HbA1c improved from 7.8 to 5.4 along the way. She has shared her journey with us on YouTube and has allowed us to use her real name so that others may benefit from her story.

She knew that 2024 would be the year when her numbers will move out of prediabetes and into the normal range. She succeeded by using the lifestyle car and fasting approach described in this book. It makes me wonder what if all we had done for her in 2021 was follow the algorithm that tells doctors which medicine to prescribe if someone comes with uncontrolled diabetes plus kidney damage? And what if her lifestyle had not changed course? What if?

Remember how Elora had some fun?

I played tough cop and asked Elora to check what was really going on when they "indulged a little." We walked through questions similar to the questions-and-answer exercise from Part 8.2.

The conversation took up the entire thirty-minute session.

I told them that increasing medication would have taken me all of two minutes, but I wanted to hold space for them to introspect on what turning diabetes around really meant to them. Did it mean zigzagging forward and backward in the emergency service lanes, going in circles? Or did it mean actually going ahead on their life's up-and-down journey on the highway, gripping the steering wheel in order to become a more experienced driver, with more skillful navigation of their decisions?

They promised to get back to me within the next ten days.

For me, whenever I have to play tough cop, I always do an internal check to scan that I am working from my heart in the patient's best interest, not from my ego. I'm looking for a win-win. A zero-sum game is never acceptable, and it's important for both sides to be able to respectfully speak their truth if we want to deliver better health care.

In the meantime, I gave them an affirmation to try whenever the possibility of "choose fun or choose diabetes" arose. I asked them to see how it felt and what ideas came to mind if they told themselves that they didn't have to choose one over the other, but rather affirm: *"I know how to balance my choices to enjoy celebrations in life while also managing my diabetes. I know how to take care of my emotional needs and physical health. I am open to new possibilities."*

They came back with some ideas. They decided they didn't want more medication to hide the "mistakes" of the wedding and other fun events inside the closet. They truly wanted to have better health with less medication, every day. Not just when life was convenient. They made a commitment to themselves to listen to their self-talk a little more and also went one step deeper into self-understanding, self-care, and self-compassion.

Learning a new way of self-managing diabetes is a massive life skill. I reminded Elora how learning something as simple as the twenty-six letters of the

English alphabet takes so much repetition, acknowledging that I saw that they'd decided that the learning curve was worth it.

As they realized they were being too rigid and too hard on themselves when learning a completely new habit, repetition became key. From there, it took a few months of therapy, journaling, and step-by-step baby steps toward their goal of maintaining healthy glucose levels–*especially* when they wanted to have some fun!

And finally, Mustafa

Now, there were multiple reasons for Mustafa's postmeal glucose to be above target, including the postop pain, recovery from surgery, and stress of lying in a hospital bed.

His carbohydrate-heavy tray was simply not helping.

So what helped him succeed during his hospital stay?

For starters, *he felt supported by having access to a responsive healthcare team,* which reassured him that his requests were not crazy. After all, he was going against the grain and creating more work for his hospital team that was chronically overworked. Because he had experienced the success of his low-carb lifestyle for many months before the procedure, his confidence in *medical nutrition therapy* came from knowing how different foods affected his body. He insisted on enough protein to support all the tissue repair needed to recover. He had just had an artificial knee installed in his body after cutting through skin, muscle, and bone.

Since he had worn CGMs in his early days of working with us, he had seen how carbs spiked his levels but good-quality protein did not. He knew his HbA1c before admission was 5.8 percent, so he also knew the hospital reading of 190 mg/dL (10.5 mmol/L) was not his normal state. *The data supported his position* that the most powerful medicine would be insisting they fix his food tray.

The support of his care team and the data he had gave him the confidence to insist on getting the assistant orthopedic surgeon to write an order that allowed his family to bring food from home. They also wrote for the hospital tray to provide more protein and less carbs. The dietitian was surprised by this, but cooperated with the doctor's orders.

He also *had a deeper understanding of medication, insulin resistance, and metabolic syndrome than his doctor, nurse, and hospital dietitian.* He knew insulin therapy was wrong for him because his body was already making insulin, so adding more insulin would make everything worse. Sad, but still common. Hopefully, this will change over time, as doctors from all fields will be inspired by the victory of Dr. Gary Fettke, orthopedic surgeon, and Professor Tim Noakes, MD, who successfully defended their careers after being persecuted for advocating low-carb diets.

Thankfully, he did not need further insulin injections from the nurse because he was able to keep his carb intake below 100 grams a day. Moreover, he'd also seen the impact of movement on his postmeal levels, so he was always motivated to walk down the hospital corridors with his physical therapist.

He wore an eye mask to give him better-quality sleep in the strange hospital environment full of bright lights, foreign sounds, and people entering the room at odd hours.

Healing started, and his postmeal levels started coming down.

He got clearance for discharge by the end of the second day because he was doing better than his team had predicted. A reduced hospital stay correlates with better long-term outcomes and less risk of needing readmission. People with diabetes experience almost twice as many readmissions after discharge than people without diabetes. Thirty percent of people with diabetes who are hospitalized need two or more hospital stays, and these admissions contribute to over fifty percent of hospital costs attributed to diabetes.[13] Readmission is exponentially expensive, painful stuff. It's worth doing whatever we can to avoid it. Mustafa came home and worked on a smooth and steady recovery with his brand-new knee. His postoperative period was uneventful, and he didn't have to wear hospital gowns again.

Part 8 summary

- You deserve to be treated by a healthcare professional who can support your healthcare goals.

- There is more to cardiac health than cholesterol and more to kidney health than creatinine.

- If you want healthier organs with less medication, say that explicitly to your care team so different specialists can coordinate and support your lifestyle change efforts.

- It is okay to tell your hospital team about your expertise at self-managing diabetes. You might teach them a thing or two.

For Bonus Materials, Visit the Website Here:

PART 9:

DIABETES IN WOMEN AND CHILDREN

9.1: Women's health: prediabetes, type 2 diabetes, PCOS, and patriarchy

As insulin is a hormone that has effects on the entire body, the relationship between diabetes and being a female can have unique consequences like polycystic ovarian syndrome, diabetes in pregnancy, and even complications postpartum and postmenopause.

If you have prediabetes or type 2 diabetes, you might also have PCOS. The common link between PCOS, prediabetes, and type 2 diabetes is insulin resistance, which we've addressed throughout this book. The insulin-resistance epidemic can affect you in different ways at different stages of life.

Polycystic ovarian syndrome (PCOS) is becoming one of the most common hormonal imbalances in young women. *Polycystic* means "having many cysts," and *cyst* just means a sac, usually filled with fluid. To understand what these cysts are, visualize an apple tree during harvesting season. Imagine that something is stopping the apples from ripening to be fully ready. The tree would gradually become full of lots of half-ripe apples. The branches become heavy and the tree gets bulky, full of immature apples that cannot be harvested because they are not ripe enough. Each has the potential to form a new apple tree but is not ready to leave the tree. A similar thing is happening with the cysts accumulated in the ovary.

The hormone imbalance of PCOS causes the follicles (eggs) to reach a certain stage of development and then get stuck. They don't become mature enough for ovulation. This does not mean the woman is infertile. She has plenty of immature eggs. She is just not releasing mature eggs (ovulating) in a regular rhythm; this explains the symptom of reduced fertility. These partially ready eggs start accumulating in the ovary, causing other hormonal features of PCOS.

I want to note that I don't call it PCOD, as it is sometimes referred to in India, where the D is supposed to stand for disease. It's a syndrome, which means *it is a varied collection of symptoms.* The word *disease* has a strong negative, unhelpful

365

connotation to it. It's called PCOS as the symptoms show up differently in different women.

Maybe you were diagnosed with PCOS **in your teens** before you developed diabetes. In your teens, *you may be more concerned with the cosmetic implications* of facial hair and acne. Wanting to look good is a healthy and natural human instinct.

In your twenties or thirties, however, *you might have body image concerns, feeling like something is wrong with you. You might think about fertility* and your ability to plan a family. If you are South Asian or Indian, your parents might be wondering if PCOS will reduce your ability to find "a man willing to marry you."

Then, **beyond your mid-thirties,** there's an increased risk of developing diabetes and other metabolic imbalances linked to insulin resistance, such as heart disease, high blood pressure, increased risk of certain cancers in later years (particularly endometrial cancer), and more.

PCOS is considered to be a form of insulin resistance at the ovarian level, but insulin resistance is not part of the criteria to be diagnosed with PCOS. Regardless, a majority of women have some form of insulin resistance, even if their blood insulin and glucose levels are normal.[1]

To be diagnosed with PCOS, your doctor needs to establish any two of the following three findings (the Rotterdam criteria):[2,3]

1. **Polycystic ovaries on sonography/ultrasound:** The radiologist needs to see *more than twenty follicles* (immature eggs) per ovary in either ovary and measure *the ovary to be larger than ten cubic centimeters* in volume. Many women get afraid when they hear that their ovaries are full of cysts, but if you recall the apple tree analogy, it's not as dangerous as it sounds.

2. **Infrequent periods due to lack of ovulation** (anovulation): *Fewer than eight periods per year* or menstrual cycles more than thirty-five days apart. In the apple tree analogy, this means less than eight apples are ripening completely per year instead of twelve.

3. **Symptoms or blood tests showing excess male hormone** (hyperandrogenism): *Excessive facial hair, acne,* and *male-pattern balding* are some of the common symptoms. In the apple tree analogy, the unripe apples stick around and create chemical imbalance. Blood tests may show elevated testosterone, dehydroepiandrosterone sulfate (DHEAS), androstenedione, and dihydrotestosterone (DHT) levels. Your doctor will need to rule out other rare hormonal conditions that can cause similar symptoms.

Again, you only need two out of the three in order to qualify for a diagnosis. Most of my patients have seen improvement in symptoms and return of natural, spontaneous monthly periods through lifestyle change alone. There is growing evidence for lifestyle change improving PCOS with less medication:

1. **Nutrition:** Keeping carbs below 100 grams a day has been shown to have a better effect on the hormonal imbalance and irregular menses than the traditional low-fat diet.[4]

2. **Sleep:** We are beginning to realize that poor sleep may reduce the benefits of improved nutrition and exercise in women making lifestyle changes for PCOS.[5]

3. **Stress management:** An eight-week randomized trial showed that offering a mindfulness stress management program reduced scores for depression, anxiety, and stress in women with PCOS.[6] The participants reported improved quality of life. Hormonal testing showed improvement in the levels of the stress hormone cortisol, measured in the saliva.

4. **Exercise:** Resistance training has been shown to reduce testosterone, insulin resistance, and fasting glucose levels in PCOS, and aerobic training has been shown to improve body image.[7,8]

5. **Body composition:** Many people associate a higher weight with PCOS, but it's not that simple. Even "skinny" women can suffer from a version of PCOS called **lean polycystic ovarian syndrome.** Women with abdominal obesity benefit as they lose inches (visceral fat) from the waist. Lean women don't need to lose weight; they may benefit from the opposite.

    Lean women with PCOS have insulin resistance in common with overweight or obese women with PCOS.[9] As you know from previous chapters, having more muscle improves insulin sensitivity. The lifestyle approach in lean PCOS includes gaining lean muscle tissue using strength training to build muscle mass, which may cause healthy weight gain in someone who is underweight. You may need medications to help with symptoms as you work on lifestyle changes, especially since it can take six to twelve months to change hair-growth or hair-loss patterns, build muscle, and see changes in hormone-sensitive areas of your skin.

6. **Fasting/time-restricted eating:** Women with PCOS and a body mass index (BMI) of twenty-five who followed a 16:8 fasting proto-

col for six weeks observed increased sex-hormone-binding globulin (SHBG), improved waist-to-hip ratio (an indirect marker of visceral obesity), and improvement of their BMIs into the normal range.[10] Further, the free androgen index, total and free testosterone, and DHEAS show reduced male hormone levels alongside an improved metabolic profile with reduced insulin resistance (Homeostatic Model Assessment for Insulin Resistance [HOMA-IR] index), reduced triglycerides, and increased high-density lipoprotein (HDL).

Notice anything? All the lifestyle changes you have learned in this book to address insulin resistance for diabetes have been proven to improve PCOS, too. It's drastically reduced my need to prescribe medications for PCOS over the years as we intensify lifestyle changes.

If you're interested in exploring prescriptions for PCOS, most drugs seek to impact metabolism, control ovulation, balance hormones, and improve cosmetic symptoms.

When it comes to **addressing the metabolism**, *metformin*, the diabetes drug that reduces insulin resistance, addresses the root cause. There is also growing interest in supplements like *myoinositol* and *berberine*. These supplements are used for their possible effects on metabolic parameters in women with PCOS, although we don't have large-scale clinical trials yet.[11]

When it comes to **excess male hormone**, *contraceptives* provide combinations of estrogen and progesterone and induce withdrawal bleeding (this is not a natural period). They suppress spontaneous ovulation, reduce the accumulation of immature follicles, and reduce the secretion of excess male hormone. As PCOS is associated with an increased risk of endometrial cancer, *intermittent progesterone prescriptions* might be given instead of contraceptives to induce withdrawal bleeding (this is not a natural period). Shedding the uterine lining (endometrium) intermittently prevents it from getting too thick or precancerous (hyperplastic) from uninterrupted estrogen exposure. It's important to visit your gynecologist regularly to check on the health of your endometrial lining.

While contraceptives are typically a blend of female hormones, that's not the only way they differ from **male-hormone-blocking drugs** like *spironolactone, finasteride,* or *flutamide*. Influencing your hormones and controlling reproduction are two different things, and I specify this because you have to use contraception when taking male-hormone-blocking drugs. *You don't want to conceive while taking these* because of the possibility of severe side effects, birth defects, and malformations in the fetus.

For those who are looking to address the cosmetic concerns associated with PCOS, specific localized treatment from your dermatologist is available. These treatments are specialized to help acne, hair loss, and excessive facial hair and will usually give better results with the support of metformin, contraceptives or male hormone blocking drugs.

The treatments that target male hormone production and work locally on the skin can reduce symptoms of irregular periods, acne, male-pattern balding, and excessive facial hair, but *they do not address the source of the hormonal problem at the root.* In fact, some of the side effects of contraceptives can include a worsening metabolic profile, sexual dysfunction, mood swings, nausea, vomiting, migraine headaches, weight gain, and increased blood glucose levels. As always, work with your doctor on the same lifestyle changes that we have discussed for diabetes and insulin resistance throughout the book, and your PCOS symptoms will improve.

I can't write a section on lifestyle change for women's health or move onto loaded topics like fertility, pregnancy, babies, and children without commenting on **patriarchy as one of the social determinants of health** (SDOH) outcomes of diabetes in women. Society as a collective whole is responsible for dismantling gender inequality.

I have spent almost half my life in the United States, and the remaining time in India. With two amazing daughters of my own, I feel compelled to call out the patriarchal belief systems that women have been exposed to. My female patients have unconsciously internalized certain belief systems that show up when I try to dive deeper into women's health issues with them. Too many people start believing the negative things that others say. I hope that you are seeking treatment that aligns with your goals first. After that, it's okay to consider the thoughts of your extended family, neighbors, parents, or in-laws. You come first.

Parents may say things like "Our daughter is too big;" "Our daughter being unmarried at the age of thirty is an embarrassment, stress, and burden for our family;" "Our daughter has PCOS, so she is less fertile, so we need to marry her off urgently;" or even "She has diabetes. Can we keep it a secret till after the wedding?"

Hearing your parents talk like this is bad enough but when your in-laws join, it can feel like the walls are closing in. It hurts to hear patients say things like, "My in-laws are unhappy that I got my period this month because that means I didn't conceive. They don't see my periods coming once a month as a sign that my PCOS is getting better." Multiple women have said to me, "My husband doesn't say anything when my in-laws speak badly to me because he knows they just want a grandchild". I would never want someone to speak to my daughters like that. After being spoken to like this for years, many women have adopted these limiting beliefs for themselves, negatively impacting their confidence and self-esteem.

I have seen the same thing from the other side, too. I've had the mother of a grown man tell me, "My son has diabetes, and I took care of him till he got married, so the responsibility is now with his wife. I hope she feeds him properly," and her son internalized it. It's the same thing when I hear men say that, "I'm a bachelor, so I can't get home-cooked food," and that's why "I need to find a wife because I can't cook." Or, it extends to family stereotypes and expectations in a double-income home, when someone tells me, "I don't get time to exercise because I have young kids and a working spouse." It's great that this man shares the responsibilities at home, but would that be the way a woman says she can't exercise?

Hearing extended family say things like, "She has PCOS. She should stop being so career oriented and have the baby before she becomes infertile," and doctors saying "Either take medication to fix your skin or have a baby. You can't do both," can make a woman start to believe that their only role on this planet is to produce a child.

And maybe that's not the worst of it. Hearing a woman come into my office and say, "I have to lose weight so that my parents can search for a groom for my arranged marriage," because "I am getting rejected by good guys because of my weight," indicates that she believes it, too. Although they suffer from body shaming, too, very few men say this to me. People of every gender need a safe space to feel comfortable in their body.

Even after a woman has found the person they wanted to marry, I hear things like "I am a housewife and can't sleep well at night because my husband comes home late from work. He needs to watch TV in our bedroom. He works so hard at the office that TV is the only way he can relax," or something like "I can't cook separately for my diabetes needs because I already cook different food for my husband's and kids' preferences." These statements show that not only are they internalizing the thoughts of everyone around them, but that those sentences have begun to negatively impact their relationship with their body and their diabetes goals.

Statements and beliefs like these have been spoken so frequently over the years that we've come to consider them as acceptable ways of thinking. Patients share these sentences with me without realizing that *none of these things are acceptable to say to any girl, boy, or person exploring their identity*. They come from a deep-rooted patriarchal, misogynistic, and disempowering culture toward women. It's time for outdated, limiting beliefs to be discarded. I don't know about feminism, woke culture, or cancel culture—I only know about kindness. Let's empower our children to create a more balanced future where everyone has access to health.

Just because a toxic culture is familiar doesn't make it right. The fact is, you get to decide how you express your sexuality, and you get to decide whether you want to get married or become a parent–or not.

If you choose to get married or find a life partner, you deserve a partner who cherishes you for the human being you are. That means you get to decide whether cooking is your responsibility or not. If we believe girls deserve an education, then we know they are spending the same amount of time in school as the boys. They don't attend cooking classes after school. They're doing homework and getting good grades. Putting food on the table and changing nappies are co-ed responsibilities in a world that values education and financial independence for all. Sure, each family can find its own healthy way to divide the work and help each other; so find yours.

Because these thought patterns are so widely accepted and because **polycystic ovarian syndrome** (PCOS) is becoming more common in young women, I want to remind you that you don't have to seek pregnancy just because of external pressures to conceive.

9.2: Pursuing pregnancy (or not) is your personal choice

I had a 34-year-old patient with uncontrolled diabetes and PCOS suffering from years of irregular menstrual periods and unpredictable ovulation. Having irregular periods from PCOS means you are ovulating *intermittently*. This means you might end up conceiving if you are sexually active and not using contraception!

By the time we met, however, she had given up on trying to conceive. She decided to turn her diabetes around through lifestyle changes with us. She changed her nutrition, started exercising, and started thirty-six-hour fasts on alternate days. Her diabetes improved rapidly.

Her periods had been irregular for years, so she didn't realize she had conceived until she went to get a magnetic resonance image (MRI) for low back pain. The highly surprised radiology technician told her it looked like the cause of back pain was that she was pregnant! More than half of the pregnancy had gone by, and she had absolutely no idea.

No matter what, you don't deserve to be stigmatized or shamed because of PCOS. If you don't plan to have a baby, that's only between you and the ones you want to discuss it with. If you want to pursue pregnancy, however, please be reassured that the world's most common hormone disorder in reproductive-age women is PCOS, and the world population is only going up—so, PCOS can't be stopping that many pregnancies!

If an "oops" pregnancy happens, it may catch you off guard in terms of your baseline metabolic health or mental readiness. If you have prediabetes, diabetes, or PCOS and are planning pregnancy, work with your healthcare provider before you conceive if you can, as preconception counseling can build up better metabolic health to provide your fetus the healthiest internal environment possible. It's a very short nine months during which your diabetes has a direct impact on your baby's long-term health and risk of diabetes when they are an adult, but I'll discuss epigenetics in Part 9.5.

I have never had to send a patient of mine with PCOS for infertility treatment, but if you have PCOS and do conceive, you're at increased risk of developing gestational diabetes.

Gestational diabetes and diabetes in pregnancy

Overweight women and women of South Asian and Indian descent are at high risk for developing gestational diabetes mellitus (GDM) because of the tendency to develop insulin resistance and diabetes. Gestational diabetes affects 6 percent of pregnancies toward the end of the second trimester as the placenta secretes pregnancy hormones that reduce insulin sensitivity by up to 60–90 percent.[12]

If you are at high risk, your gynecologist will probably screen you for preexisting diabetes at the time of diagnosis, then check you for GDM by ordering an oral glucose tolerance test (OGTT), usually around the start of the third trimester (around 27–28 weeks). This can be done in many ways, but the usual approach is a nonfasting 75 g OGTT, where you are given a sweet syrup to drink in the doctor's office. The diagnosis is made if the glucose level crosses 140 mg/dL (7.7 mmol/L) two hours later.

Having GDM puts you at a much higher risk of developing type 2 diabetes within the next five years, although the risk persists for *more than thirty-five years* after your baby is born. There is also an increased risk of cardiovascular disease in your later years.[13]

In comparison to GDM, *diabetes before pregnancy* is when you are found to have diabetes either before you conceive or in the first two trimesters (before the 27th week) of pregnancy. Regardless of your status, work with your obstetrician and endocrinologist to prepare your body for as healthy a pregnancy as possible. You may want to take special care to discuss an ophthalmology screening because pregnancy can worsen diabetic retinopathy, in addition to a review of vaccinations, exercise, and alcohol and smoking cessation. Also, if you have type 1 diabetes, you may want to discuss hypoglycemia and diabetic ketoacidosis (DKA) prevention strategies. Lifestyle intensification and a review of hemoglobin A1c (HbA1c) and medications before conception can help reduce insulin resistance in particular.

GDM, undiagnosed diabetes, or type 2 or type 1 diabetes before pregnancy, come with increased risks related to maternal health and delivery complications, while the baby can suffer from complications of their own.

When it comes to **maternal health**, risks include excessive weight gain in pregnancy, increased blood pressure (preeclampsia), *worsening diabetic retinopathy* (so it's ideal to get the dilated eye exam before pregnancy and in every trimester), and almost one-third of women with GDM *develop full-blown type 2 diabetes* within five years of delivery. Breastfeeding has been associated with a lower risk of diabetes later in life.

In regards to **labor and delivery**, complications during delivery include *prolonged labor, tears in the vaginal wall, traumatic childbirth, and increased chance of a cesarean section. After delivery, there's a heightened risk of postpartum depression, posttraumatic stress disorder* (PTSD) from a traumatic birth, along with the potential repercussions of a *cesarean section.*[14] While it *deprives the baby of the natural vaginal bacterial flora* during normal labor, there's also potential for a *prolonged hospital stay* and an increased chance of *formula-feeding replacing breastmilk* due to less natural stimulus for the mother's lactation to start.[15]

But that's not all.

In the newborn baby, exposure to high glucose and insulin concentrations can cause an increased risk of *birth defects* and also a birth weight heavier than usual (*macrosomia*, meaning close to 9 lb or 4 kg). Macrosomia can be correlated with different short-term and long-term risks. Short-term risks include the risk of *difficult labor* as well as *birth trauma.*[16] Things like *neonatal low glucose* (requiring supplemental feeding instead of the mother's milk), *preterm labor,* and *breathing difficulties* after delivery could lead to an *increased need for the newborn to need intensive care unit* (ICU) *support* after birth.[17]

There is growing interest in long-term metabolic risks, too. It's possible that long-term programming of fat cells and fat storage in the baby may be influenced by the maternal womb environment. Her internal environment is impacted by her nutrition, her stress levels, and her external environmental exposures. The time spent in the mother's uterus can impact the sensitivity of the baby's fat cells to *weight gain later in life* through influencing the baby's DNA. This has implications because it can cause a higher chance of the newborn developing obesity *and type 2 diabetes themselves* decades later in adult life.

Epigenetic effects are the effects of behaviors or the environment on DNA expression. These effects don't change the DNA code, but they affect the way genes are read and expressed by the body. I will cover this in more detail in a few chapters. The most important thing to know here is that many of these complications can be prevented by turning around type 2 diabetes before pregnancy, controlling your glucose levels before and during pregnancy if you have type 1 diabetes, and preventing GDM.

9.3: Pregnancy in progress

When it comes to nutrition and weight gain in pregnancy, **the same nutritional approach from this book can be used in pregnancy in consultation with your doctor.** A low-carb, protein-sufficient diet using healthy fats helps prevent excessive weight gain. There is no need to intentionally "fatten up" the expecting mother with high-carb treats.

I see so many women who tell me that they never lost the "baby weight." In reality, the baby doesn't need the mother to gain much weight. Mother Nature wants to make sure the human race survives and has the intelligence to give the fetus what it needs. Of course, it is up to us to make lifestyle choices that support a healthy pregnancy.

The growing fetus takes the nutrients it needs via its connection to the mother's placenta. The expecting mother ends up naturally gaining the required weight in pregnancy even if she doesn't forcibly consume extra carbs all day long! If you are starting pregnancy with a normal weight, you only need the equivalent of 300 extra calories during the last three months of pregnancy. If you are overweight before pregnancy, you don't need to intentionally gain weight.

A normal healthy pregnancy can result in around ten to fourteen kilograms (twenty-two to thirty pounds) of weight gain over nine months, which includes blood, water, fat, uterine mass, the placenta, and of course, the growing baby. Remember, an average healthy baby weighs around 2.8–3.8 kg (6 to 8.5 pounds) at birth.

The **glucose targets in pregnancy** are to keep fasting glucose levels below 90–95 mg/dL (5 mmol/L) and two-hour postmeal readings below 120 mg/dL (6.6 mmol/L). Wearing a continuous glucose monitor (CGM) can help you keep a close watch on your patterns. The HbA1c is falsely lowered during pregnancy as a result of changes in circulation and red blood cell (RBC) life span. So, you need to monitor actual glucose readings.

If a low-carb approach is not sufficient to achieve normal glucose levels, then prescriptions will be necessary. You will need to work with your obstetrician and endocrinologist during this time, every few weeks, to quickly achieve glucose control. Remember, we only have nine months, and time flies quickly. So, it's important to have your progress reviewed at least every 2 weeks to ensure the glucose levels come into normal range as soon as possible. Metformin is generally considered safe in pregnancy, but you will need to review these decisions with your doctor. If that is not enough, the basal (slow-acting) insulin to be used in pregnancy is glargine at bedtime to control fasting levels.[18] A quick-acting insulin taken before meals will help achieve the best control of postmeal levels. Remember that insulin causes weight gain, so we want to achieve the best glucose control with the lowest insulin doses.

These can be continued during breastfeeding if the glucose levels remain high after delivery.

Regarding exercise during pregnancy, a research study showed that various combinations of moderate intensity resistance and aerobic training for twenty to thirty minutes–two to seven days a week–resulted in better glucose levels, reduced need to start insulin, and reduced insulin doses in women with GDM.[19]

If you have already been exercising regularly before pregnancy, you can safely continue most of your baseline exercise for the first two trimesters. By the third trimester, you probably need to modify the movements that require you to spend a long time lying on your back. This is because the growing baby can compress your large blood vessels and affect your circulation. As always, talk to your obstetrician to see what exercise you can continue in pregnancy, and only undertake an exercise regimen with professional supervision to ensure correct form.

An athletic, strong woman will go through pregnancy and labor with less back pain, maintaining high levels of activity until the very last moment, with fewer complications during delivery and a quicker recovery to baseline postpartum. Exercise also has a protective effect against postpartum depression. So your best bet is to get active and fit before you even conceive!

9.4: Postpartum and postmenopausal health

After the baby is born, *breastfeeding* **is the most natural way to lose pregnancy weight.** If the baby is exclusively breastfed, this burns the equivalent of around 500 calories a day for the mother, using the body fat she accumulated in the pregnancy. This calorie demand makes the nursing mother more hungry than normal, but if the nursing mother is being excessively "fattened up" by loving relatives and grandparents, that would prevent her from losing the pregnancy weight. This is why when it comes to **postpartum nutrition**, it's important to *focus on a low-carb, protein-sufficient diet* so that you can reduce your risk of diabetes in the long run.

Check your 75 g OGTT at three months postpartum to make sure the GDM is resolved, and monitor your blood work for diabetes annually. You just had a baby, are healing from delivery, and will now be sleep deprived, too! Be sure to talk to your doctor about resuming your prepregnancy fitness routine, but also about giving yourself the rest and space you need to recover.

Especially if you suffer from postpartum depression. **Postpartum depression** can affect one in seven women—that's a lot of mothers and newborns. It is one of the greatest causes of maternal suffering and mortality, and it also affects the baby. Tell me if you notice a theme here: *we think a combination of genetic, hormonal, and environmental factors* likely contributes to postpartum depression.

Does that sound familiar at all?

Scientists are investigating whether insulin resistance plays a direct role in postpartum depression.[20] This seems plausible since insulin resistance is linked to depression in the general population. Ask for help if you are struggling or wondering why you aren't enjoying being a new mother. It's not your fault and you don't have to do this alone.

It's not just the child-bearing age, either. When it comes to the effects of hormones and insulin, postmenopause has its own set of challenges.

After menopause, you lose the protective effect of female hormones that give younger women lower rates of cardiovascular death compared to men below the age of 45. Menopause has been associated with an increased risk of insulin resistance, inch gain around the waist, and decreased muscle mass.[21] The good news is that the drop in estrogen and progesterone doesn't have to mean an inevitable increase of excess body fat or a permanent decline in mental or physical performance. We don't have to accept the normal process of menopause as a justification for worsening diabetes or unavoidable weight gain.

Postmenopausal women's health includes being able to enjoy a fit and athletic life by focusing your attention on bone and muscle health. Guess what? *The same tips from the earlier chapters are your way forward.* Get enough protein, perhaps even more than your previous intake, to counter the declining efficiency of amino acid absorption and accelerating muscle and bone loss that increase the risk of postmenopausal osteoporosis.[22] Postmenopausal women with diabetes have higher fracture rates than those who don't have diabetes, suggesting that diabetes itself might be reducing bone microarchitecture. Continuing your resistance training to preserve muscle will help you enjoy a healthy metabolic rate and health span far beyond menopause.

Lifestyle change can help reduce some cases of postmenopausal urinary incontinence and some may benefit from correcting the estrogen deficiency. Keeping the glucose levels normal helps prevent recurrent urinary infections.

Outside of recalibrating your lifestyle wheels as you go through the stages of menopause, *hormone replacement therapy* (HRT) is a safe option in the right candidate and should be discussed with an endocrinologist or gynecologist who understands the mortality, cardiovascular, bone health, genitourinary, and cognitive benefits of HRT, especially in the first few years of menopause or perimenopause.[23]

The experience of turning around diabetes through your journey as a woman, whether it's menopause, pregnancy or childbirth, isn't something you have to deal with alone. I'm here to remind you that the job of your care team is to make your experience less stressful.

Let's also help you navigate the epigenetic effects of diabetes and GDM on your baby's future health as *they* enter childhood and adolescence.

9.5: Children, epigenetics, nature, and nurture[24]

Why did your child develop type 2 diabetes? Yes, some of it can be genetic, meaning the tendency is in their DNA. Patients tell me, "It's hereditary." Yes. That's nature.

But kids can't refund their parents. They are given your genetic code at the time of conception through one strand of DNA from each biological parent. After that, the embryo is exposed to the maternal environment. So besides getting Mom and Dad's DNA, the developing fetus has nine months of exposure in the womb to the metabolic health and chemical exposure of the mother. **Epigenetics** *is the effect of our behaviors and environment on the expression of our DNA.* While these effects don't change the DNA code, they affect the way genes are read and expressed by the body. If you remember the printer analogy from Part 2.4, epigenetics is the influence of the environment on what files on the laptop get clicked open and sent to the printer (or not).

The maternal womb environment potentially influences the epigenetic long-term programming of the fat cells and fat storage in the fetus. This is important, as it can cause a higher chance of the newborn developing obesity and type 2 diabetes themselves decades later in adult life. After they are born, your kids also "inherit" your lifestyle and your habits, which is also part of the environment influencing their DNA.

In terms of "**nature versus nurture**," the *DNA code represents the role nature has* in causing an inherited tendency to develop diabetes in children. *Changing the environment that influences the expression of that genetic code is a way to hopefully nurture* more positive outcomes from our inherited biology.

The changes discussed earlier in this book will help all families who want to create a healthier environment for their child who has type 2 diabetes. This can positively influence and nurture their diabetes outcomes, even with the same family tree and DNA.

In order to benefit from the lifestyle changes discussed earlier, children need the adults in their life to provide emotional security and create a healthy learning environment. For this reason, I've made changes to the order of the lifestyle wheels in this chapter and renamed them a bit. First, we start with what would be considered the "stress management" wheel, but when it comes to children, I like to think of it as **the relationship and emotional well-being wheel.** This wheel *centers around healthier family dynamics, communication, and safe expression of emotional need.* Here, we want to focus on *developing emotional self-regulation skills and self-esteem* (a healthy body image is at stake here, and therapy may be needed, so the adults may need to work with a professional who understands). This first step will help *set up a healthier division of responsibility* as the child gets older.

When the family dynamic is centered, then we move on to **the nutrition wheel**. Just like with adults, our concerns are *fixing protein malnutrition and reducing overall carbohydrate intake.* However, in regards to children, we also want to *pay attention to role modeling, mindfulness, and balance* when consuming addictive foods.

Then when we move into sleep, I actually refer to this as **the sleep, growth, and learning wheel** which is centered on *helping children improve their duration and quality of sleep* to support physical, mental, and emotional growth.

Finally, in lieu of the exercise wheel, for children we have **the play and movement wheel.** This wheel is all about making physical activity and movement fun. We want to encourage children to enjoy play, celebrate fitness, and exercise to feel strong—not to lose weight.[25]

This does happen.

I had been working with Priya on her weight concerns. She asked if I would have a chat with her husband, Alok, and their nine-year-old daughter, Maya, because they had just found out Maya had type 2 diabetes. This came as a shock to the whole family.

The girl had been gaining weight, and the grandparents noticed darkening of the skin at the back of her neck. The family assumed she had not been scrubbing properly during her bath, but her friends were already bullying her, making fun of how she looked. They visited the pediatrician for the thick, dark skin patches and were surprised when the test results showed she had type 2 diabetes. The parents were seated on either side of the child, and I sensed a rift between the adults. The kid was seemingly oblivious, scribbling on her tablet.

They were an Indian family that lived in a vegetarian multigenerational home with Maya's paternal grandparents; and when I asked the family what they wanted to do, it became clear that they wanted me to get their child to "behave," somehow.

They shared their thoughts as we sat in the office.

Alok said to Priya, "I've been telling you both that she's getting too big for the last two years, but neither of you will do anything about it . . . I'm not home all day and I can't cook—the kitchen is your responsibility. I should be able to celebrate with my kid with sugar once in a while since I barely see her during the week. It's the breakfast and lunch that you are messing up . . . and you can't expect my eighty-year-old parents *not* to want to pamper her!"

Priya shared her complaints when she replied to Alok and said, "She refuses to eat more than a few bites of the protein and says she hates whatever healthy recipes I plan on the menu. It's exhausting because she is difficult to please, and I can't hide the vegetables in her favorite dishes anymore. I have to think of everyone's likes and dislikes in the house. I am going crazy, and your parents don't support me when I force her to eat her vegetables first. They sneak her favorite treats to her afterward."

As if that wasn't enough, she continued, "She promises me she won't throw a tantrum for sugar until our designated treat day on Sunday. But by midweek on Tuesday or Wednesday, she is begging me for something sweet and knows exactly where we keep it in the kitchen. Finally, I get so frustrated by her whining that I just give it to her and let her know she broke her promise to me. Other times, she fakes it and tells me she is hungry in between meals, just so she can have a snack. She has started lying to me, and that's breaking my heart."

Maya had a different take on all of this.

She looked up at me and said, "The doctor says I have diabetes because I am fat. ***Daddy tells me every day that I am fat, so now I want to lose weight.*** I get on the scale every morning before I go to school. My favorite foods are restaurant food, and my home food is very boring. Mumma keeps yelling when it's time to eat, so it's more fun to eat in my bedroom."

Like I mentioned, when it comes to living with diabetes, we want children to aspire to feel strong, not lose weight or look thin; the same thing goes for teens. On occasion, I have worked with families who are wondering how to help their teenage children with type 2 diabetes.

Jay was one such teen.

His parents wanted him to work with us while he was still living at home because ***everyone knew how kids gain weight when they go to college.*** Working with a child on lifestyle change basically means working with the whole family, and I learned a lot just by listening to how the parents spoke about the situation.

Jay's mom had this to say: "Jay has always been a big eater. He could eat more than us ever since he was eight years old, and he just loves soda and sweets. If it's on the table, he can't resist. When he was little, he would sometimes get overtired and not realize he was hungry. I had to keep feeding him every few hours to avoid tantrums. When he was very little, he didn't chew his food. He would keep it in his cheeks, and I had to distract him with cartoons and airplane games so that he would open his mouth." After that bit of background, she continued, telling me that "He doesn't eat enough vegetables and I only let him have dessert after he eats something green, but now he's never interested in eating with us. He just orders in and buys junk food outside. I'm so worried about him, Doc! These days, even my dirty looks aren't enough when he picks up too much from the buffet."

Jay's dad, on the other hand, declared that "All he does is sit around all day and play games on his phone, but he knows he should stop eating so much junk. He just needs someone to set him straight."

Jay just shrugged.

As you can see from Maya and Jay's examples, telling the kid what is "right" for them usually backfires.

9.6: How to help your child turn type 2 diabetes around

As we just learned from Maya and Jay's parents, forcing all of the "right" choices onto your child can have the opposite impact. Let me explain with a happier analogy from your imaginary kid's childhood.

Imagine your child is five years old and you have arranged a birthday party for them, with the highlight activity being a treasure hunt. You have carefully hidden the goodies all around the party venue in ways that the kids can discover them and feel like explorers, triumphantly raising their trophies to show off to their friends. Because you organized the treasure hunt, you know exactly where all the goodies are. Wouldn't it just be easier and faster for you to pick up the items and distribute them out into the kids' hands? You naturally realize how this would ruin all the fun because *the whole point of the game is for the kids to go through the discovery process* and locate the treasure themselves. It's the same when teaching your child a healthy relationship with their food and their body. They will feel connected to the decisions and have a sense of ownership when they discover them through their intrinsic motivation and strengths. Soon after they are out of diapers, *knowing their parent believes in them and has their back* is the support they need.

You have probably experienced this already. Just because you tell your teenager what's right for their health doesn't mean they will immediately embrace it. In health care, there is a name for this urge to tell people what they should do when "we know what's best for them." The founders of motivational interviewing call it the *righting reflex*.[26] Even though the advice may be 100 percent correct and well intentioned, it doesn't cause long-lasting behavior change. So, forcing your adolescent to exercise or restricting their diet in the house doesn't prepare them for adult life.

As parents or educators, the best way we can set a young adult up to be prepared for life is to help them develop the habit of *self-directed learning*.[27]

Disclaimer: I am not a pediatric endocrinologist or a child psychologist. I don't prescribe type 2 diabetes medications to kids. I am lucky to be a mother to two amazing daughters and am an endocrinologist for adults. This section is to help you think about what lifestyle changes you want to work on as a family that can help your child achieve better glucose levels with less medication. If your child has type 2 diabetes, this section does not replace working with your pediatrician or pediatric endocrinologist to review medication, puberty, height, and overall development.

With that, there are five pillars of parenting a child with type 2 diabetes in a way that supports their health goals and sets them up for long-term success.

1. Division of responsibility

Ellyn Satter describes the division of responsibility when it comes to feeding.[28] As a parent, your responsibility changes as your child grows and their mind develops. In their infancy and toddler years, they are fully dependent on you for their food supply. They learn their eating behaviors from your parenting style. When the child is very young, the parent is responsible for *what* food is on the menu (providing healthy and tasty options that the whole family eats), *how* it is presented, where the family eats, when food is offered (mealtimes), and keeping a *pleasant* eating environment. The child is responsible for *whether* they eat and *how much*.

As they approach adolescence, they want more independence from you in all of their decisions, still needing reassurance that you have their back. At each stage of your child's mental development, you empower them when you work as a team and gradually hand them more responsiblity.

2. Consistent messaging is how kids learn.

What message do you want to give?

If Jay was storing food in his mouth as a toddler, he probably wasn't hungry at family mealtime. In that case, it is his autonomy to decide whether or how much he eats. If his mom thinks he didn't eat "enough," that's Mom's opinion. A child who has developed type 2 diabetes and is overweight has definitely been eating.

If Maya's mom's anxiety made her offer compensatory snacks in between meals and chase Maya around the house, begging or bribing her to eat, Maya learned to ignore her own appetite signals. Negative attention was still attention.

3. Trust yourself as a parent and trust your child

Can you trust that a hungry child will eat, especially if mealtime is a pleasant social family bonding time? The next eating opportunity will be the next time the family sits for a meal. There are no snacks in between meals.

Do you trust that your kid's taste buds can be trained? With consistency, creativity, and curiosity from you, the child will learn.

4. Parents are the first teachers

Parents are role models, so most often, kids establish their relationship with food, exercise, and sleep habits by modeling you. If your child needs to change, then you, as parents, need to change, too. They listen to your self-talk and take mental notes from you when you frown at your body, grabbing your own body fat in the mirror.

Our kids learn more from what we do than what we say. Are you in this parenting role to win one plate battle at a time? Or do you want to teach your child how to self-regulate their relationship with their food and their body as a lifelong skill? Here are some lessons you may want to consider working on with your family in order to build healthy habits and support your child as they move into adulthood.

1. **If every meal is a prolonged attempt at distraction . . . *you may be enforcing mindless eating.*** Parents sometimes trick kids into eating by sticking them in front of a digital screen, turning mealtime into staring time so that the kid becomes conditioned to open their mouth to accept food, just so the cartoon doesn't stop. Eating beyond natural satiety becomes a Pavlovian response. Parental guilt and anxiety might cause kids to learn mindless eating early in life, before they can even develop any memory of it. The trigger to overeat is then transferred in adult life to other external cues, like all-you-can-eat buffets, cruise ship food extravaganzas, movie popcorn tubs, and jumbo combo deals. The trigger to reduce eating is transferred in adult life to external interventions like diet plans, medication, and anyone selling weight loss.

2. **If every meal is stressful for the parent . . .** *it's probably stressful for your kid, too.* I have seen adults who learned complex coping styles and limiting beliefs from their childhoods. These are oversimplified and not so linear in reality, but believing or thinking things like:

    a. Family mealtime means battle (unhealthy family dynamic)

    b. Food means power struggle (unhealthy relationship with food)

    c. I am not capable of doing this on my own (low self-confidence)

    d. I am not good enough (low self-esteem)

    e. I have a sweet tooth (low self-regulation)

    f. I am not good enough (perfection)

    g. I overeat (unhealthy relationship with body)

    h. I am "too big" (inadequacy, low self-worth, body dissatisfaction)

    i. My parents don't believe me (insecurity, approval seeking, or people pleasing) can become mindsets that stay with you all through childhood into adulthood. We want to stop that from influencing *parenthood*. At the extreme end, I have seen adolescents develop binging and purging tendencies, bulimia, and other self-harm tendencies. We've had to involve professional help, not just for the child, but equally for the parents. It becomes a very difficult problem to solve.

3. **If kids have to eat predetermined portions of vegetables to earn dessert, they learn that** *sugar belongs on a pedestal as a prize, ignoring my body's fullness signals and stuffing myself earns me a reward, and someone else gets to decide how much I eat.* Right now, it's parents; later on, it's the food industry.

    One thing I did when we traveled with our kids when they were young was walk them through the buffet, showing them what foods had protein and how many grams of protein their bodies needed to take in per day. They were then encouraged to walk through the buffet with full permission to pick some high-quality protein sources.

Depending on the vegetarian options, we would sometimes all have a protein shake in the hotel room before visiting the buffet, then have a serving of dessert if we were still hungry. Now my kids know how to self-regulate their food, enjoying sugar in balance and finding it nauseating to eat in large quantities. I chose not to police them but to empower them.

4. **If parents feel like they have to serve junk food, soda, cupcakes, and refined carbs at every celebration . . .** *they are modeling how to respond to the peer pressure of society.* And society has gotten pretty crazy. They don't realize that by giving their children sugar-sweetened beverages, fructose-containing processed food, and sugar-laden sweets, their children are experiencing biochemical changes in the brain similar to addiction.

If cocaine tasted sweet, would you say it's cute to give it to your child because they really wanted it? Although cocaine was removed from Coca-Cola in 1903, the sugar and caffeine were not.[29]

Parents should be aware that there is a money trail while our kids get sick. The same society that condones selling brightly colored marshmallow cereal and soda to kids is seeing rising rates of children with obesity suffer from not just type 2 diabetes but conditions like sleep apnea, high blood pressure, eating disorders, fatty liver causing organ damage, and mental health disorders, such as attention deficit-hyperactivity disorder (ADHD), anxiety, and depression. Occasionally, obesity and type 2 diabetes become severe enough that kids need bariatric surgery because their bodies can't cope.[30,31,32]

It's not easy to resist the pressures of society, and I know it's not easy to always do what's "best" for your family and their health. It's not possible to live like a monk in the middle of this modern world, and it's not necessary or sufficient to wait for a global 100 percent ban on sweets in order to turn around diabetes. At this point, you might be wondering whether my kids even enjoy a "normal" life.

The trick here is to start the conversation at home, helping our kids by modeling a balance between eating for pleasure as well as health, and to build our children's confidence so that they can learn these skills without feeling "uncool." We do celebrate mindfully with a little bit of sugar every once in a while, knowing how to balance our intake while caring for our bodies. Sure, a little bit of sweet every now and then doesn't kill anyone—when it's consumed in balance. Their taste buds get satisfied with a small amount of sugar because they don't eat it every day. If they have dessert, they prefer it to be made with much less sugar than the industry standard.

With junk food constantly available at the press of a button, it's urgent that we teach our boys and girls to navigate the food landscape and learn to cook whole, unprocessed foods for themselves. Their lives depend on it.

5. **That's why insisting toddlers "should eat more" and teenagers "should eat less"** *is confusing.* An outside professional can't really "fix" the teenage "rebellion."

Parents flip their position when they realize it's not cute anymore, but it's toxic if the same parents who taught the kid to overeat, then start judging and body shaming the teenager when they continue the habit. We suddenly expect the kid to drop the bad habits we gave them just because they look tall enough to be adults.

6. **Body shaming starts at home—***no teen is overeating or gaining weight on purpose.* No teen wants diabetes. No teen wants medications or doctor visits. Complaining to the doctor that your child is too big or overweight is unhelpful. Shaming the child in front of others is hurtful. All kids want to look good, just like adults. Developmentally, good looks around puberty increase your chances of finding a mate, creating offspring, and continuing your species.

7. **That's why the responsibility of your children's health can be** *gradually handed over to the child.* As the child gets older, they can take on more responsibility, sharing their input on meal planning. I involved my kids in planning their meals from before they were ten. As a family, you can find a balance, with all mealtimes being pleasant and food being tasty; with close to nine out of ten meals being healthy; and with one out of ten foods being purely for taste or enjoyment, without much nutritional value. Nagging the child with your anxiety and constant need to control will defeat the very independence you want them to display, making it more difficult to embrace adulthood and teach healthy eating habits to your grandchildren.

8. **Drop the blame, guilt, shame, and drama** *by drawing boundaries and communicating as a team.* Healthier communication is possible and will require mindfulness from the adults. It will take a lot of work from you, but this is a learning experience for the whole family.

If it's grandparents "spoiling" your kids, have the conversation.

I have not met any grandparent who wants to make their precious grandchild sick. I know you believe that preventing the next generation from suffering is worth it. Use the Drama Triangle conversation steps from Part 4.11 if it helps.

5. And finally, it's okay to take professional help.

Recognize that a healthcare professional gets maybe an hour per session with your child. Parents get much more time with their kids and have far more influence on them than anyone else. Change will be needed from everyone at home to make it work, but if you need help with addressing old thought patterns from your past, be sure to seek professional help for yourself, too. Raising children is not for the faint of heart, and it takes a village. There's no shame in reaching out to that village to help you, your family, and your child build and maintain healthy habits over the long run.

Being a parent is hard work, and raising a child with diabetes doesn't make it any easier. Over the years, I've met with so many families, and I can tell you with certainty: everyone's case is different. Instead of stressing yourself or your family out by trying to be perfect, you can focus on trying to teach your family more effective self-care habits using the adjusted wheels from this chapter.

9.7 What could Maya and Jay's parents do?

Ican't say it was easy for me to witness the familial interaction as Maya's parents went back and forth, before Maya told me that she wants to lose weight. I could see dysfunctional communication between the adults, and the child was being left to her own devices. I knew that leaving insulin resistance unaddressed in a nine year old was putting her at a five-fold risk of not only the complications of diabetes, but also mental health disorders like schizophrenia or bipolar disorder by the time she turned twenty-four.[33,34]

I felt bad for Maya, but was not equipped to be their family therapist.

I asked the parents if they could work on their communication first, and I recommended a few books that had helped me improve my parenting style a few years earlier. All parents want the best for their child and unknowingly make mistakes when they don't know better or haven't experienced better themselves. Priya was already working with me on her own weight, so she understood and trusted my line of thinking. She knew she had to work on herself, her self-talk, and her communication with Alok.

Maya was just nine and dependent on the grown-ups.

Priya started attending therapy to address her own emotional baggage and heal the relationship she had with her own body. She had to work on forgiving herself. There was tremendous guilt for having allowed the frustration from her married life to prevent her from supporting Maya's health. Still, she was able to find the courage to accept what had happened in the past and put one step forward, one day at a time.

Surprisingly, **the battles with Maya evaporated once Priya changed the way she engaged with her daughter.** Maya loved being involved with her mom in planning meals for the week. All she probably wanted was to feel a sense of belonging and connection with her parents.[35] The quality time helped them both. Priya had to find more effective ways of expressing her needs to Alok and her in-laws.

Slowly but surely, the family rallied together for the sake of supporting Maya. By the time Maya was eleven, the family had won against type 2 diabetes, and her blood reports were fine. She didn't need the weighing scale and enjoyed participating in dance and sports events in school with her friends.

But what about Jay's parents?

Since Jay was almost 18, I asked his parents' permission to work with Jay directly. They agreed and were happy someone was willing to take over coaching him. I knew Jay wanted to be treated like an adult, so that's what I did.

I asked him what mattered to him most and what he thought was happening with his health. He was resentful of his parents' double standards around controlling his food versus expecting him to show independence–but he didn't talk to them about it. It was easier to just forget about it by eating whatever he wanted when they weren't around.

Jay was a very intelligent kid.

He was studying to get into engineering college, and he responded well to logic. I explained the concept of carbs, insulin resistance, and protein malnutrition. He didn't like being overweight and wanted to understand why he kept gaining weight. His parents didn't know and couldn't explain it to him. After working with us, he started understanding why he was always hungry and wanting large amounts of food to feel satiated: **he wasn't getting enough protein.**

Because he was going to be on a college campus beginning the following year, he asked to learn how to navigate restaurant menus and count his nutritional intake himself. He asked me to tell his parents that he needed to get more chicken in the house for himself and permission to order more fish when they ordered in. He enjoyed eating more meat and planning his meals around protein. He wanted the diabetes and extra body fat to be gone before he started college.

So that's what he did. Because he had only had type 2 diabetes for a year, he was able to put it into remission within six months. He now lives on campus, eats mostly animal protein, and is able to focus on student life.

Now that we've covered all of the lifestyle wheels and fasting, and applied that knowledge to women and children, it's time to talk about how to approach type 1 diabetes. Much like type 2, type 1 diabetes can start in childhood, but affects adults as well.

Part 9 summary

- Women with polycystic ovarian syndrome can get pregnant if they want to.

- Insulin resistance plays a role in PCOS, gestational diabetes and post-partum depression. This book has shown you what you can do about it.

- Kids are more likely to succeed at diabetes self-management and weight management around parents who believe in their ability to gradually take more responsibility.

- Consistency, trust, respect, body positivity and role modeling all help children focus on developing a healthier relationship with their food and their bodies.

For Bonus Materials, Visit the Website Here:

PART 10

HOW TO HANDLE TYPE 1 DIABETES, TURN AROUND INSULIN RESISTANCE, AND ACHIEVE MORE STABLE GLUCOSE LEVELS WITH LESS INSULIN

10.1: Approaching Type I Diabetes

Accoding to a blog by Stanford University, people with type 1 diabetes have to make around 180 additional decisions per day, over and beyond people without type 1 diabetes.[1] The good news is, all of the lifestyle changes mentioned in this book till this point can help you prevent or reverse insulin resistance so that you can manage your glucose levels with the lowest possible insulin doses.

We covered the differences between type 1 and type 2 diabetes in Part 1, **but can someone with type 1 diabetes also get type 2?**

To answer this, let's look at my client, Natali, who was frustrated about her type 1 diabetes.

"Doc, I have not logged anything in your app this week. It's been too much. I eat randomly throughout the day, and it messes up the data. And no matter how many units I inject, the glucose just doesn't come down! I'm spending hours hovering around my glucometer, getting nothing else done at work. Finally, I just inject twenty units to push it down and get on with my day. Now I feel bloated and look like shit in these pants, my work clothes don't fit anymore; the buttons don't close. All this weight around my tummy looks disgusting. I weigh myself three times a day, and it just keeps going up. How can I even put any of this into any app?"

Natali had type 1 diabetes; this most often involves an autoimmune attack on the pancreas. The body's immune system mistakenly targets the beta cells that produce insulin; this autoimmune destruction leads to insulin deficiency. Insulin is crucial for allowing glucose to enter cells, and without it, blood sugar levels rise significantly. In type 2 diabetes, of course, loss of insulin sensitivity is the concern, beginning with the prediabetic stage of insulin resistance.

Did you know that even if someone doesn't have type 1 or type 2 diabetes, everyone goes through normal, or physiological phases of insulin resistance in life?

We tend to notice and talk about these phases in people with type 1 diabetes because of the intense monitoring, but **physiological insulin resistance** is normal for everyone *during the growth spurt of puberty*, when growth hormone levels increase; *every morning around 4:00–6:00 a.m.* as a result of the normal process of the "*dawn phenomenon*"; *premenstrual days*, followed by a tendency for lower glucose levels once the menstrual periods start; and *in the third trimester* of pregnancy. These are normal healthy situations when the glucose level is slightly higher than baseline.

Outside of those situations, insulin resistance is something that should be addressed, and here, we are considering it in the context of people with type 1 diabetes.

If you are facing worsening insulin resistance as an adult with type 1 diabetes, all of the previous lifestyle chapters can help you achieve more stable glucose levels with lower insulin doses. If we consider twenty-five units to be the approximate amount of insulin released into the circulation per day by a person without diabetes, then progressively needing more than forty units per day, or more than one unit of insulin per kilogram body weight might suggest you are heading toward insulin resistance.[2] What tends to frustrate people is that their dawn phenomenon starts to break through their overnight slow-acting (basal) insulin dose, and they start the morning by waking up with a high glucose. It feels like they have lost a battle first thing in the morning before they even had a chance to fight. **Signs that you should probably see your doctor due to potential insulin resistance along with type 1** include *worsening acne, hypoglycemic events becoming less frequent, rising HbA1c with the same insulin dose and same lifestyle, gaining weight* (especially around the belly), and *needing higher doses of insulin to keep glucose levels stable* (crossing forty units per day).[3] By working with your doctor and applying the lifestyle approaches throughout this book, you can keep your glucose and hemoglobin A1c (HbA1c) levels within range with the lowest possible insulin doses, and avoid the problems of type 2 diabetes.

10.2: Brittle type 1 diabetes: Swinging too high and too low

Liva was nine when she was diagnosed with type 1 diabetes. By the time I met her, she was twenty-six, and she had pretty much given up on having a normal life. In spite of taking sixty units of insulin divided across four injections per day, with pain at her insulin injection sites, her glucose levels would fluctuate within a twenty-four-hour period, swinging from a low of 40 mg/dL to a high of 400+ mg/dL (2.22 to 22.2 mmol/L), giving her HbA1c of 8 percent.

She was eating six times a day, taking the shots after the main meals as advised.

She was told to stop playing outdoor sports, even though that was the only thing she enjoyed.

She came from a religious family, and people said she got diabetes because she didn't pray enough. She prayed harder, but nothing improved. She felt pretty convinced as an angry tween that "God" would not do this to little children. She lost faith.

It felt pointless to even bother checking her level because it was never in the target range. She would spend days without using her glucometer, which also saved money on testing strips. For months, she took just enough insulin to stay out of the hospital. The only thing she looked forward to was sensing the occasional hypoglycemia (hypo), which was her opportunity to gobble down some chocolate to get the level back up.

Despite her mother being a family physician and reaching out to multiple endocrinologists, none of the experts had been able to stabilize her levels. The extent of her treatment plan for years before we met was, "Take more insulin when it's high; eat something sweet when it's low."

When a doctor sees this situation, they unfortunately sometimes label it as *brittle diabetes*. **This is absolutely incorrect and harmful language.** To understand what I mean, let's come back to the analogy of driving a car.

Have you ever watched a Formula One car race? The racers achieve speeds of up to 350 kilometers per hour (220 miles per hour), maneuvering turns while experiencing thirty kilograms (70 pounds) of force pulling their head to one side. They have to be ready to hit the brakes to bring an 800-kilogram (1,760-pound) car to a complete stop within seconds.

High acceleration. High deceleration. High wear and tear. High risk.

That's what patients tell me living with type 1 diabetes on a high-carb diet plus high insulin doses can feel like. Starting with a high-carb meal causes the glucose to rise rapidly; this is chased with high insulin doses, causing the glucose to fall steeply. When you overcorrect with too much insulin, however, you crash into hypoglycemia. Then, you need to correct the low glucose with quick-acting carbs, and you obviously don't take insulin for these carbs because you need the glucose to rise. Often, you overcorrect with emergency correction carbs. So then?

The high-speed chase starts again.

Like Formula racing, the hormone imbalance of type 1 diabetes is tricky. Prescribing insulin to mimic a pancreas is tricky, doctor-patient communication can be tricky, and human behavior and coping mechanisms are tricky.

It can be a very exhausting experience, both mentally and physically, to see your numbers bounce up and down. Going through these highs and lows can feel like you are being thrown around in a foosball machine. *Even so, I want you to know that there can only be mismanaged diabetes, not brittle diabetes.*

It's not easy and it's not fun, but I have witnessed hundreds of people resolve "brittle diabetes" as we focus on the changes discussed in this book. They end up needing less insulin, and life becomes just a little bit easier than before.

If we continue our driving analogy, I want you to compare Formula One driving to being stuck in bumper-to-bumper traffic while driving through a busy market. The speeds are so slow that if your bumper did touch someone else's, the damage would be minimal, repair would be easier, and the aftermath would be less painful. You might even pull away without a scratch.

That's what living life with type 1 diabetes on a low-carb diet with adequate protein intake, personalized insulin dosing and sufficient muscle mass is like. One survey of 288 people living with type 1 on less than fifty grams of carbs per day showed that 87 percent of respondents were either satisfied or very satisfied with their diabetes control, with an average HbA1c below 6 percent and low insulin requirements.[4]

10.3: Matching your insulin to your activity

You might be struggling to get the glucose to stay in the normal range. **Two common causes for this** are a *mismatch between your exercise and insulin regimen, or hypoglycemia unawareness.* I'll be sure to cover both of these causes. Let's begin with exercise and type 1 diabetes, starting with Gurmeet.

My patient Gurmeet was a state-level tennis player.

He was on 70/30 premixed insulin twice a day, and hypoglycemia kept interrupting his practice sessions. He worried that the low glucose would reduce his performance during competitive games. He carried chocolate to every match, eating some all day and taking higher insulin doses to fuel his game. The energy boost provided explosive power that he used to win crucial points.

Ria, on the other hand, was a senior ballet student in the best dance academy in the city.

When rehearsals got more intense, she had to sit on the sidelines for hours because low glucose levels would make her shiver and feel so weak that she had to huddle on the floor, hugging her knees, until her glucose levels came back up. Her parents and doctors told her to give up on the idea of being a professional dancer. She should "take up a safer hobby, like chess," they said, but she knew she was an excellent ballerina and wanted to make a career out of dance.

We'll come back to Gurmeet and Ria a bit later, but their stories are examples of doctors telling people with type 1 diabetes what they "can't do." When I hear such tales, I wonder what gives such doctors permission to do what they do.

I have to remind myself that they mean well and are just trying to protect their patient from harm as best they know how, but they are probably suffering from the unconscious cognitive bias called the Dunning–Kruger effect.[5] This can be particularly harmful in healthcare situations where patients come to the doctor trusting that they are getting the best professional advice possible. Everyone with type 1 deserves to exercise and be active if they want to. Although many people have observed that cardio (aerobic) activity drops glucose levels and strength or high-intensity interval training raises glucose levels, this may not always be the case.[6]

There are examples of people with type 1 completing long endurance efforts, like running 100 miles on a five-day fast, or explosive strength training, so it's a matter of adjusting your insulin accordingly.[7,8] People with type 1 diabetes have reached Olympic and Grand Slam levels of excellence in sport, and you can, too.

Work with your doctor to assess how your body responds to aerobic, high-intensity, low-intensity, and strength-training workouts to create a plan that works for you. You may want to take account of timing of exercise in relation to the last meal eaten, as it may be playing a larger role in post-workout glucose fluctuations. Research suggests that perhaps working out in a fasted state has more effect on glucose responses than the type or intensity of exercise.[9] Additionally, the ketogenic diet has been used by endurance athletes to experience glycemic stability during endeavors like cycling 4,000 kilometers over twenty days.[10]

A 2023 trial looked at the effect of different exercise modes on glucose levels in people with type 1 diabetes and found that the glucose levels were lowered across all types of exercise, so you deserve to do what you like to do, instead of giving up ballet or any other active hobbies![11] Gathering all the data can feel like a lot of effort; knowing that you won't need to give up what you love can make it seem more worthwhile to work with your doctor. The incentive to decipher how your body responds to different workouts and meals, is that your insulin dose can be adjusted to prevent hypoglycemia and keep glucose levels stable for longer periods of time.

10.4: Paying attention to hypoglycemia

L et's go to the second cause of struggling to get the glucose to stay in the normal range: **hypoglycemia unawareness.**

Hypoglycemia unawareness, impaired awareness of hypoglycemia (IAH), and hypoglycemia-associated autonomic failure (HAAF) are important, serious, and potentially life-threatening side effects of aggressive insulin therapy in type 1 diabetes. This happens when the glucose *level is so low that the brain is not functioning properly, but the person isn't aware* of the problem, so they don't take corrective glucose, and the level keeps dropping. Throughout this guide to turning your diabetes around, I have shared patient success stories, but not all of them started out so smoothly. I've worked with many people who live with type 1 diabetes and develop hypoglycemia unawareness, and their experiences range from highly concerning, to terrifying, to downright heartbreaking.

One **particularly concerning** situation was with a man with type 1 diabetes who worked as a personal trainer, assisting and spotting people lifting weights. His client told him he was acting strange while supervising the client's heavy barbell set. The trainer didn't realize his glucose level was dangerously low until after the client's workout had ended. It was very risky for him to be handling heavy weights *while being unaware he was in the middle of a severe hypoglycemic event.*

Another person I know is a fitness enthusiast who loves hiking, cycling, and running. She went out on a mountain hike with her family and her father later told me about her strange behavior during the hike. He narrated how it was unusual to see her binge eating two packets of biscuits and quickly chugging a box of juice in the middle of the hike without taking any insulin dose and without telling anyone she was hungry. When her dad insisted on checking her blood glucose, it was still normal, *meaning she had corrected a severe hypoglycemic episode.* That sounds like a win, right? The concern is that she had no memory of doing any of this; her brain probably went into survival mode and could not register what happened.

Then, there were some people whose stories had put them in severe danger and left their loved ones horrified —I couldn't imagine living either of the experiences they described.

For instance, a patient once told me that *her partner found her unresponsive, lying stiff* as a log in bed with her jaw clenched tightly shut. Even though he was much stronger than her, it was almost impossible to get glucose gel into her mouth, placing her on the verge of having a seizure that night.

Another patient was cooking in the kitchen and chopping vegetables when her husband noticed she was acting strange. He suspected she was probably hypoglycemic. When he tried to get her to eat something, *she came toward him with the kitchen knife in anger.* It was a struggle to disarm her and force in some glucose.

At least these patients had someone to administer glucose, because in other stories, they weren't as lucky. I had one man tell me *how he had collapsed at the bus stop outside his house, lying unresponsive on the street* as a result of hypoglycemia, till a neighbor recognized him and activated help.

Similarly, I met *a man who was discovered unconscious on the floor in the back of his office.* His colleagues (who knew he had diabetes), assumed he had a low glucose level and luckily revived him with juice. That's when he decided to change his insulin protocols by finding a new doctor. He was a single father, and his aging mother was helping raise his eight-year-old daughter. He wanted to be in the best possible health for the people he cared so much about, and realized he needed to take hypoglycemia seriously.

Not taking it seriously, however, can cause **some of the most heartbreaking incidents** I've heard. One in particular belongs to a receptionist who was close to retirement. She was overweight and insulin resistant, and one day, she missed her bus stop and got off at the wrong one. Due to hypoglycemia, she was lost and disoriented only a few stops away from her home. Although she made it home safely, we heard about the incident a few days later through her husband who kept wondering what would have happened if she had gone too far away from home.

Because she had special learning needs and struggled with math, I'd tried giving her a simple low-carb diet plan to follow that would require lower and more consistent insulin doses, with a reference chart on how to decide the insulin dose for different types of meals. Living with type 1 was putting a huge strain on her retirement savings, but carbohydrate-dominant foods fit her limited budget. She kept choosing the familiar foods instead of following the plan.

When she got tired of seeing high glucose levels after a high-carb meal, she would get frustrated and inject a large insulin dose without any calculation. This caused very volatile glucose levels, with prolonged hypoglycemia and hypoglycemia unawareness. *One major risk of such repeated hypoglycemic states is that it can cause loss of cognitive function.*[12]

When she was not experiencing a severe hypoglycemic episode, she was a pleasant, friendly, and kind colleague who was loved by all. I suspected the repeated episodes had reduced her memory and ability to learn what I was trying to teach. We live in an imperfect world with a broken, fragmented medical system, and it breaks my heart that there isn't more we could do to help her.

The most devastating of all, was a lab technician who had type 1 diabetes. He was this really nice guy who used to take insulin through an insulin pump without checking his glucose levels for days, and the last time I saw him was when I had strictly warned him and told him in writing that he was at risk of hypoglycemia unawareness. He was instructed to always check his glucose before driving; otherwise, he was not authorized to drive. I told him I would have to involve the hospital legal team, and they might have to inform the driver's license issuing agency. I would refill his insulin prescriptions as long as he followed the required safety measures. He could be dangerous on the road to himself and others. Indeed, severe hypoglycemia is related to motor vehicle accidents and is a known public health risk in people with diabetes.[13] He stopped seeing me.

He was found by the police one morning, unresponsive in his car on the side of the road–his head resting on the steering wheel. He must have pulled over after perhaps feeling unwell or tired on his way home after the night shift. The insulin pump was still delivering insulin, and his glucose level was undetectable when the ambulance arrived.

He never made it home.

His face has not left my mind, and I can never forget my last conversation with him. I often wonder what else we could have done to help him. ***Insulin was lifesaving and, tragically, deadly for him.***

As sad as it is, it doesn't have to end that way. Not all scary experiences with hypoglycemia end in a tragedy.

One lady I worked with with type 1 had just returned to the boat after scuba diving in the Philippines. As the divers were taking off their gear on the deck, she insisted on being served juice. *While she was waiting for the juice, she fell over and started having a seizure on the boat.* Her companions were totally caught by surprise and somehow managed to keep her safe until the seizure subsided. They gave her a soft drink, and even after two cans, her glucose level was only 80 mg/dL (4.44 mmol/L). If this seizure had happened just a few minutes earlier while she was still in the water, she would have drowned.

Luckily, she is completely fine and recovered from the event, with a painful tongue bite and jaw pain that took a few weeks to completely heal. Being underwater and swimming around must have made her glucose level drop more quickly, and she may have been more distracted than usual to notice the hypo symptoms. She can't remember the last insulin dose before the dive, and this suggests that she may have already been heading for a low-glucose event before entering the water.

A year and a half later, her pump settings have been reconfigured, and she continues to enjoy water sports without further events.

Like everyone referenced here, when your high blood glucose determined that you had type 1 diabetes, insulin was lifesaving. As the lifesaving insulin dose is started, glucose levels start coming down. The first time you get hypoglycemia, you physically know it is going low.

Sweating. Shaking. Nervousness. Irritability. Hunger.

Knowing intuitively that something is wrong.

Hypoglycemic awareness comes from these warning signs that are created by the sympathetic nervous system (SNS), or the fight-flight-fright system. This emergency alarm system tells you to get food to bring up your glucose levels immediately. Your endocrinologist needs to know urgently if you are no longer experiencing these symptoms as your glucose drops.

"High glucose damages your organs" has been drilled into people's minds for decades, and *you might have been conditioned to fear the high glucose levels*. On the other hand, a hypoglycemic event can be corrected with glucose (or choco-late!), so it might not feel as scary.

The problem is, high glucose levels cause harm over decades.

A low glucose level can cause severe harm immediately—like, right now. Today. We know that prolonged hypoglycemia can harm brain neurons within hours, so when we combine the severe hypoglycemia *with* hypoglycemia un-awareness—we have an extremely dangerous situation that needs to be corrected as a top priority.

Understanding hypoglycemia unawareness

To understand **hypoglycemia *unawareness***, think of a night-shift security guard in a multistory building. Their job is to keep the building residents safe by keeping watch at the main gate of the building overnight. One night, a new visitor shows up. The guard will request identification, then ask where the visitor is going and the purpose of the visit. After all the questions have passed scrutiny, the visitor is allowed inside the building.

Suppose the visitor comes every night. After a while, the person becomes fa-miliar, and the guard lets them in without any questions. No more security checks.

What if the visitor is a dangerous criminal who has now breached the normal security protocol just by visiting frequently?

That is exactly what hypoglycemia unawareness is. If the hypoglycemia keeps happening, the dangerous phenomenon becomes familiar, and the alarms from the SNS become less intense. The health of your brain depends on the SNS generating those physical security alarms to make you eat and quickly bring the glucose levels up. Repeated hypos blunt the warning symptoms that keep you safe.

When the glucose drops *really* low with hypoglycemia unawareness, the stress hormones are still pumping through the system, without the sweating and anxiety. It might even feel like an adrenaline rush or a buzz. I have an unproven theory about this. It's just a theory because I have never experienced this myself, and patients don't remember the event clearly enough to walk anyone else through what happened. It's like the amnesia after a concussion.

Is it possible that the combination of impaired judgment from the brain getting less glucose plus the underlying buzz from stress hormones rushing through the system causes people to sometimes behave aggressively, as if they don't want to come out of that bad hypo state? Close family, friends, or loved ones might be the ones to notice your hypoglycemia and feel 100 percent sure you're having a bad low because you begin acting so strange.

Paradoxically, when they ask you to check your glucometer reading, ask you to eat food, or approach you with sugar, you might not react well. We've heard multiple frightening accounts from terrified relatives of how scary it got when the person with severe hypoglycemia was refusing treatment and getting angry, hostile, and even potentially violent.

The bad news

It's difficult to know for sure what the experience is like because most people don't remember their event afterward; they often insist after coming out of the hypoglycemia that it wasn't as bad as the witnesses are describing. The patient may think others are exaggerating because they themselves didn't fully register what happened. Their brain resources were diverted to emergency survival mode, instead of memory or learning. It can make it hard for them to understand or learn what their friends and family are fussing about. Sometimes they take it personally.

If the hypoglycemia lasts all through the night, repeatedly, you may be so tired that you sleep through it without correcting the low all night. *The dangerous visitor has been invited for a sleepover.* You might wake up with nightmares or a headache, but you might be glad to see a morning reading of 50 mg/dL (2.77 mmol/L), not realizing that your counter-regulatory hormones saved your life in the night and barely pushed the level up by the morning. Now the night security guard thinks this dangerous visitor is a welcome member of the family!

In people at risk of nocturnal hypoglycemia, *I have them set an alarm to check the level at 3:00 a.m.* which is when the glucose is likely to be at its lowest. Basically, we want to retrain you to catch the hypoglycemia when the level is falling from 80 to 70 mg/dL (4.44 to 3.88 mmol/L) by restoring the physical warning alarms (of hunger, sweating, and shaking) set by the SNS. We don't want you to go straight to the neurological symptoms at which point your ability to make decisions about self-correcting low glucose levels is impaired.

If the hypoglycemia continues, your brain gets less and less glucose, and you are at risk of losing consciousness or having a seizure. The negative effect of low glucose in the brain is called **neuroglycopenia**. It's very dangerous to you in the short term if you are alone, and also dangerous to people around you if you are driving or operating heavy machinery or equipment.

The good news is, restoring hypoglycemia awareness has been shown to improve circulation in crucial areas of the brain.[14]

The good news

Sometimes people feel relief when the SNS symptoms have stopped, even though it's a very dangerous complication of diabetes management with serious consequences. These risky events are avoidable and preventable. Please talk to your doctor if you don't notice physical symptoms when your levels fall from 80 to 60 mg/dL (4.44 to 3.33 mmol/L). Waking up with a reading of 50 mg/dL (2.77 mmol/L) is not acceptable if it means you slept through hypoglycemia all night. Prioritize urgent restoration of hypoglycemia awareness because unawareness is also linked to an increased risk of having a heart attack or stroke.[15] This takes close follow-up with your endocrinologist to reset the glucose targets and insulin doses to strictly avoid hypoglycemia for a few weeks.

What does restoring hypoglycemic awareness take?

It looks like resetting the alarm systems, and retraining all the security staff about who is allowed to enter the building and who needs to be stopped at the gate.

Staying between 120 and 180 mg/dL (6.6–10 mmol/L) for two to four weeks usually restores some awareness in my patients. You will need close follow-up and insulin adjustments—do not try this unsupervised or alone. Work with a professional; plan with your doctor to spend *at least two weeks with all glucose readings above* 120 mg/dL (6.6 mmol/L).

There is new research to support that in severe cases, it can take up to two years to restore awareness. Anecdotally, I have seen hypoglycemia awareness return in much less than that when we work closely with people. The first six months seem to make a very big difference once we help the person understand how insulin works in the body and how the body responds to hypoglycemia. Wearing a continuous glucose monitor (CGM) has been shown to reduce hypoglycemic events. We use glucometer data to change insulin doses to prevent hypoglycemia while also aiming for an HbA1c below 7 percent.

The smart treatment for hypoglycemia, is working with your doctor

If you are experiencing hypoglycemia unawareness or severe hypoglycemia, and your HbA1c is high; we have to *fix the hypos first,* before we go after the high HbA1c.

The logic is that a high HbA1c needs lifestyle change and *maybe* more insulin. If you do both of those things without fixing the hypos, then the hypos will get worse. So, we have to fix the lows before we fix the highs. This takes a lot of coordination, data gathering, and communication between you and your medical team. Find someone who understands the importance of fixing both problems (lows and highs) at the root.

Remember, the hypos are *iatrogenic,* meaning they have been caused by prescription insulin. You deserve a medical team that is interested in and capable of helping you stop hypoglycemia while addressing insulin resistance so that you can manage type 1 diabetes with the lowest and safest insulin dose possible. ***You deserve better advice than "more carbs for the lows, more insulin for the highs."***

When you work with your doctor, treatments will vary based on your level of hypoglycemia. Hypoglycemia is officially defined as a glucose level, confirmed on glucometer, of below 70 mg/dL (3.8 mmol/L). Not every low glucose is life-threatening.

For mild hypoglycemia; use the 15-15-15 rule. Take *15 grams* of readily available glucose by mouth in any ONE of these forms: 100 mL of juice; 200 to 250 mL of plain, unsweetened whole (full-fat) milk; glucose gels or three to four glucose tablets, each being four grams of glucose. I recommend that you choose a liquid source as the first preference because we want the glucose to start getting absorbed from the mucous lining inside the cheeks before it even reaches the stomach. Some gels come in travel-friendly packaging like a ketchup sachet. After *15 minutes,* recheck the glucose level. It should rise by 15 *mg/dL* (0.83 mmol/L). If it does not come up by that much, then consume another 15 g of glucose until you see it rise by that much, or see it come above 70 mg/dL (3.8 mmol/L).

Then you need to eat a small mixed meal (without quick acting insulin) that has complex carbohydrates, protein, and fat. I have patients who panicked and chugged bottles of soda or gobble a whole packet of biscuits or chocolate. This becomes an overcorrection that keeps levels volatile for longer; a balanced meal will give you a more stable result. Monitor your levels closely, depending on the number and type of insulin units taken that caused the hypo, and *take this information to your doctor* so that they can adjust the insulin dose that caused the hypoglycemia! If you are on a pump plus CGM, you can suspend the pump. ***Always confirm the actual level with glucometer readings*** because these rapid

411

fluctuations are what give the largest CGM errors. I have seen a margin of inaccuracy of up to 100 mg/dL (5.55 mmol/L). Newer closed-loop pumps have predictive technology that automatically suspends insulin delivery before you reach a severe hypo and automatically resumes when glucose levels start rising again. This technology has given people with type 1 diabetes more time in range (TIR), better HbA1c, and less time spent in hypoglycemia.[16] This is as close to a widely available artificial pancreas as we have at the time of writing. Researchers are developing dual-hormone closed-loop systems that deliver both insulin and glucagon. Alerts can be sent to parents and healthcare providers via the cloud to integrated dashboards and devices.

A severe hypo is often preceded and followed by blood glucose disturbances in the twenty-four hours before and after the event.[17] **For recurrent severe hypoglycemia: a glucagon intramuscular injection should be part of your emergency kit.** Think of it like an epi pen for someone with severe nut allergies; you still need to be evaluated by a medical team if you use glucagon to get out of immediate danger. Glucagon seems to be less effective if you had a recent severe hypoglycemic event, so it is very important to work with your doctor to *reduce the insulin dose that caused the hypo.*[18] In terms of a glucagon shot, both you and your friends, family, and caregivers will need to be educated on how to give an instant shot because you will most likely be unable to give it yourself. Obviously, we would like to avoid severe hypoglycemia at all costs, but we all have to start somewhere on the path to restoring hypoglycemia awareness.

Now that we have covered how insulin can cause hypoglycemia and how it needs to be adjusted to suit your lifestyle, let's discuss the commonest insulin regimens in type 1 diabetes.

10.5: Achieving more stable glucose levels with less insulin

Since the first young boy to receive bovine (cow) insulin in his buttocks on January 11, 1922, insulin delivery technology has improved drastically,, giving millions of people with type 1 diabetes their lives back through subcutaneous insulin.[19,20]

When you first got diagnosed with type 1 diabetes, you were probably sent home from the medical system with a prescription for multiple daily injections (MDIs) of insulin. There are three different ways to plan those multiple injections; different insulins cover both slow-acting (basal) and quick-acting (bolus) insulin needs:

1. **Fixed-dose premixed insulin:** A mixture of slow plus quick insulin such as Neutral Protamine Hagedorn (NPH) or degludec plus aspart/lispro/glulisine in a 70/30 or 75/25 ratio. At two shots per day, there is no flexibility of mealtimes, as missed meals can cause hypoglycemia. Carb counting is not used, so the quick-acting dose is not adapted to the meal.

2. **Fixed-dose basal-bolus insulin without carbohydrate counting:** A mix of slow-acting basal glargine/detemir plus quick acting bolus aspart/lispro/glulisine usually totalling four shots per day; the slow-acting injection is once a day and one quick-acting dose is taken for each of the three major meals that have carbs. While there is no carb-counting to adjust the number of bolus units, there is *flexibility when it comes to meal timing.*

3. **Flexible basal bolus with carbohydrate counting:** This is also a mix of slow-acting basal glargine/detemir plus quick acting aspart/lispro/glulisine that is usually given across four daily shots. The basal

injection is taken once a day. Carb-counting is a part of this approach, so it provides maximum stability, safety, and flexibility. The bolus can be adjusted based on the amount of carbs being eaten, and is taken ten to fifteen minutes prior to the meal, offering *flexibility to eat varying amounts of carbs*. The number of bolus injections is reduced when you eat a very low-carb meal or skip a meal.

As you can see, the most effective way to manage type 1 diabetes using MDIs is basal-bolus therapy with carb counting.[21] The basal-bolus approach acknowledges two types of insulin needs.

Basal insulin needs cover the background requirements, even when you're not eating, which means that *it is not used to correct high glucose*. It is *affected by the time of day* (like the dawn phenomenon), *exercise, fasting, illness, menstrual patterns,* or *stress,* and is then treated with either slow-acting insulin as part of a multiple daily injection plan or by using quick-acting insulin released continuously via an insulin pump. *In a pump, the basal rate can be changed on demand.* The dosing accuracy for basal insulin is assessed by fasting glucose readings, or when there's a gap of more than six hours since the last meal or bolus dose. In multiple daily injections, the slow-acting insulin effect typically lasts for about twelve to twenty-four hours in the body. We will come to pumps shortly.

Bolus insulin needs, comparatively, **cover meals** and is used **for the correction of high glucose levels**. Quick-acting insulin is used here. The number of units needed is *affected by the type of food* eaten; the higher the carb, the higher the bolus needed. The dose is also *affected by the starting glucose level* before the meal; you would add more units to correct a high reading. On a pump, different types of meals can be covered by a dual-wave, square-wave, or extended bolus, and *quick-acting insulin delivery is increased on demand in the form of spurts above the basal dose.* Quick-acting insulin lasts for two to six hours in the body, and the dose accuracy can be determined by the two-hour postmeal readings.

In addition to glucometer readings, a continuous glucose monitor (CGM) adds value when making an insulin pattern switch. It keeps you informed of your blood glucose trends as you learn what works for you and your body.

Basal injections on MDI

If you are taking insulin injections, your slow-acting options are NPH, glargine, levemir, and degludec. Many people achieve reasonably stable glucose levels with a **once-a-day basal insulin injection**. You may face some challenges at specific times because the once-a-day injection releases basal insulin at a fixed rate throughout the day.

For example, twelve units of glargine insulin would deliver approximately half a unit of insulin every hour, for twenty-four hours. With once-a-day injections, there is no way to increase the basal amount between 4:00 a.m. and 6:00 a.m. to cover the dawn phenomenon. Some of my patients work around this by taking an early-morning small dose of bolus insulin.

There is also no way to temporarily reduce the basal during vigorous exercise or when a meal is skipped. Some people work around this by taking a small snack before exercise, or they keep eating at regular intervals. Ideally, the basal rate should not cause hypoglycemia just because a meal was skipped. If this keeps happening, you should see your doctor to adjust the basal insulin dose.

When taking MDI, the basal dose adjustment has to wait till the next slow-acting dose is due, which typically has a twenty-four-hour dosing schedule. If you take a higher basal dose injection by mistake, the risk for hypoglycemia remains for the duration of the type of insulin used, so you will have to monitor your glucose levels closely every few hours. Panicking and quickly eating massive amounts of carbohydrates happens to the best of us and may feel necessary in the moment, but will perpetuate the "brittle" diabetes experience; this is where diabetes self management education and support (DSME and DSMS) helps.

Bolus injections on MDI

While your quick-acting options are human regular insulin and the newer insulin analogs (aspart, lispro, or glulisine), there are two types of bolus doses you will need to know about.

First, there is the *mealtime bolus*. This is administered when you eat, but you can choose between a **fixed bolus**, or a **flexible bolus based on carb count and insulin-carb ratio** (ICR). In a **fixed bolus**, *the doctor tells you how many units of quick-acting insulin to take per meal,* regardless of what you plan to eat. For example, they might tell you to take five units of aspart before each meal, three times a day. This causes fluctuations in glucose levels if each meal has different amounts of carbohydrates, and/or your body has different carbohydrate tolerance at different times of the day. People on fixed meal boluses end up force-fitting their lives to survive the dose. If the dose is too high, they have to compensate and eat more carbs. If the dose is too low, they have to take more correction insulin. They might feel like they are always chasing and reacting to a number.

A **flexible bolus based on carb count and ICR** *has the advantage of the mealtime insulin bolus* (quick-acting dose for the meal) being *adjusted based on the carbohydrate count* of that particular meal. This means the dose becomes fully flexible and customized based on what you are eating at that moment.

I compare this to getting a custom tailor-made shirt stitched just for you. The tailor who is going to create this fancy shirt for you *claims* to give you a personalized fit, only to hand out a cookie-cutter, one-size-fits-all, you-have-to-fit-into-my-measurements-no-matter-what, ready-made version. If the tailor did that, they might go out of business.

Similarly, prescribing fixed-dose insulin without an insulin carbohydrate ratio and carbohydrate counting sets a person up for "brittle" diabetes. We know that "brittle diabetes" is not the best name for it, because I have found it to always be iatrogenic, which means caused by the prescription or treatment itself. An endocrinologist competent at managing type 1 diabetes will be able to decipher your insulin carbohydrate ratio (ICR). This formula specifies how many grams of dietary carbs get covered by one unit of quick-acting insulin at various times of the day. I have said this here in one neat sentence, but it can take a few months of intense data gathering and analysis. Doctor-patient teamwork can identify an accurate insulin dose amidst the noise of wide fluctuations. It is laborious and time-consuming, but it works. The body has patterns and rhythms that are waiting to be deciphered. It wants homeostasis, not daily roller-coasters.

Once you know your formula, all you need to do is calculate your dose based on how many carbohydrates you plan to eat at a particular meal. For example, if your doctor sets your ICR at lunch to be twelve, that means they have calculated one unit of quick-acting insulin will cover twelve grams of carbs at lunch. If you plan to eat twenty-four grams of carbohydrates for lunch (two small thin slices of bread), you would take two units of quick-acting insulin ten minutes before that meal. If you are on a pump, the doctor would program your ICRs into the pump corresponding with your usual mealtimes, and then all you have to do is tell the pump how many carbs you are eating. The pump does the math using the ICR, calculates the insulin dose, and delivers it after your permission.

So, your meal timing and insulin dose are in your hands, just like your food and your life are! This gives you more flexibility because the doctor has no idea what or how much you plan to eat at what time, or what is happening in your life. You are better off knowing how to adjust your insulin in a safe, calculated, and scientific way rather than making it a never-ending guessing game. There are free carbohydrate counting courses available online; a recently published book by Ashwini Wagle from San Jose State University addresses the complexity of carb counting South Asian foods.

The second type of bolus insulin dose is a ***correction bolus for high glucose based on the insulin sensitivity factor*** (ISF).

The ISF is the formula for correction doses, meaning the number of mg/dL or mmol/L glucose we expect to be lowered by one unit of correction insulin bolus. I always have my patients take their ISF along with the ICR before meals. Not after.

There are some formulae people use, such as dividing 1,500 by your total daily insulin dose to calculate the ISF and dividing 500 by your total daily insulin dose to estimate your ICR. I have found through years of practice that calculating the dose based on actual data from analyzing a well-maintained glucose log, CGM, and food log is a much more accurate, safe, and quick way to get to the right dose. Setting ICRs and ISFs has helped people achieve stable blood glucose levels within months after having lived with fluctuating "brittle" levels for years.

Sometimes people want to take their mealtime bolus after seeing the plate, checking how hungry they are, and doing the carb count after getting halfway through the meal. This is like *getting on a train that has already pulled away* from the railway station. You are chasing something that is speeding away, and you might get hurt. Some of you may have been taught this, like Liva was, as a "treatment" for "brittle" diabetes. The logic may have been, "If we chase it after it's already going high, then at least it won't go low."

Tempting, but wrong. That advice comes from a limited understanding of insulin physiology. It's much safer to board a train while it's waiting for you on the platform.

We generally advise patients to take the ICR + ISF ten minutes before a meal. This reduces the risk of hypoglycemia and mimics normal physiology because the pancreas would have released insulin when the brain anticipates a meal (the cephalic phase). That is like a passenger who is already on the railway platform with their luggage *waiting before the train pulls into the station.* They are ready to board smoothly, settling down inside the train before it departs. You can set a complex bolus like a dual wave or square wave if you're having a meal that is high in fat and carbohydrates; this applies when the blood glucose is expected to rise a little initially and then rise again later or it stays high a little longer because of the delayed absorption of the meal. Your pump specialist can work on different combinations with you to find what works best.

Similarly, if you take a correction bolus two hours *after* a meal when you see a high postmeal reading, you may experience a low-glucose reaction because the glucose level is naturally on its way down after the meal has been fully digested. The peak glucose is settling down anyway. That's *like jumping off a moving train too early* while it's slowing down to a stop. You might hit the concrete with your face.

Insulin pumps or continuous subcutaneous insulin infusions (CSIIs)

As per the 2024 American Diabetes Association (ADA) *Standards of Care in Diabetes,* everyone with type 1 diabetes should be considered for being managed on a newer-generation insulin pump with automated insulin delivery. Technology has made impressive strides in type 1 diabetes management in the century since Leonard was first treated in 1922. Work with an endocrinologist who knows how to help you navigate this. It's an art as much as a science, and you deserve to be treated by someone competent. This is a rare skill, so it's likely you know more than many doctors do about pump therapy.*

When it comes to **basal insulin on a pump**, the same quick-acting insulin molecule is used for basal and bolus needs, usually a newer analog (lispro or aspart).[22] To cover the basal requirement, the quick-acting insulin is given at a certain hourly rate, which can be set at different rates for different times of the day and can also be set to different preprogrammed patterns for weekends, fever, premenstrual insulin resistance, exercise routines, and so on. You can even set a temporary basal where the pump can deliver a certain number of units per hour or a percentage of the default basal for a certain number of hours, based on the situation. For example, for vigorous exercise, you might set a 60 percent basal for the duration of the workout, and 80 percent for the next two to three hours as the muscles continue to lower the glucose levels during the post-workout recovery period (remember that muscle is the glucose taker among our three musketeers).

For a mild walk, you might set the basal at 90 percent of regular, just for the duration of the walk. Additionally, for "dawn phenomenon," you might set the hourly rate to be higher from 4:00 a.m. to 6:00 a.m., whereas the basal for the rest of the day is set lower. You can even suspend the pump or temporarily disconnect it for brief periods.

There are so many possibilities on the pump. You will be able to find the right settings by taking your detailed lifestyle data to a pump specialist who can help you interpret the patterns and change the pump settings. Newer pumps, when paired with continuous glucose monitoring technology, can predict a hypoglycemic event and automatically suspend insulin delivery, which will resume when glucose levels start rising again.

In regards to **bolus insulin on a pump**, the pump still uses the ICR and ISF like MDIs do. I calculate the insulin carbohydrate ratio (ICR) by looking for paired glucose readings before and after a meal that have remained stable. Then I check how many units of quick-acting insulin worked for the carbohydrates in that meal. Let's say the glucose level remained normal before and after taking five units for a cup of brown rice which is forty-five carbohydrates. That gives me an ICR of nine for that time of day. Benefits of taking boluses via the pump include the absence of needle pricks for multiple boluses (which can be delivered at the press of a few buttons), and active insulin time is factored in.

To understand active insulin, let's say you had lunch at 1:00 p.m. and decided to add another small snack an hour later. The pump would calculate how much of that lunch bolus is still active in your body, based on the active insulin settings your doctor has programmed into the pump. It would subtract a portion from the

---

* I found one parent blog that shows me it is possible for people to learn how to manage this better than many physicians can: https://link.medium.com/dTuE5uAgrob.

estimated snack dose so that you don't get "insulin stacking." Stacking is when you have multiple active insulin boluses piling on top of each other until they suddenly add up to a severe hypo.

Let me explain. Say your active time is programmed into the pump as four hours, but in reality your bolus takes five hours to fully wash out of the system. The pump will be willing to give you a new full bolus too soon, and you may experience a hypo when you take a second bolus within five hours of the last one.

Conversely, let's say your active insulin time is set at six hours but your insulin bolus only works in the body for around four hours. You will feel like the pump is refusing to give you a sufficient bolus soon after the last one, and you will see the glucose coming down frustratingly slowly despite requesting a correction dose. You will have to gather quite a bit of data for your doctor to determine whether it's the ISF or active time that needs to be changed. The trick is to figure out if the insulin dose feels too slow only when you are correcting a high reading (then you need to adjust ISF) or it it's too slow whenever you request a dose for small frequent meals with a normal glucose level (in which case you need to adjust active insulin time).

Newer pumps can auto-deliver micro-boluses to correct high glucose, based on the target glucose range, insulin sensitivity, and active insulin time set by your team. Sometimes patients notice the bolus setting is not right in the pump and "lie" to the pump about carbohydrate intake just to fool the pump into delivering additional insulin. Inform your doctor about this so that they can fix the settings and let the high-tech software hopefully make life a little less difficult.

Pro Tip: I have seen people with uncontrolled glucose levels in spite of investing in a pump. They made the switch from MDIs understandably to get away from the hassle of so many needle pricks; but nobody taught them how to carb count or how to activate any of the pump software. They were relieved that needles were replaced by buttons and would take occasional manual boluses through the pump often without checking their glucose levels. At best, that's like buying the world's most high-tech smartphone and using it only to make calls; you would be missing out on the benefits of activating the data plan, installing life-changing apps or customizing features, all of which would make your life much easier. At worst, it's like Formula One driving with your eyes closed. If your team doesn't know how to teach you to harness the power of the pump, you deserve better.

But what if the pump has sorted out my glucose levels and then suddenly stops working? It's happened before!

- **Patient 1:** Help! I am in Japan on holiday and absent-mindedly jumped into the water with the pump! Now it is completely dead!

- **Patient 2:** I am in the mountains, and my pump has stopped working!

- **Patient 3:** What do I do? I am in Goa for my own wedding – my reception starts in two hours – and my pump is saying "No delivery"! I am going to send all the guests home and rush to Mumbai now!

- **Patient 4:** Grrr! My pump display has gone dead. I am in lockdown, spending my birthday at my vacation home away from the city, and the nearest pump replacement is a boat ride away!

What do all of these have in common?

They're all actual calls and messages that I have received over the years! All of these people are warriors, champions, and successful, intelligent people. They are high-functioning individuals. They actually take very good care of themselves and are committed to health.

Yet, s*** happens sometimes. It can be scary and frustrating.

I can only speak from the physician side of this. Contact your healthcare professional to individualize these ideas; this does not count as medical advice. In the rare event that something like this happens, you want to be prepared.

Always keep fresh, high-quality batteries with you. Some pump problems are caused by old batteries. If you have a replacement pump, just load the same settings and contact your doctor to let them know.

Always keep a copy of your current pump settings saved somewhere on the cloud, carry a printout, and share a backup copy with your loved ones and your doctor's office. That can be used to start a temporary pump or switch to MDI. If your current pump settings have been working well due to years of close fine-tuning with your endocrinologist, you are better off sticking to those settings! The information you will need includes your *total daily dose* (TDD) in terms of *average number of units of insulin used per day; basal settings* (standard, pattern A/B, or if you have named the patterns for exercise, premenstrual, etc.) and *which basal you use the most;* target blood glucose range; and active insulin time tells the pump how many hours each bolus is expected to last in the system. Additionally, you should include the ICR, or how many grams of carbohydrate are covered by one unit of insulin at various times of the day, and the ISF, or how much of a reduction in glucose in mg/dL or mmol/L is expected per unit of insulin given as a correction factor for high blood glucose at various times of the day.

By having this information easily available and shared with your care team, **your endocrinologist and pump manufacturer support team should then be able to help you in an emergency.**

If you need to switch to injections, your doctor will have you take a percentage of the total basal dose. For example, if your total basal requirement was, on average, twelve units per day of basal on the pump, then your doctor might have you take eighty percent, that's $0.8 \times 12 = 9.6$ units of slow-acting insulin, like glargine. The pump was giving you the basal as an hourly rate of short-acting insulin, so this means you need to separately purchase slow-acting insulin if traveling to remote places, just in case.

Because it's difficult to inject 9.6 units, you would take 9 units because it's safer to err on the lower side and make adjustments upward from there. Let me explain why.

High glucose levels cause harm over the years; low glucose levels cause harm over minutes and hours. It is safer to tolerate two to three days of hyperglycemia than severe hypoglycemia during the temporary phase without a pump, especially if you are in a remote location. Remember, when you switch from a pump to multiple daily insulin injections, *there is no way to suspend insulin delivery* like you can on the pump. Once you take a slow-acting dose, it's with you for close to twenty-four hours. Also, *the pump might have been set with a different basal rate from hour to hour*, so the pump might have been delivering less basal insulin around 2:00 a.m. and more around 4:00 a.m. for the dawn phenomenon. The slow-acting dose delivers at a constant rate across the twenty-four hours. You don't want to be overdosing the slow-acting insulin during a window that needs less basal insulin. Remember, prevent lows *and then* correct the highs.

In this example, the slow-acting insulin shot will just give you 9 units equally over twenty-four hours, that is, 0.375 units per hour all day, twenty-four hours a day, versus, let's say, 0.250 units per hour at 2:00 a.m. and 0.4 units per hour at 5:00 a.m. These are just hypothetical examples, and these numbers are not meant to serve as prescriptions for anyone. Do NOT adjust your pump on your own based on this information, but take it to your doctor to discuss your treatment plan.

Additionally, if you switch to injections, *the short-acting insulin is used for boluses at mealtime.* Since the pump used to calculate the units for you if you were using the software correctly, now you will have to count this yourself. Divide the carb count of each meal by the relevant ICR to get the meal coverage and if the pre-meal glucose is high, divide the required glucose correction by the ISF to get the correction coverage. Taking the ICR and ISF added together as a pre-meal dose, ten to fifteen minutes before the meal will reduce volatility. Skip the bolus if eating to correct a low glucose, just like you would if the pump was on.

Finally, *be sure to avoid taking repeated quick-acting insulin corrections back-to-back* within four hours. If you take multiple doses one after another, you are at risk of "insulin stacking," where the previous dose has not yet lost its effect, and then the new dose starts acting on top of it. This puts you at risk of sudden, severe hypoglycemia. The pump would have locked you out from repeated boluses, saying "Active insulin."

By taking these precautions, you should be able to give yourself some peace of mind in the event of an emergency. Each of my four patients managed to stay safe by following these steps, and they were able to continue their holidays without major disruption. Eventually, they got themselves a working replacement pump and went back to their routines. As always, this section does not replace working with your doctor to create the right plan for you.

10.6: Safety checklist to reduce diabetes distress in type 1

Because you are reading this, you know more than I do about how living with type 1 diabetes can sometimes be tough. Depending on your age when you were diagnosed with type 1 diabetes, the level of psychological distress you experience can vary. It also vary afterward, as life throws different situations at you. When you are very young, your parents are vulnerable to caregiver diabetes distress; as an adult, your significant other can experience distress, too.

It might feel like a tightrope walk as you aim for perfect glucose levels, also known as *time in range* (TIR). Too high or too low, both are dangerous in their own way. All you are trying to do is live your life and be as healthy as possible. The unique daily decisions you have to make when living with type 1 present a large cognitive load, and can cause some amount of emotional burnout or fatigue.

But what can you even do about it?

In my practice, I look for a repeating pattern over at least three days before making a change in the insulin dose. *When you see a high glucose reading despite taking insulin and can't explain it, consider using my mechanic's checklist* so you can look for what needs to change.

1. Lifestyle

a. Nutrition: Carbs, hidden sugars, unknown food industry additives, excessive salt, dehydration

b. Sleep: Reduced quality or quantity

c. Stress: Physical or emotional

d. Exercise: Different workouts can raise glucose levels differently.

Work with a knowledgeable healthcare professional to plan the insulin doses for exercise.

e. Body clock: Travel across time zones, intermittent fasting, duration of fasting[*]

2. Testing related[23]

a. Faulty or expired glucometer strips, faulty glucometer battery, faulty glucometer hardware

b. Inaccurate coding of strips with meter as per manufacturer instructions

c. Contamination on the fingers

d. Pump-sensor-glucometer mismatch: due to faulty sensor filaments or glucometer, or sensor calibration issues

e. Using only CGM, not verifying on glucometer, or faulty CGM sensors

3. Insulin not being delivered

a. Air bubbles in pen/syringe/pump tubing

b. Lipodystrophy at site (scar tissue in the fat under the skin)

    i. To prevent this, you can rotate your injection sites in a W or M pattern around the navel so that you don't return to the same site for another few doses to allow the injection site to heal. You may get a clue by looking or feeling for bumps under the skin.

c. Skin inflammation at the pump site

    i. A large insulin bolus through the cannula can reduce the lifespan of the site. I learned this from a patient, not a book. Liva has figured out how to get her pump site to work beautifully for longer than six days, even though the typical life of a pump site is three days. When you think about it, this makes sense. It's unnat-

---

[*] Insulin will need adjustment if you switch time zones because your body doesn't know you got on a long-haul flight!

ural to have more than five units of insulin suddenly arrive under the skin all at once. A working pancreas would have delivered all of its insulin via the portal vein to the liver, which would have then been delivered all across the body in the bloodstream. Delivering a high amount of insulin into the subcutaneous tissue for a high-carb meal probably causes a local inflammatory response, which causes the site to malfunction.

d. Injection into muscle: if there's pain during injection or blood on the tip of the needle after injection, these can be clues that the dose went into muscle instead of the fat under the skin (subcutaneous fat), causing variable absorption.

e. Injection technique issue, not reaching the fat below the skin: due to needle being too short, too long, too slanted, or not slanted enough, or perhaps the skin is not being pinched away before injecting.

f. Faulty pen or malfunctioning pump

g. Low pump battery or a kink in pump tubing (the pump should alert you)

4. Insulin delivered but less effective

a. Denatured insulin as a result of extreme temperature: If you are not sure if the insulin is bad, open a new vial/pen. Do not refill your syringe or pump from the same source.[24]

ii. Extreme cold: People have sometimes made the mistake of putting their insulin into the freezer, on ice, or into checked luggage on an aircraft. Insulin is a protein and gets denatured if it freezes. Store unused insulin in your refrigerator and travel using a dedicated insulin cooling case or pouch in your hand luggage. Carry a doctor's note for airport authorities.

iii. Extreme heat: Insulin is stable at room temperature as long as your room is 59°F–86°F (25°C–30°C). Many tropical regions are too hot for these "room-temperature" cutoffs; wearing an insulin pump outdoors for a prolonged period on a very hot day or leaving the insulin in a vehicle or in the sun on a hot day can also cause insulin to denature and lose potency.

b. Expired insulin

c. Medications like steroids, antibiotics, decongestants, antipsychotics, and cholesterol- or blood-pressure-lowering medications that raise glucose

d. Insulin resistance (you know what to do about that now that you have read this book)

5. Medical/surgical illness

a. Severe pain, fever, viral infection, bacterial infection like food poisoning, toothache

b. Any surgical emergency or physical injury/trauma

c. Diabetic ketoacidosis (DKA), which is a medical emergency and is completely different from nutritional ketosis or ketosis from fasting.

   i. If you are feeling unwell, with unexplained malaise, vomiting, or generally not feeling OK, it's safer to assume you have DKA and visit the nearest emergency room without delay. Don't rely only on home ketone testing. Untreated DKA can be fatal.

In addition to this checklist, there are questionnaires that can help you score your psychological distress levels related to living with type 1 diabetes. These can help identify if the burden is accumulating at a level that might be reducing your quality of life. There are separate surveys for you, for parents of teens with type 1, and for partners of people with type 1 diabetes. There are also surveys to measure hypoglycemia and device confidence, too. Dr. William Polonsky and Dr. Lawrence Fisher at the Behavioural Diabetes Institute are pioneers in this field. Take the survey and discuss it with your healthcare professional to see if you might benefit from additional help and support.[25]

While researchers are working hard to find a cure for type 1 diabetes, many individuals face the reality of living with type 1 diabetes day in and day out, nonstop. The possibility of burnout is valid and real. I just want you to know you are not alone, and there are many people out there who can help if it feels like too much.[26]

10.7: Circling back to Natali, Liva, Gurmeet, and Ria

So, what happened to these patients who were struggling with the effects of type 1 diabetes? If you recall, Natali and Liva were struggling with getting simple solutions and answers to their glucose problems, while Gurmeet and Ria didn't want to give up their favorite activities as a "simple" solution.

In Natali's case, her frustration was understandable; it seemed pointless. She came from a wealth management and finance background and had invested in portfolios that looked promising. I asked her if she kept staring at balance sheets as the only way to assess whether a company was on the right track or not.

"Of course not," she said. She looked into day-to-day operations to make sure the right processes were in place. Improving the inputs gave better outputs.

So we used a similar approach. I needed to help her to have more confidence in herself than in the number on the weighing scale. We handled each issue step-by-step over a period of many months.

I also requested her to stop fat-shaming herself. Would she talk about her best friend that way? Of course not. Sometimes when we feel low or powerless, it's "easier" to take out our rage and negativity on ourselves. I asked her how she felt when she looked in the mirror and said she "looked so fat." Did that make her want to take care of her body? Not really.

This self-care mindset took a while to sink in. Slowly but surely, she became aware that her carb intake was reaching 200 grams a day and her weekend alcohol binges were worsening her insulin resistance.

The biggest task for her was to log her data so that we could look for patterns in her glucose and insulin fluctuations. She sometimes stopped seeing us over the holidays and resurfaced in January. She realized that we were not judging her "absenteeism" from our appointments, and she mustered the courage from within to show up for herself.

Now she understands the power of carb counting, and how being low-carb helps her insulin bolus doses stay low. Eventually, her TDD came down from over sixty units of insulin a day to forty, and she has signed up for strength-training workouts. With data from her, we were able to decode patterns of how her body responded to strength-training workouts versus cardio sessions. We have been working together for over three years now. She is finally losing inches from her waist thanks to lower insulin needs, and she has shown fierce determination to show up for herself by looking her battles more squarely in the eye.

Returning to Liva

We know that "brittle diabetes" is really just mismanaged diabetes, so our first step was to correlate her carb intake with her insulin doses and observe the glucose patterns. The use of a few CGMs with meticulous data in her diary helped us identify her patterns. She started taking her bolus before meals, and we taught her how to count carbohydrates. Her anger toward diabetes started to settle as she finally saw glimmers of stability coming, and she felt empowered knowing that her bolus dose was in her hands. Moving to an insulin pump gave her even more flexibility with her basal rates, and she figured out different needs during her menstrual cycle.

One time, after things had stabilized and her early diabetic retinopathy had returned to normal, she came for an appointment and asked me to increase her insulin dose. By then, I knew we had ironed most things out. The high readings were not revealing any pattern that I could respond to.

I told her I thought she needed to work on her stress management because this fluctuation was not coming from an inaccurate carb count, carb ratio, or any other pump setting. I told her increasing insulin would be the wrong treatment. I would have been causing her harm by just giving her more insulin without exploring other causes for the fluctuations. By then, I had earned her trust, and she took this feedback seriously.

She embarked on a spiritual journey, learned self-help meditation practices like emotional freedom technique (EFT) and reiki, and unearthed another layer of self-awareness. Over the more than ten years that I have known Liva, she has taken up one challenge at a time, whether it was to embrace low-carb or add resistance workouts, marry the love of her life, move to the United Kingdom, come out to her colleagues about her type 1 diabetes diagnosis, experience love and joy in her family, and more. She lives a life full of gratitude and faith now, and always messages me on her "diaversary" with a note of appreciation for the work we did together. She doesn't really need insulin adjustments from me anymore because she has understood her patterns, and she makes this world a better place every day. She was kind enough to allow the use of her real name, so that others may derive hope from her story.

Remember Gurmeet?

Gurmeet's 70/30 (NPH/lispro) insulin was denying him the flexibility he needed to be active on the court every day. He needed both cardio (aerobic) training for endurance and explosive muscular strength to win long, grueling championship games. He was able to afford the latest closed-loop pump that had predictive technology. This meant the pump would be able to halt insulin delivery if the sensor detected that he was approaching a low glucose level and resume delivery once the levels started to rise.

This prevented him from hitting bad hypos.

We taught him how to set different temporary basals for competitions and practice sessions. He felt better on a low-carb approach and stopped needing chocolate to power his muscles. His insulin requirements came down, and in spite of taking less insulin per day, his severe hyperglycemic events completely resolved.

Lastly, Ria

We switched Ria from premixed 70/30 degludec/aspart, to multiple daily injections with glargine and aspart. This way, she could skip her mealtime bolus insulin when she wasn't eating, and she prevented hypoglycemia during long dance rehearsals by munching on nuts or cheese.

She was underweight when we first met, and she lost more weight as her total daily insulin dose came down. There was a brief phase where I was concerned she might be developing an eating disorder, with hints of anorexia nervosa in the way she thought about food and her body.[27,28] I had to make sure that she was not intentionally skipping insulin to lose weight.[29]

I reminded her how having enough body fat would help maintain regular periods and keep her bones strong. She had learned that skipping insulin caused high glucose levels with unhealthy weight loss; now she wanted to build muscle to be a stronger dancer. So she focused on healthy eating habits and added strength-training workouts to put on lean muscle. She eventually applied for financial aid to get an insulin pump.

Once her glucose levels settled and she was able to move forward in her dance academy, her mental health improved rapidly. She has started seeing a therapist for the negative thoughts about diabetes and is a champion in her life everyday, pursuing a career as a professional dancer.

Part 10 summary

- High glucose levels in spite of high insulin doses point to insulin resistance along with the insulin deficiency of type 1 diabetes.

- "Brittle diabetes" can be stabilized by a low carb approach along with basal bolus insulin or an insulin pump.

- Carbohydrate counting to calculate meal time insulin bolus doses provides the most flexibility and safety.

- Hypoglycemia and hypoglycemia unawareness need to be corrected before increasing insulin doses for an elevated HbA1c.

For Bonus Materials, Visit the Website Here:

PART 11
THE JOURNEY AHEAD

11.1: Navigating the ups and downs of life

It has been my life's greatest honor to be able to serve people with diabetes as they come forward and take a stand in how their lives will turn out. Theory and practice are two different things, and what they have done goes beyond diabetes. It has been nothing but awe-inspiring to see their wisdom light up their lives with self-care, creativity, and confidence.

I wish these tips were in medical textbooks.

Hopefully, this book will help people push healthcare workers to discuss lifestyle change more openly and will enable health workers to have those conversations with more confidence. In this closing section, I want to talk about how you can use the information in this book to adjust to things in life that may have otherwise been an obstacle for you while managing your diabetes. While I review different applications of this knowledge, I also want to present you with a boiled-down version of the solutions I have seen everyday champions apply in their lives, starting with Zaineb.

Zaineb wanted to resume mountain trekking and hiking after her diabetes stabilized. She knew most camping trips involved carb-heavy meals, so she carried her protein and healthy fat along. She figured the extra weight in her bag would serve as her rucking weight and would prepare her to lift her own equipment on her dream hike to Everest Base Camp.

She had put the idea off for years, when diabetes had looked like it wasn't going to leave. But after she learned the power of low-carb workouts, she focused on powering her mitochondria with healthy fuel and consistent endurance exercise. Gaining muscle wasn't just for diabetes; it was to climb her next mountain, both figuratively and literally.

She turned into a fat-burning machine and turned her type 2 diabetes around, building muscle, doing the outdoor activities she loved, and setting higher goals for herself every year. Age was not stopping her. At sixty-two, she climbed the highest peak in her state, and she plans to visit Everest Base Camp soon. She won't be needing her insulin prescriptions on that trip because she has gotten off insulin and is doing fine on just metformin.

I hope servicing your own lifestyle car will support your journey of turning around diabetes so you can reclaim your health, just like Zaineb.

In her case, her illness (diabetes) was holding her back from the life she wanted to live, and she's not the only one. I'm sure you agree that there is so much more to life than managing diabetes. Let me ask you, **what do travel, holidays, weddings, celebrations, meetings, buffets and work travel** all have in common?

Someone else made the menu.

The food and travel industry wants you to eat cheap, processed carbs and have allocated million-dollar budgets to make it happen. Failing to plan is planning to fail, so plan ahead. Don't let them win, because you work hard all year. You deserve frequent breaks and holidays to rejuvenate yourself mentally *and* physically. When it comes to events where the food is provided for you, there are a few ways to take charge of the situation.

First, *consider how you will ensure protein at each meal.* Do you need to carry a protein supplement or protein-rich nonperishable foods along? Since my family is vegetarian, we often ensure each of us gets twenty-five to thirty grams of protein from our hotel room and then step out to try new food experiences. My family will sometimes give a scoop of their whey protein to the hotel staff and request the kitchen to add it to a banana milkshake. I carry my plant-based protein shake or request cage-free eggs or a tofu scramble. The service industry is usually more than willing to honor special requests.

If renting a place with a fridge, you can carry nuts, seeds, nut butters, protein shakes (single ingredient), cheese, yogurt, unsweetened jerky made the traditional way (read the label), canned meats, sardines, or fish soaked in brine (read the label to make sure it's only pure meat and salt—no seed oil, starch, or sugar!), or freshly-sliced, unprocessed deli meat in your luggage. You could purchase these locally; there are many options to support your protein needs.

Once that's settled, how will you keep the body active, even without access to your gym, your weights, or your trainer? Do you need to pack a small foam roller, resistance bands, or TRX® bands in your luggage? What experiences will help you get in some walking and movement every day? Is it possible to stimulate your muscle groups till failure at least once every three to four days on the trip? It doesn't have to be the full-fledged workout you always do.

There are five-minute full-body, no-equipment workouts, mobility routines, and hotel room workouts on YouTube. Wearables like continuous glucose monitors (CGMs), Oura rings, Whoops, handheld Lumen devices, and Apple or Garmin watches help you get feedback on how different choices like late nights, alcohol, and restaurant food are affecting your body. You don't really want your doctor upping your prescriptions just because you had a good time. The food, sickness, and pharmaceutical industries benefit from that. Not you.

Additionally, **remind yourself why and what you are celebrating**. You might have different feelings about a work-mandated luncheon as opposed to your sibling's wedding, and that's okay.

When it comes to meetings, conferences, and clients the sponsors may provide a packaged lunch that's mostly carbs because it suits the budget. Does it suit you? Are you obliged to eat it? You didn't arrive at the corporate event without considering how this meeting was going to advance your career. Are we considering the effect of this meeting on your body? Remember, nobody is going to prioritize your health or diabetes more than you. If you are leading the meeting, you can ask the meeting organizer to remove the bowls of candies and biscuits from the table. Nobody needs them. Nobody.

I had a patient who decided to fast to skip dealing with the pressure to eat at a networking event. He sipped on fasting fluids, and nobody noticed. Less decision fatigue. His mind stayed sharp, and he got more networking done.

If you feel obligated to wine and dine your clients and alcohol must be served, you can tip your server ahead of time to serve you soda, lime, and water which make it look like you are sipping liquor. As long as your guests are being served free alcohol, they won't really be paying detailed attention to your drink. I've even made it through rounds of shots just chugging virgin lime water while everyone got progressively tipsy. You get to decide what "moderation" means when it comes to alcohol. In any case, the best practice is to tell people the truth. They can handle knowing that you are working on healing your liver and are abstaining from alcohol. Statistically, it's highly likely that some of them need to work on their metabolic health, too. What working professional really wants their business partner, boss, or employee to make their diabetes or liver worse?

If you are at an event where there is a menu or buffet, where options have been preselected for you to decide among, there are some tips to making decisions for your diabetes.

When presented with a buffet, go ahead without your plate and walk around to survey the options first. I find this helps me calm the mind, plan my choices, and avoid putting unnecessary stuff on my plate just because it looks eye-catching and new. What's the rush? When you come back the second time with your plate, the food doesn't look as mesmerizing. As vegetables and protein sources are usually an option for most lunch or dinner buffets, there are some protein and low-carb foods you can usually find at a breakfast buffet. Foods like *nuts, seeds,* and *milk* at the cereal counter (do you need the cereal?); *nut butters; whole eggs* cooked in butter, not refined oil; *fresh cheese, brined olives, chickpeas or beans,* and *fresh meats at the salad counter;* and *yogurt on ice,* be sure to look or ask for plain unsweetened (you can carry unsweetened Greek yogurt or request it ahead of time). Sometimes we visit the local convenience store to stock up on protein options in our hotel room fridge. Additionally, at the egg station, vegans can request a tofu scramble instead of scrambled eggs. This may require some advance planning, like carrying tofu along or requesting the chef to arrange for tofu for you. Indian hotels give you a cheela (lentil pancake) option; you can ask them to add an egg to this if it fits your beliefs.

In the event that you are not provided with a buffet, but instead **given a pre-selected menu**, you can request the server to skip serving the bread basket, nachos, or papad while you are hungry and waiting.

For *vegetarians*, *you need to plan your protein options.* With Indian food, you will get paneer and pulses (lentils). If choosing pulses, do you really need roti or rice?

Indian and Italian food will always be carb-heavy. Indian food is often too spicy to eat alone when you don't dilute the masala with carbs.

Asian food has plenty of low-carb vegetable options, coconut curries, peanut curries, and tofu. Paneer works if you are okay with dairy.

Middle Eastern food has falafel, hummus options, and mezze platters with olives. Do you need the pita or can you use a spoon or crudites to scoop the hummus? Greek yogurt dips might be on the menu, too. Burrito bowls keep all the fun ingredients of Mexican food without the tortilla. Be generous with the guacamole, beans, fajita vegetables, cheese, sour cream, salsa, and lettuce. The rice and corn are more starchy. The beans and corn can be your carb of the meal.

For people who eat animal protein (non-vegetarians in the Indian context), a protein-focused entree is much easier to find. You can use all of the previous tips and add the animal protein of choice. You can skip the lentils and starchy vegetables because animal sources like eggs, fish, poultry and red meat provide enough low-carb, high-quality complete protein.

When it comes to applying this guide to your reality, you will run into choices quite often.

If you **travel for work**, chances are you have eaten in an airplane, airport or hotel lobby on your way to a conference or work event. My client Vijay was just like that.

Vijay was a jetsetter. His business required him to travel every month, and he spent two-thirds of his time on the road. Before working with us, he would enjoy the free juice and wine on every flight, stop at fast-food kiosks, and always be on the go. His sleep was constantly disrupted by all the travel. As he gradually recognized how he was working his way into sickness, he realized he had choices. He realized there were alternatives that he had never considered before.

For example, the juice was totally unnecessary. He had seen it spike his levels up to 200 mg/dL. No thanks. He would plan his three meals to be focused on animal protein. He asked the chef to stop at his table and put in his low-carb request.

Colleagues liked his idea and opted for what he was having. For times when nothing was available, he now carried his protein shake as a backup. He asked for a hotel room near the pool or on the same floor as the hotel gym so that he could just walk around the hallway and get in some movement before his meetings started. He realized that being in a hotel, airplane, or airport didn't define what happened to his diabetes—he did.

Eventually, he was able to hire an assistant to lighten his load. He split his travel commitments with another colleague so he was able to spend more restorative time at home. He realized there was really no point in earning all that money if he was spending all of his time away from his family and away from his health.

He turned twenty-two years of diabetes around by addressing his insulin resistance through more balanced nutrition, better sleep habits, exercise, and connection with family. All I had to do after that was reduce his diabetes, blood pressure, and uric acid medications.

If you travel like Vijay, and you're comfortable knowing what to order off of a menu, then you can try to look for additional opportunities to manage diabetes by arranging walking or treadmill meetings, and seeking standing-desk options. Leaning forward while seated at a desk loads the spine in ways that you really don't want for eight hours a day. Leaders think differently and do things differently. Have the courage to make that special request and turn it into an office wellness conversation. You might just inspire someone who has low back pain, sciatica, and disc issues to change their posture, too. Lifestyle disease is more of an epidemic than you might think.

Most people who travel for work often visit the same location more than once. If there is a place where you have become a frequent flyer, the hotel likely values you as a repeat customer. If you have a healthy experience at a corporate hotel and talk about it among your colleagues, other executives will prefer that hotel. Traveling for work can be rough on the body, and most executives wish their hotel experiences could be healthier. The hotel also wants to keep you happy—it's a win-win-win if the hotel entertains your request. The change starts with you. Flip the script again and own it.

Instead of feeling sheepish or worrying that others might feel like you are being fussy, assert what you require to take care of your health when you travel for work. You aren't doing anything wrong by making a special request. Your health is worth it. Someone with peanut allergies would speak up, right? What's the difference?

Now that we've covered the "ups" in life, where we are living life on our terms, let's talk about the downs.

When it comes to navigating through stressful patches or illness, *what is your emotional support system? Be sure to keep nourishing foods on hand;* what are the healthiest things you can buy that support recovery when it feels difficult to cook? Additionally, it can be *helpful to redefine comfort food.* What does your body *need* to pull through? For ideas, here are some comfort fluids you can have when sick:

- **Vegetable broth:** Consider ginger; garlic; and umami flavors such as nutritional yeast, mushrooms, mushroom powder, or miso paste. Add a dollop of healthy fat plus a few aromatic herbs of choice, such as coriander, lemongrass, or kaffir lime. Just steep the ingredients together in hot water for a few minutes and you're done.

- **Rasam:** This South Indian hot soup is a comfort food for many. It takes a little while to prepare and has some essential spices and in-gredients, but it can be a welcome warm feeling down your throat when you aren't feeling well. Skip the jaggery. I've seen people bulk prepare it and keep some in the freezer for rainy days.

- **Bone broth:** Homemade takes many hours to make, which might not be practical when you are sick. Nowadays ready-made bone broth is available, too. This provides minerals, collagen, gelatin, and marrow.

- **Paaya soup** is the equivalent traditional South Asian/Indian broth made from trotters (*paaya* means "foot"). This is rich in collagen and gelatin.

All this is great, but you are unlikely to want to go grocery shopping in the middle of an illness. So what can you stock up in your pantry, to help you be pre-pared for the ups and downs?

11.2: Stocking the pantry: organic, or not?

Narain and his wife Seetha were both overweight and had diabetes. Both of their sons were overweight, and they couldn't bear the idea of seeing their innocent kids go down the diabetes road with a lifestyle disadvantage. Prevention was their only option.

Narain and Seetha knew the whole family needed to redefine their relationship with food and their bodies. The couple decided to turn around their diabetes to give a different environment to their kids. They made a family activity out of cleaning the home pantry and turned label reading into a game to find protein. The kids realized it was cool to do things differently from their peers and show their friends how junk-food labels were sneaky.

The pediatrician confirmed both kids had fatty liver, and the entire family switched gears to get to the bottom of insulin resistance in their home. By drastically reducing their intake of refined sugar and junk food, the children reversed fatty liver within a year.

Previously, every celebration revolved around food. Now they replaced junk time with quality time. The parents took the kids outdoors, planning outings with extended family that included movement and contact with nature. The couple now goes to the gym together. Surprisingly, everyone loved it.

Their extended community and friend circle noticed the transformation in the family after they adopted a low-carb, active lifestyle—three generations benefitted from a husband and wife deciding it was time to take their health into their own hands. They don't want any more kids to fall prey to preventable disease, and are champions in their social circle, spreading awareness and confidence that even vegetarian Indians can reverse insulin resistance and metabolic disease.

Narain and Seetha took a hard look at their habits, and started asking the right questions.

Why store junk like crackers, juice, cookies, chips, soda, marshmallows, instant noodles, and candy in the house? Who needs to eat these?

If you are getting enough animal protein at your main meals, you are unlikely to feel hungry between meals, but protein deficiency in vegetarians is the most common reason I see for people feeling hungry between meals. Here are some vegetarian additions to your pantry that can provide variety, texture, flavor, and protein to each main meal and reduce the need for between-meal snacking.

Savory	Neutral	Fresh/ Organic Dairy	Umami	Fermented	Sweet
-Frozen edamame -Chickpea salad -Lentils -Organic hummus -Pesto sauce -Unsweetened marinara sauce -Tofu/ tempeh -Whole soybean salad	-Hemp hearts -Chia seeds -Pumpkin seeds -Sunflower seeds -Nuts (not roasted, sweetened, or salted): macadamia, pecans, almonds, cashews, pine nuts, peanuts, etc. -Nut butter (unsweetened) -Avocado	-Cottage cheese -Cream cheese -Greek yogurt, unsweetened -Icelandic yogurt (skyr), unsweetened -Ricotta cheese -Mozzarella cheese -Any fresh soft or hard cheese	-Nutritional yeast -Tempeh -Miso paste -Mushroom powder	-Kefir, unsweetened -Sauerkraut -Kimchi -Kombucha (make sure they haven't added sugar / sweeteners back after fermentation)	-Blueberries, unsweetened -Strawberries, unsweetened -Local berries in season -Low-carb keto unsweetened trail mix with unsweetened berries -Organic honey in moderation -Organic maple syrup in moderation -Natural cinnamon -Natural vanilla -Fresh fruit, whole

This is not an exhaustive list, but these options have a wide range of textures and flavors and could help you diversify more than just your protein sources.

But should you stock your pantry with organic options?

The word *organic* is expected to mean that the farm has not used pesticides or chemical fertilizers, but the soil, air, and water might still have preexisting pollutants from months or years ago. Herbicide endocrine disruptors like glyphosate are already in the soil, water, and air; avoiding all of this may require us to move to the moon, considering how many chemicals are everywhere.[1] So what can you do? The idea is not to get overwhelmed but to make one small, manageable change at a time.

We don't have strong scientific long-term data showing that buying organic produce creates measurable differences in exposure to pollutants or translates to better long-term health outcomes.[2] I am not an expert in farming, but I still buy organic when I can for peace of mind, and if nothing else, for the placebo effect of knowing that I am doing "something" to reduce our chemical exposure. In addition, we buy produce from my local organic farmers' market, which could be an option for some people. In my mind, at the very least we are supporting a local business, and farm-to-table foods hopefully come with less hormonal manipulation or genetic modification. Obviously, eating out when we socialize means we are probably ingesting some chemicals from conventional farming methods, so we try to reduce that load when eating at home, for what it's worth.

11.3: Pollution and endocrine disruptors in our environment

S aid technically, there are chemicals in our environment that enter our bodies and create reactive oxygen species, which trigger inflammatory chemical (reduction oxidation or redox) reactions that exert epigenetic effects.[3]

Say what?

Said simply, we live in a highly polluted world. The pollutants in our environment might be affecting our gene expression and interfering with hormone messaging.

Junk food is purposely loaded with endocrine disruptors that epigenetically hijack our natural appetite regulation and expression of hormones that cause natural satiety. All of this potentially sends fake news to our appetite center about how much energy is available, triggering endocrine problems like obesity. What can we do about it?

Everyone is doing their best to live on Earth in spite of all our urbanization. It will require government will and policy to stop these pollutants from entering our lives. The idea of this book has been to help you be informed so that you can do as much as you can for your and your family's health. This section is no different. When it comes to addressing the endocrine disruptors in our lives, the goal is to approach it without becoming neurotic.

For me, there were two easy ways to do this.

First, **invest in clean food storage and preparation**. We threw out all our nonstick and aluminum cookware and replaced it with *glass, stainless steel*, and *cast iron*. That includes food preparation, processing and storage. I can't really measure the impact this had on my family (or didn't), but at least we are using less reactive materials for cooking, and I don't stress over it anymore. Next time you get the chance, you can look into replacing nonstick cookware, as it can leach the plastic coating into your food. Get rid of anything with bisphenol A (BPA), as it's a proven endocrine disruptor that was used in baby bottles, food, and beverage packaging until 2008. Avoid plastic food and water storage.

In addition to your kitchenware, you can try opting for cleaner fast-moving consumer goods (FMCGs) and consumer packaged goods (CPG). The closer you look, the more you will notice ingredients with possible hormone effects in our daily lives.

In India, most dishes are still washed by hand. Dish detergent residue is possible, especially when dishes are rinsed in a hurry. We stopped using regular dish detergent because I didn't want to be eating soap after all the effort to clean out my fridge! Who knows what dish soap does to my gut microbiome.

We now use dish soap made from the most natural ingredients possible, including the Indian soap nut (areetha). This is gradually possible with bath soap, shampoo, lotions, chemical sunscreens, fragrance, hair dyes, cosmetics and creams too, but we have not made the switch, yet. Dr Vanita Rattan is a doctor and cosmetic formulator who puts out free educational content on YouTube to help people learn to read skincare product labels. The "Think Dirty" app helps you check labels for ingredients in over-the-counter goods whose effects you may not be aware of; for ease I opt for shorter ingredient lists and try to minimize cosmetic use.

While endocrine disruptors are a part of the food supply, there are other aspects of our environment that are polluted, potentially causing harm. *Negative news, noise, artificial light, poor air quality,* and *toxic family environments* are just some aspects of **environmental pollution.** If you recall from Part 4.6: ***experience = the experiencer + that which is experienced.***

Again, most of this book focuses on what you can change about yourself without needing your environment to change, but still—the environment does epigenetically affect your DNA, as well as your thoughts, emotions, and state of being. We don't live in impermeable bubbles.

We are wired to coexist with the environment using all our senses. Most of us can't just pack up and move to a place without pollution, even if these affect our quality of life. Perhaps it will make us more mindful of what we consume on TV, the news, or social media. Air filters and water filters may help, but I'm not an environmental safety expert, so do your research if investing in filters. Placing healthy boundaries and filtering out toxic relationships is easier said than done; consider it as a form of pollution management, too.

11.4: List of questions and conversations for your doctor, topic-wise

In Part 8, we addressed how to work with doctors and hospitals, and before that, we discussed all of the different screenings and labs you may be offered or requested. But sometimes, just because you know what you need, it doesn't mean you know how to ask.

Below you can find some questions to ask your doctor based on the different components of the lifestyle car—by topic.

Nutrition:

- Can you help me, as I want to reduce my carbohydrate intake?

- Please check my medication to confirm low-carb is safe so that I won't develop hypoglycemia or low blood pressure as I reduce my carbs.

- Will you help me reduce my medication as I reduce carbs?

Sleep:

- I took a sleep survey (STOP-BANG) and want to get tested for sleep apnea.

Stress management:

- I want to work on my relationship with food and stress management skills.
- Can you recommend well-known therapists in our area who help access the subconscious emotions and go beyond just talk therapy or medications alone?

Exercise:

- Do I need a cardiac evaluation before advancing my aerobic and strength training?
- I want to address my pain and mobility limitations through physical therapy so that I can safely increase my muscle mass and strength.
- I'm interested in longevity and increasing my health span through fitness.

Fasting:

- Please check my medication to confirm fasting is safe so that I won't experience hypoglycemia or low blood pressure as I fast.

Tests/medications/healthcare providers

- Can you test my C-peptide so that we can be sure I don't need to be on insulin?
- Please tell me which of my medications are causing weight gain, brain fog, or __[symptoms you are facing]__.
- What monitoring do I need quarterly and annually to screen for complications of diabetes?
- Please order my dual-energy X-ray absorption (DEXA) with body composition analysis so that I can track that I am gaining muscle and losing fat over time.
- Should I be doing a coronary artery calcium score?
- Can you walk me through your thinking about the data on statins and how they apply to my health?

- Are you willing to have a conversation with my physiotherapist/cardiologist/nutritionist to coordinate my care so that I can safely make lifestyle changes to achieve better health with less medication?

- I read this book on how to turn around diabetes. Are you willing to discuss some of the things I learned from it?

11.5: If you are a healthcare provider

© Glasbergen/ glasbergen.com

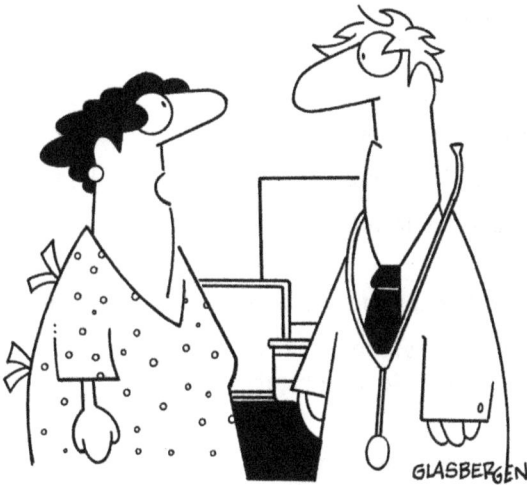

GLASBERGEN

"You don't make patients feel guilty about cancer.
You don't make patients feel guilty about Parkinson's.
You don't make patients feel guilty about Alzheimer's.
Why are you making me feel guilty about diabetes?"

From cognitive dissonance to community

If you work in health care, you may have felt uncomfortable at some point while reading this book. I get it. I felt it, too. I suspect cognitive dissonance is one of the leading causes of physician burnout in diabetes care. More than half of diabetes and endocrinology doctors have reported burnout in the United Kingdom, and close to half of endocrinologists in the United States have reported feeling burned out.[4,5] Why are diabetes doctors burning out? Well, here are some possible reasons:

- Feeling ineffective in making a meaningful difference in someone's diabetes journey

- Patients are dissatisfied when hearing they need more medication, but that's all you have been trained to give them when diabetes gets worse.

- They want less medication, but all you have is the words "lose weight; exercise more."

- The American Diabetes Association (ADA) guidelines say to provide person-centered care and motivational interviewing, but you have no idea how to do so.

- The ADA guidelines say to assess goals of care, assess 24-hour physical behaviors, and offer weight-management programs, but don't know how this can be done efficiently.

- Tons of electronic records and billing sheets to fill out.

- Tons of messages to reply to, labs to review, and prescriptions to rewrite.

- Each person with diabetes has a long list of items to be checked.

- You have barely eight minutes per patient because the diabetes epidemic is exploding, leaving barely any time for empathy or connection.

- Daring to ask the patient about stress, social determinants of health, or lifestyle change opens up a conversation you aren't equipped to have.

- You have performance targets to achieve to justify your income.

- Patients with diabetes just don't get better; complications are inevitable, so it feels pointless after a while.

From discomfort to change

The world needs an army of health professionals who mobilize into action and change. Stepping away from the mainstream takes courage. Luckily a revolution is already mounting, and more and more healthcare workers are becoming beacons of hope for their patients.

Organizations like Diet Doctor, The Fasting Method, Low Carb MD, The Society of Metabolic Health Practitioners, LowCarbUSA, The Nutrition Network, Low Carb Denver, Low Carb Down Under, Lifestyle Medicine, Functional Medicine, Motivational Interviewing Network of Trainers, and so many diabetes reversal organizations in India are saying no to the status quo of just prescribing more medication and chasing chronic progressive diseases downhill.

Each country now has metabolic health champions. India has seen over a dozen health-tech diabetes reversal startups enter the market. People have traditionally been open to "alternative therapy" in India like acupuncture, accupressure and home remedies to turn diabetes around with less allopathic medication. Do your research before blindly consuming health giving powders that might have heavy metals or liver toxins in them, under the label of "all natural." Look for tried and trusted providers in your local network and check their actual coaching style, patient feedback, testimonials and long term patient outcomes. The list of individual providers trailblazing this work worldwide is growing. Reach out. Grow the tribe. Work together. Help your patients reclaim their health through lifestyle change.

Computerization

Diabetes care is going digital. Wearable glucose-monitoring technology and health-tracking are here to stay. We have built our own Electronic Health Record (EHR) that integrates with our patient mobile app. We have leveraged low-code solutions to increase our touch points with patients in a continuous care model. Diabetes cannot be turned around in a ten-minute consultation.

Health-tech companies want to touch lives at scale, and artificial intelligence (AI) will disrupt many established norms, but the need for human empathy and personalized hand-holding will remain. We use learning management systems to hold patients' hands so that they learn the things that help them turn their health around. They can consume this content asynchronously, in their free time outside of the medical consultation. Get creative with what the world of technology can do to help you help your patients.

Build the technology that solves your problems.

Careers

The joy and reward you experience from helping people at the root is something that can't be experienced just by reading this book. If this book has inspired you in any way, are you ready to make a shift in your practice? Because you have made it to the end of the book, chances are you sense the truth in these pages, and now you can't unknow it. This is a good problem to have.

I was bitten by this bug around a decade ago, and I can tell you, there might be no turning back. You *know* this is why you entered health care in the first place. Your patients will bless you for the change they see in your practice.

Are you ready? Do you want to join a team that has been doing this for years and is in love with what they do? We have tripped over plenty of the stumbling blocks of building a lifestyle-first practice and are always looking to grow our team of passionate professionals.

Reach out to us if you feel inspired about changing the way you want to show up for your patients. We are developing training courses for healthcare professionals so that they benefit from my gray hair. If working along the guidelines you read in this book means something to you, we would love to hear from you. And we are never burned out. We love what we do and could not imagine providing health care any other way. It's how we would want to be treated.

11.6: Call to action now that you know how to turn around diabetes

Now that you have gained the knowledge you need to change your life—you can change the lives of other people living with diabetes, too. By connecting to what you want and communicating all you've learned, you can build a community of people who support you and want to see the world deal with diabetes by turning it around and putting insulin resistance into remission. I've done my part in sharing all I know with you, and now it's your turn to share with others.

Connect to what matters to you most

Why does it matter for you to take the trouble to change your habits and turn around diabetes? What makes it worth the effort?

Communication

Check your self-talk here. Do you call yourself a diabetic? Or someone with diabetes who is learning to achieve better glucose levels with less medication? Is your language limiting or expansive? Language matters.[6]

Community

China, India, Pakistan and the United States are the top four countries (in that order) with the highest number of people with diabetes as of 2021.[7] This ranking is projected to continue into 2045, even though the United States is the country with the highest number of people with obesity as of 2022.[8] Diabetes can be deadly, and this book has shown you how suffering from progressive diabetes can be optional. If something can be both deadly and optional, that means we have an awareness opportunity. We need to come together and address grassroots solutions for diabetes in locally relevant ways. Talk about the ideas from this book with people in your life. Perhaps you might get them thinking. Start a grassroots revolution within your circle and we can actually turn around this lifestyle epidemic in this generation. Spread the word. Find your support system. Human connection keeps us alive.

Continuous learning

Learning the twenty-six letters in the alphabet took repetition; learning how to turn around diabetes is an ongoing process. The journey never stops, and by the time this book reaches its one-year publication anniversary, there will be more information I will be wanting to add to its pages. That's science. We just keep learning.

Bonus chapter

Now that you have completed this book, I want to give you access to my upcoming bonus chapter, which is going to be a compilation of extra material that didn't make it into this final manuscript. Tell me what you want to see in the bonus chapter. What do you still want to know?

Contact us

Sign up for our newsletter on our website: www.reisaanhealth.com to stay in touch and up-to-date on our live events and updates. We can always improve how we strive for better health with less medication, so feel free to ask us questions (and tell us what you think of this book!).

Connectivity, app, and course

If you enjoyed this book and want to take these learnings deeper, I am developing a follow-along video course as well. This will help you move step-by-step through the lifestyle changes that we have covered. In the videos, I will walk you through the concepts you read about here. Sign up for our newsletter to be the first to know when the online course is live. Of course, you will need your doctor to manage your medication so that you can safely apply what you learn.

Consultation and coaching

The most high-touch way to incorporate the concepts I have outlined here is to work directly with a coach. If you want more, you always have the option of reaching out to me and my team. We would love to help and serve you.

Part 11 summary

- Travel, weddings, meetings, stress patches and holidays are part of life. Advance planning, packing and pantry changes can help health remain a constant part of your life through the ups and downs.

- Making the switch to safer food storage and cooking materials and reducing packaged food consumption might reduce exposure to chemicals and environmental factors that disrupt hormonal balance and trigger inflammation.

- Stock your pantry with protein-rich options, healthy fats, and low-carb whole foods.

- You have the power to positively influence your community through your success.

- Turning around diabetes starts with the first step. If you're ready to get started, let's go!

For Bonus Materials, Visit the Website Here:

Epilogue

It's been over ten years since I first met Dinesh. I had the diabetes educator knowledge stored away in the back of my head for two years, from 2011, till that first meeting with him in the fall of 2013.

What made me willing to switch roles from doctor to educator and from prescriber to listener? Was he the very first person I met who was unhappy about going on insulin? Certainly not.

Was he just "stubborn" enough to catch my attention? I doubt it.

He was as concerned for his own well-being as anyone else would be. The desire to thrive is a universal human need.

What changed, then, to make me listen? As I mentioned in Part 4, I hit the rock-bottom moments of my own personal life in 2013; I was drowning in victimhood. My emotional turmoil was giving me prediabetes and also making me a stressed-out mom around my two little daughters, who were six and three at the time. That was my wake-up call. It was now or never.

On one of those extremely dark nights, I had shown up distraught at the home of my friend Rukhmini, with no idea why she was the one I reached out to that evening. Thank goodness she opened her doors for me that night. After hearing me out, she said, "Rosh, you are ready for reiki." I remember being so internally broken by that point that I knew I would have done *monkey* if she had said I was ready for it. I would do whatever it took.

I was determined to turn my life around. I knew I was meant to do more in this lifetime. I ended up learning two levels of reiki from her that summer. Between 2013 and 2016, my medical practice grew, but so did my spiritual practice. I was changing on all levels internally, healing inner child wounds, attending various spiritual and self-help trainings, participating in meditation workshops, reading books on psychology and the tendencies of the mind, while remaining intensely curious about how people were driven to show up in life. It was unavoidable that this inner self-work transformed how I showed up externally at work. So, what happened?

I stopped identifying so much with my roles, titles, stories, and presumptions about anything. I was willing to open my heart in more areas of my life. I was willing to listen. Whatever it took to experience peace and connection with the positive people in my life. I was able to come back more quickly to the present moment, recognizing unhappiness, thought loops, or disturbances in my body as a clue that I was getting triggered and swept away.

Reiki said to have gratitude. So I worked on gratitude.

Bhairavi, one of my therapists, said to work on forgiveness. I worked on forgiving some early childhood memories.

Lawrence, my hypnotherapist, helped me throw light into shadows that had been buried in my subconscious. I was able to take charge of the narrative through reframes.

Many thinkers have influenced me over the years.

Eckhart Tolle said in his book *A New Earth* that our children come into this world through us, but they are not ours. They deeply want to be seen and heard. He said it was possible to see the "Being inside the Human." And at the level of Being, we are not older or bigger than our kids. We are equals. This changed my parenting style forever.

Michael Singer said in *Untethered Soul* (paraphrasing) that the mind can flip around, saying it likes certain things, and then immediately flop back and say it doesn't like those things. He taught how identifying with that incessant chatter inside was a sure way to unhappiness. I realized that as a lifestyle doctor, I can take a patient's behavior personally, or I can accept the truth. They are already doing what they are doing, with or without my "permission." The question is, do I want to be fully present to them so they can become more present to themselves?

Michelle May spoke about emotional eating and gave me tools no trainee doctors were given in internal medicine residency or endocrinology fellowship. I learned to help people heal their relationship with food by beginning with mindfulness.

Dr. William Miller and his colleagues taught me motivational interviewing (MI), where we recognize that the person with the most expertise about the patient is the patient, even if they may not recognize it. MI taught me that feeling two ways about something and feeling internally conflicted or ambivalent is a completely normal part of the human experience. By judging it, we are shutting down the very communication we seek to establish as healthcare professionals.

James Clear, in his book *Atomic Habits,* said that meaningful change happens at the level of identity. If that's true, then can I help my patients take a look at what needs to change in their description of themselves?

Daniel Kahneman said there is the lazy, fast, intuitive, irrational system 1; and the effortful, slow, deliberate, and thoughtful system 2. To make a better society, we have to stop manipulating the quirks of system 1 for corporate greed and help people make better use of their system 2.

Brené Brown said there is power in vulnerability and that shame thrives in the shadows—so we're throwing on the lights.

Simon Sinek said to start with *why*. The *what* and the *how* follow outward from that. The *why* often comes from the nonverbal emotional experiences we all go through and sometimes cannot be fully explained in words. If we accept that, can we accept that people may sometimes do things that they can't fully explain?

Jason Fung opened my eyes to the possibility of fasting as a medical treatment. My scientific and logical mind was willing to challenge previous knowledge if more convincing data came along. I followed the "strong convictions, loosely held" approach to keep learning and updating my understanding.

When I was nine, Michael Jackson's "Man in the Mirror" gripped me. He said, "If you wanna make the world a better place, take a look at yourself and make a change." Mahatma Gandhi said to become the change we wished to see in the world.

Vedanta, reiki, and quantum meditation taught me that we are all One, and the spiritual teachings of the Indian sages said the idea of separateness is an illusion, or Maya.

There seemed to be a common reality that circled around consciousness and love as universal constants of life.

Truth seemed to be coming at me from all angles. I could see the same pattern everywhere. We are all one. We are all the same.

The diabetes educator curriculum taught me the patient empowerment model, and this resonated more than the patient compliance model. I didn't see any benefit in a power dynamic with a patient. We are equals.

In 2016, I left the hospital environment, so that I could provide comprehensive and multispeciality care in a holistic, integrative, and functional way. In India, a doctor's clinic is referred to in Hindi as a "Dawakhana" which translated literally means, "the place for medicine, or the place where you get medicine." Dawa means medicine, or treatment.

"Khana" as a suffix means "the place for" and by itself means "to eat." I jokingly started playing with the words and came up with a pun that stuck. My clinic became a place for "dawa-kum-khana, or dawa-mat-khana." This meant, "eat less medicine or no medicine," by achieving better health with less medication through medically supervised lifestyle change and deprescription. The lifestyle car came to be. The inexhaustible fuel that powered its engine was self-love.

I don't live in a transcendental state. I am pretty flawed, and my mind is a neurotic work in progress. I get upset. I participate in the daily humdrum of life, enjoying it and actively engaging in it. But I come back to center often because it nourishes me.

The world is a reflection of what I put into the universe.

If someone would have told me in 2012 that I would be writing an important book that might help someone turn around diabetes, I wouldn't have believed it. I didn't think I had anything special to say.

After more than two years of pitching agents and publishing houses to get this book to you, a door opened in late 2023 to take the manuscript to the version you are holding now.

The universe wanted this book to reach you, and so it has.

The undeniable force of life is what has made me the physician, mother, wife, daughter, sister, friend, and person I am today. It took one leap of faith, and I have been guided ever since.

May you get the clarity, guidance and support you seek to turn around diabetes.

-Mumbai, May 2024

Acknowledgements

Thank you Neeraj, for being my friend. You are my rock, and my partner in everything. I am thankful everyday that you decided to spend your life with me. You don't know it but I got the luckier end of this partnership. The opportunity to raise our daughters together was the most beautiful blessing we could have asked for. The world is a better place with them in it and it's so exciting to watch them grow. To both of my amazing daughters, I love you more than words. I hope this book inspires you to create the world you want to see. Being Aashna's mumma and Aanya's mama is my favorite thing in the world. You are intelligent, kind, unique and strong individuals and I am so proud of you. My hugs and kisses are always with you.

Thank you to the original startup incubators and angel investors in me: my parents. Mom, you taught me about unconditional love and forgiveness. You taught me about prayer and faith. Dad, you taught me to believe in myself and to speak my truth. You taught me about the power of the mind and Consciousness. Both of you are the perfect parents for me in this lifetime. I love you. To my in-laws, Rashmi and Natavarlal Sanghani. You are living proof of what it means to be pure channels of unending love. You have lived your entire lives focussed on the most important thing. Family. To Meera didi. You care for me and my family in a way that lets us focus on our life purpose. Your daily devotion to your work and your prayer is a blessing that raises the vibration of our home.

To my brother Ravi. My thoughtful, intense and caring brother. I see a reflection of my own intensity in you. Similar, yet unique. May you, Divya and the boys laugh and love everyday. To my brother Ram. My loyal, creative and funny brother. I have come to rely on your ever positive outlook and lifelong trust. You genuinely believed in me, propelling this book to the finish line. You and Shipali have taught me how to not take everything so damn seriously. May you both always have access to a warm cup of chai whenever you want it.

To childhood friends. Dhruv, Satchit and Charuta. You actively taught me what friendship is, through your non-judgemental acceptance of me through the ups and downs. You put up with me talking non-stop about the book over the last year.

To my teachers in medicine. My first patient in Mumbai, Mr I.F. and my first patient in the States, Mrs. J.M. Thank you for placing your trust in trainee doctors and healthcare workers like me. It is a trust that we need to earn, uphold, and respect. I have learnt from each of my patients over the years, who placed their health in my hands. It is the greatest act of vulnerability, to ask for help. I strive to always honor that space, and keep my heart and mind open to every patient I meet. At KEM hospital during medical school: Dr Supe and Dr Karnad, Dr Manu Kothari, Dr Natarajan. At Jefferson psychiatry: Dr Kenneth Certa. At County Internal Medicine: Dr Rudy Kumapley, Dr Brendan Reilly, Dr Maurice Lemon, Dr John O'Brien, Dr Susan Glick, Dr Peter Clarke, Dr David Goldberg. At County Endocrinology: Dr Ambika Babu, Dr Evelyn Lacuesta and my bestie Judy Kolish RD, CDE. The endocrinologists at UIC and Christ hospital and CDE's at UIC Kari Kohrs and Christina Moy. For your support during my private practice at Christ, Dr Marc Silver, Bridget Gibbons, Lubina Hernandez, Sha-Tonnya Reid and CDE David Kats. To Rukhmini, my friend, spiritual teacher and guide. I am sure I have known you across lifetimes. Thank you for shining the Light so I could find my Truth. To my colleagues at Hinduja hospital who noticed and supported the lifestyle approach as I innovated along the way. To colleagues from private and teaching hospitals, private practices across Mumbai and India. To all the staff prior and current, at Aasaan Health Solutions and Reisaan Health. You have been part of creating something new in diabetes care and lifestyle medicine. To the early readers of this book, when it could not even be called a draft. David Jacobowitz, Anne Mullens, Dr William Miller and Manas Rath. You read through pages and pages of my initial rambling while I worked my way to find the final version we have now. Your early support and honest feedback helped me chug along and not give up. I suspect you believed in me more than I did myself and you wanted this book to succeed. For that, I am forever grateful. Dr Miller, the gift of motivational interviewing that you, Dr Rollnick and Dr Moyers have given the world changed me as a person and a professional. Having the foreword of this book written by you is a dream come true for me. To Dr Divya, Dr Kruti and my trainer Dhiraj Bediskar for helping clean up the exercise sections. To my endocrinology friends, classmates and colleagues who helped me reference and source articles from e-journals and reviewed technical parts of the book. To Dr Phil Ovadia who took the effort to reach out and ended up introducing me to Joshua Lisec. To Joshua, your professional guidance helped me extract the core message from multiple previous manuscripts into one that effectively flowed and delivered what I had been trying to say. Your book, courses, consultation and editing services have made all the difference in making this a book I am proud of. To Vijay, for designing a thoughtful and beautiful cover. To Neha, Anup and Pooja for the photographs. To Ashdin, Ankur and Noel for the audiobook. To Dr Jason Fung, for being an early supporter of this book, purely on its merit. Your nod means a lot to me, considering your own pioneering work in changing how the world thinks about insulin resistance.

To Life itself, for what the Universe has continued to unfold in front of me at every step.

All you needed me to do was have faith, surrender and take one step forward.

To not give up, despite the odds.

To believe the inner crazy voice that says we can change the diabetes epidemic in this generation.

To entrust me with this responsibility and message.

To believe that this introverted shy person with stage fright and frizzy hair can increase awareness around self-care for diabetes.

All You wanted me to do was put in my best.

I submit this book to You and lay my keyboard to rest.

I allow myself a few moments to soak in the sense of completion.

But wait–

What's next?

What's next?

If you're like me and you just can't get enough, here is the official further reading list of Dr. Roshani Sanghani:

Part 1: The Science

- Fat Chance by Robert Lustig, MD
- Always Hungry by David Ludwig, MD, PhD
- Good Calories, Bad Calories, Why We get Fat and What to do about it and Rethinking Diabetes by Gary Taubes
- Why We Get Sick by Ben Bikman PhD
- The Obesity Code by Jason Fung, MD
- The Diabetes Code by Jason Fung, MD

Part 2: Nutrition

- Eat What You Love, Love What You Eat by Michelle May, MD
- Nutritive Value of Indian Foods by the National Institute of Nutrition NIN and Indian Council of Medical Research ICMR
- The Hacking of the American Mind by Robert Lustig, MD, MSL
- Hooked: Food, Free Will, and How the Food Giants Exploit Our Addictions by Michael Moss
- End your Carb Confusion by Amy Berger and Eric Westman
- Keto Clarity by Eric Westman, MD

Part 3: Sleep

- The Sleep Solution by Chris Winter, MD
- Why We Sleep by Matthew Walker, PhD

- Breathe: The New Science of a Lost Art by James Nestor
- The Circadian Diabetes Code by Satchin Panda, PhD

Part 4: Stress management, self-talk and spirituality

- The Autobiography of a Yogi by Paramhansa Yogananda
- Words of Grace and Who Am I? by Sri Ramana Maharishi
- Lessons in meditation by Jyotish Novak, presented by Ananda Sangha worldwide
- Bhaja Govindam by Adi Sankaracharya
- The Untethered Soul by Michael Singer
- A New Earth by Eckhart Tolle
- Forgiveness the greatest healer of all by Gerald Jampolsky
- Taking the Leap by Pema Chodron
- The Four Agreements by don Miguel Ruiz
- You Can Heal your Life by Louise Hay
- You are the Placebo by Joe Dispenza
- The Biology of Belief by Bruce Lipton
- When the Body Says No by Gabor Mate
- Getting to Yes with Yourself by William Ury
- Atomic Habits by James Clear
- Worry Cure by Robert Leahy, PhD
- The Body Keeps the Score by Bessel van der Kolk
- Man's Search for Meaning by Viktor Frankl
- Switch How to Change when Change is hard by Chip and Dan Heath
- How to Do the Work by Nicole LePera
- The Anatomy of Anxiety by Ellen Vora, MD
- Feeling Good The New Mood therapy by David Burns, MD
- Brain Energy by Chris Palmer, MD
- The Gifts of Imperfection by Brene Brown
- Change your Diet Change your Mind by Dr Georgia Ede

- Discourses by Meher Baba

Part 5: Exercise

- Outlive by Peter Attia
- Maffetone Method The Holistic, Low-Stress No-Pain Way to Exceptional Fitness
- The Art and Science of Low carbohydrate Performance by Steve Phinney, MD,PhD and Jeff Volek, PhD
- Run for your life how to run walk and move without pain or injury and achieve a sense of wellbeing and joy by Mark Cucuzzella MD
- The Art of Impossible by Steven Kotler
- 15 minutes to fitness by Dr Ben Bocchicchio

Part 6: Fasting

- The Complete Guide to Fasting by Jason Fung, MD with Jimmy Moore

Part 7: Labs, Medications, Doctors, and Screening

- A conversation with Robert Lefkowitz, Joseph Goldstein and Michael Brown https://www.jci.org/articles/view/64244/pdf
- Michael S Brown, MD and Joseph L Goldstein MD 1985 Nobel Laureates in Medicine https://pubmed.ncbi.nlm.nih.gov/8689397/
- Cholesterol Clarity by Eric Westman, MD
- Nature Wants us to be Fat by Richard Johnson, MD
- Drop Acid by Dr David Perlmutter

Part 8: How to work with doctors and hospitals

- Working with doctors to protect your body
- Awkward: Recovering from fun
- Diabetes and the hospital
- Why I stopped working in the hospital environment

- Shirin, Elora, and Mustafa: Where are they now?

Part 9: Children and Diabetes

- Prepared, What Kids Need for a Fulfilled Life by Diane Tavenner
- How to Talk so Kids will Listen and Listen so Kids will Talk byJoanna Faber and Julie King
- Fearless Feeding How to Raise Healthy Eaters from High Chair to High School by Jill Castle and Maryann Jacobsen
- How to Get Your Kid to Eat but not Too Much by Ellyn Satter
- French Kids Eat Everything by Karen Le Billon

Part 10: Living with Type 1 Diabetes

- Dr Bernstein's Diabetes Solution by Richard Bernstein, MD
- My Kid is Back: Empowering Patients to Beat Anorexia Nervosa by Daniel Le Grange and June Alexander

Endnotes

Preface: The patient who made me listen

1 "Recommended Dietary Allowances and Estimated Average Requirements: A Report of the Expert Group, 2020 (Updated 2024)." ICMR-National Institute of Nutrition, Indian Council of Medical Research, Department of Health Research, Ministry of Health and Family Welfare, Government of India. Accessed May 1, 2024. https://www.nin.res.in/RDA_short_Report_2020.html.

2 U.S. Department of Agriculture and U.S. Department of Health and Human Services. Dietary Guidelines for Americans, 2020-2025. 9th ed. December 2020. https://www.dietaryguidelines.gov/resources/2020-2025-dietary-guidelines-online-materials.

3 Chutima Talchai, Shouhong Xuan, Hua V. Lin, Lori Sussel, and Domenico Accili, "Pancreatic β Cell Dedifferentiation as Mechanism of Diabetic β Cell Failure," Cell 150, no. 6 (2012): 1223–1234, https://www.ncbi.nlm.nih.gov/pmc/articles/PMC3445031/

Part 1: The Science of Diabetes

1 J. Roth, I. Whitford, R. Dankner, and L. Szulc, "How the Immunoassay Transformed C-Peptide from a Duckling into a Swan," Diabetologia 55 (2012): 865–869, https://doi.org/10.1007/s00125-011-2421-0.

2 Matthew C. Riddle, William T. Cefalu, Philip H. Evans, Hertzel C. Gerstein, Michael A. Nauck, William K. Oh, Amy E. Rothberg, et al., "Consensus Report: Definition and Interpretation of Remission in Type 2 Diabetes," Diabetes Care 44, no. 10 (2021): 2438–2444, https://diabetesjournals.org/care/article/44/10/2438/138556/Consensus-Report-Definition-and-Interpretation-of.

3 Risk for cardiovascular disease associated with metabolic syndrome and its components: a 13 year prospective study in the RIVANA cohort https://cardiab.biomedcentral.com/articles/10.1186/s12933-020-01166-6

4 Forte, José Castela, Rahul Gannamani, Pytrik Folkertsma, Sridhar Kumaras-wamy, Sarah Mount, Sipko van Dam, and Jan Hoogsteen. 2022. "Changes in Blood Lipid Levels After a Digitally Enabled Cardiometabolic Preventive Health Program: Pre-Post Study in an Adult Dutch General Population Cohort." JMIR Cardio 6, no. 1: e34946. https://doi.org/10.2196/34946.

5 Natsuko Tsujino and Takeshi Sakurai, "Orexin/Hypocretin: A Neuropeptide at the Interface of Sleep, Energy Homeostasis and Reward System," Pharmacological Reviews 61, no. 2 (2009):162–176, https://pubmed.ncbi.nlm.nih.gov/19549926/.

6 Martin A. Katzman and Matthew P. Katzman, "Neurobiology of the Orexin System and Its Potential Role in the Regulation of Hedonic Tone," Brain Sciences 12, no. 2 (2022): 150, https://pubmed.ncbi.nlm.nih.gov/35203914/.

7 Amira Klip and Mladen Vranic, "Muscle, Liver and Pancreas: Three Muske-teers Fighting to Control Glycemia," Essays on APS Classic Papers 291, no. 6 (2006): E1141–E1143, https://journals.physiology.org/doi/full/10.1152/classices-says.00043.2006

8 Benjamin Bikman, Why We Get Sick (Dallas: BenBella, 2020).

9 Susanna Søberg, Johan Löfgren, Frederik E. Philipsen, Michal Jensen, Adam E. Hansen, Esben Ahrens, Kristin B. Nystrup, et al., "Altered Brown Fat Thermo-regulation and Enhanced Cold-Induced Thermogenesis in Young, Healthy, Winter Swimming Men," Cell Reports Medicine 2, no. 10 (2021): 100408, https://doi.org/10.1016/j.xcrm.2021.100408.

10 Lee, Paul, Sheila Smith, Joyce Linderman, Amber B Courville, Robert J Brych-ta, William Dieckmann, Charlotte D Werner, Kong Y Chen, and Francesco S Celi. 2014. "Temperature-acclimated brown adipose tissue modulates insulin sensitivity in humans." Diabetes 63, no. 11 (November): 3686-3698. https://doi.org/10.2337/db14-0513.

11 F. Johnson, A. Mavrogianni, M. Ucci, A. Vidal-Puig, and J. Wardle, "Could Increased Time Spent in a Thermal Comfort Zone Contribute to Population In-creases in Obesity?" Obesity Reviews 12, no. 7 (2011): 543–551, https://pubmed.ncbi.nlm.nih.gov/21261804/.

12 Vasudev Kantae, Kimberly J. Nahon, Maaike E. Straat, Leontine E. H. Bakker, Amy C. Harms, Mario van der Stelt, et al., "Endocannabinoid Tone Is Higher

in Healthy Lean South Asian Than White Caucasian Men," Scientific Reports 7 (2017): 7558, https://www.nature.com/articles/s41598-017-07980-5.

13 Piotr Schulz, Szymon Hryhorowicz, Anna Maria Rychter, Agnieszka Zawada, Ryszard Słomski, Agnieszka Dobrowolska, and Iwona Krela-Kaźmierczak, "What Role Does the Endocannabinoid System Play in the Pathogenesis of Obesity?" Nutrients 13, no. 2 (2021): 373, https://www.ncbi.nlm.nih.gov/pmc/articles/PMC7911032/.

14 Esmaeil Mehraeen, Faeze Abbaspour, Maciej Banach, Seyed Ahmad Seyed Alinaghi, Ameneh Zarebidoki, and Seyed Saeed Tamehri Zadeh, "The Prognostic Significance of Insulin Resistance in COVID-19: A Review," Journal of Diabetes and Metabolic Disorders (2024), https://link.springer.com/article/10.1007/s40200-024-01385-8.

15 Robert A. Rizza, "Pathogenesis of Fasting and postprandial Hyperglycemia in Type 2 Diabetes," Diabetes 59, no. 11 (2010): 2697–2707, https://diabetesjournals.org/diabetes/article/59/11/2697/16191/Pathogenesis-of-Fasting-and-Postprandial.

16 Bayrak, Muharrem. "Metabolic Syndrome, Depression, and Fibromyalgia Syndrome Prevalence in Patients with Irritable Bowel Syndrome: A Case-Control Study." Medicine 99, no. 23 (June 5, 2020): e20577. https://doi.org/10.1097/MD.0000000000020577.

17 Sroka, Natalia, Alicja Rydzewska-Rosołowska, Katarzyna Kakareko, Mariusz Rosołowski, Irena Głowińska, and Tomasz Hryszko. "Show Me What You Have Inside—The Complex Interplay between SIBO and Multiple Medical Conditions—A Systematic Review." Nutrients 15, no. 1 (December 24, 2022): 90. https://doi.org/10.3390/nu15010090.

18 Mkumbuzi, Lusikelelwe, Mvuyisi M O Mfengu, Godwill A Engwa, and Constance R Sewani-Rusike. "Insulin Resistance is Associated with Gut Permeability Without the Direct Influence of Obesity in Young Adults." Diabetes, Metabolic Syndrome and Obesity: Targets and Therapy 13 (August 24, 2020): 2997-3008. https://doi.org/10.2147/DMSO.S256864.

Part 2: The First Wheel of the Lifestyle Car: Nutrition

1 Tera L. Fazzino, Daiil Jun, Lynn Chollet-Hinton, and Kayla Bjorlie, "US Tobacco Companies Selectively Disseminated Hyper-Palatable Foods into the US Food System," Addiction 119, no. 1 (2024): 62–71, https://onlinelibrary.wiley.com/doi/epdf/10.1111/add.16332.

2 Marta Zaraska, "Food Can Be Literally Addictive, New Evidence Suggests," Scientific American, https://www.scientificamerican.com/article/food-can-be-literally-addictive-new-evidence-suggests/.

3 Molly McDougle, Alan de Araujo, Arashdeep Singh, Mingxin Yang, Isadora Braga, Vincent Paille, Rebeca Mendez-Hernandez, et al., "Separate Gut-Brain Circuits for Fat and Sugar Reinforcement Combine to Promote Overeating," Cell Metabolism 36, no. 2 (2024): 393–407, https://www.sciencedirect.com/science/article/pii/S1550413123004667?s=08.

4 RobertLusting.com, https://robertlustig.com/.

5 David S. Ludwig, Caroline M. Apovian, Louis J. Aronne, Arne Astrup, Lewis C. Cantley, Cara B. Ebbeling, Steven B. Heymsfield, et al., "Competing Paradigms of Obesity Pathogenesis: Energy Balance versus Carbohydrate-Insulin Models," European Journal of Clinical Nutrition 76, no. 9 (2022): 1209–1221, https://escholarship.org/content/qt0h84c705/qt0h84c705.pdf.

6 Eenfeldt, Dr. Andreas, MD. "How Low Carb is Low Carb?" Accessed May 2, 2024. https://www.dietdoctor.com/low-carb/how-low-carb-is-low-carb.

7 Lorenzo M. Donini, Luca Busetto, Stephan C. Bischoff, Tommy Cederholm, Maria D. Ballesteros-Pomar, John A. Batsis, and Juergen M. Bauer, "Definition and Diagnostic Criteria for Sarcopenic Obesity (SO): ESPEN and EASO Consensus Statement," Obesity Facts 15, no. 3 (2022): 321–335, https://pubmed.ncbi.nlm.nih.gov/35196654/.

8 Mohan, Viswanathan, Vasudevan Sudha, Shanmugam Shobana, Rajagopal Gayathri, and Kamala Krishnaswamy. "Are Unhealthy Diets Contributing to the Rapid Rise of Type 2 Diabetes in India?" Translational Nutrition, 2023. https://doi.org/10.1016/j.tjnut.2023.02.028.

9 Weiler, Mary, Steven R. Hertzler, and Svyatoslav Dvoretskiy. 2023. "Is It Time to Reconsider the U.S. Recommendations for Dietary Protein and Amino Acid Intake?" Nutrients 15, no. 4: 838. https://doi.org/10.3390/nu15040838

10 Denise K. Houston, Barbara J. Nicklas, Jingzhong Ding, Tamara B. Harris, Frances A. Tylavsky, Anne B. Newman, Jung Sun Lee, et al., "Dietary Protein Intake Is Associated with Lean Mass Change in Older, Community-Dwelling Adults: The Health, Aging, and Body Composition (Health ABC) Study," American Journal of Clinical Nutrition 87, no. 1 (2008): 150–155, https://pubmed.ncbi.nlm.nih.gov/18175749/.

11 Donald K. Layman, "Dietary Protein and Exercise Have Additive Effects on Body Composition during Weight Loss in Adult Women," Journal of Nutrition 135, no. 8 (2005): 1903–1910, https://doi.org/10.1093/jn/135.8.1903.

12 Nuha A. ElSayed, Grazia Aleppo, Vanita R. Aroda, Raveendhara R. Bannuru, Florence M. Brown, Dennis Bruemmer, Billy S. Collins, et al., "Chronic Kidney Disease and Risk Management: Standards of Care in Diabetes—2023," Diabetes Care 46, suppl. 1 (2023): S191–S202, https://diabetesjournals.org/care/article/46/Supplement_1/S191/148040/11-Chronic-Kidney-Disease-and-Risk-Management.

13 American Diabetes Association Professional Practice Committee, "Chronic Kidney Disease and Risk Management: Standards of Care in Diabetes—2024," Diabetes Care 47, suppl. 1 (2024): S219–S230, https://diabetesjournals.org/care/article/47/Supplement_1/S219/153938/11-Chronic-Kidney-Disease-and-Risk-Management.

14 Agnes N. Pedersen, Jens Kondrup, and Elisabet Børsheim, "Health Effects of Protein Intake in Healthy Adults," Food and Nutrition Research 57 (2013): 21245, https://pubmed.ncbi.nlm.nih.gov/23908602/

15 Robert A. Saxton and David M. Sabatini, "mTor Signaling in Growth, Metabolism and Disease," Cell 168, no. 6 (2017): 960–976, https://www.ncbi.nlm.nih.gov/pmc/articles/PMC5394987/pdf/nihms850540.pdf.

16 Donald K. Layman, Tracy G. Anthony, Blake B. Rasmussen, Sean H. Adams, Christopher J. Lynch, Grant D. Brinkworth, and Teresa A. Davis, "Defining Meal Requirements for Protein to Optimize Metabolic Roles of Amino Acids," American Journal of Clinical Nutrition 101, no. 6 (2015): 1330S–1338S, https://www.sciencedirect.com/science/article/pii/S0002916523274286?via%3Dihub.

17 Jeremy P. Loenneke, Paul D. Loprinzi, Caoileann H. Murphy, and Stuart M. Phillips, "Per Meal Dose and Frequency of Protein Consumption Is Associated with Lean Mass and Muscle Performance," Clinical Nutrition 35, no. 6 (2016): 1506–1511, https://doi.org/10.1016/j.clnu.2016.04.002.

18 Brad Jon Schoenfeld and Alan Albert Aragon, "How Much Protein Can the Body Use in a Single Meal for Muscle-Building? Implications for Daily Protein Distribution," Journal of the International Society of Sports Nutrition 15 (2018): 10, https://doi.org/10.1186/s12970-018-0215-1.

19 Jorn Trommelen, Glenn A. A. van Lieshout, Jean Nyakayiru, Andrew M. Holwerda, Joey S. J. Smeets, Floris K. Hendriks, Janneau M. X. van Kranenburg, et al., "The Anabolic Response to Protein Ingestion during Recovery from Exercise Has No Upper Limit in Magnitude and Duration In Vivo in Humans," Cell Reports Medicine 4, no. 12, (2023): 101324, https://www.sciencedirect.com/science/article/pii/S2666379123005402.

20 Frankie B. Stentz, Amy Brewer, Jim Wan, Channing Garber, Blake Daniels, Chris Sands, and Abbas E. Kitabchi, "Remission of Pre-Diabetes to Normal Glucose Tolerance in Obese Adults with High Protein versus High Carbohydrate Diet: Randomized Control Trial," BMJ Open Diabetes Research and Care 4 (2016): e000258, https://www.ncbi.nlm.nih.gov/pmc/articles/PMC5093372/pdf/bmjdrc-2016-000258.pdf

21 Mrinal Samtiya, Rotimi E. Aluko, and Tejpal Dhewa, "Plant Food Anti-Nutritional Factors and Their Reduction Strategies: An Overview," Food Production, Processing and Nutrition 2 (2020): 6, https://fppn.biomedcentral.com/articles/10.1186/s43014-020-0020-5.

22 David J. Unwin, Simon D. Tobin, Scott W. Murray, Christine Delon, and Adrian J. Brady, "Substantial and Sustained Improvement in Blood Pressure Weight and Lipid Profiles from a Carbohydrate Restricted Diet: An Observational Study of Insulin Resistant Patients in Primary Care," International Journal of Environmental Research and Public Health 16, no. 15 (219): 2680, https://www.ncbi.nlm.nih.gov/pmc/articles/PMC6695889/.

23 A. Overlack, M. Ruppert, R. Kolloch, B. Göbel, K. Kraft, J. Diehl, W. Schmitt, and K. O. Stumpe, "Divergent Hemodynamic and Hormonal Responses to Varying Salt Intake in Normotensive Subjects," Hypertension 22, no. 3 (1993): 331–338, https://pubmed.ncbi.nlm.nih.gov/8349326/.

24 Richard Johnson, Nature Wants Us To Be Fat (Dallas: BenBella Books, 2022).

25 Richard J. Johnson, Miguel A. Lanaspa, L. Gabriela Sanchez-Lozada, Dean Tolan, Takahiko Nakagawa, Takuji Ishimoto, Ana Andres-Hernando, et al., "The Fructose Survival Hypothesis for Obesity," Philosophical Transactions of the Royal Society B 378, no. 1885 (2023): 20220230, https://www.ncbi.nlm.nih.gov/pmc/articles/PMC10363705/.

26 Shavawn M. Forester, Emily M. Jennings-Dobbs, Shazia A. Sathar, and Donald K. Layman, "Developing a Nutrient-Based Framework for Protein Quality," Journal of Nutrition 153, no. 8 (2023): 2137–2146, https://pubmed.ncbi.nlm.nih.gov/37301285/.

27 Daniel Kahneman, Nobel Laureate in Economics and author of Thinking, Fast and Slow (New York: Farrar, Straus and Giroux, 2013).

28 Carlos Augusto Monteiro, Geoffrey Cannon, Mark Lawrence, Maria Laura da Costa Louzada, and Priscila Pereira Machado, Ultra-Processed Foods, Diet Quality and Health Using the NOVA Classification System (Rome: Food and Agriculture Organization of the United Nations, 2019), https://www.fao.org/3/ca5644en/ca5644en.pdf.

29 Nina Teicholz, "Junk Food Has Been Rebranded as 'Ultra-Processed,'" Unsettled Science, February 6, 2024, https://open.substack.com/pub/unsettledscience/p/junk-food-has-been-rebranded-as-ultra?r=1siaqx&utm_campaign=post&utm_medium=email.

30 Arielle Richey Levine, Joseph A. Picoraro, Sally Dorfzaun, and Neal S. LeLeiko, "Emulsifiers and Intestinal Health, an Introduction," Journal of Pediatric Gastroenterology and Nutrition 74, no. 3 (2022): 314–319, https://pubmed.ncbi.nlm.nih.gov/35226642/.

31 "Added Sugar Repository." Hypoglycemia Support Foundation. Accessed April 8, 2024. https://hypoglycemia.org/added-sugar-repository/.

32 M. Yanina Pepino, "Metabolic Effects of Non-Nutritive Sweeteners," Physiology & Behavior 152 (2015): 450–455, https://www.ncbi.nlm.nih.gov/pmc/articles/PMC4661066/pdf/nihms705238.pdf.

33 Pauline Raoul, Marco Cintoni, Marta Palombaro, Luisa Basso, Emanuele Rinninella, Antonio Gasbarrini, and Maria Cristina Mele, "Food Additives, a Key Environmental Factor in the Development of IBD through Gut Dysbiosis," Microorganisms 10, no. 1 (2022): 167, https://pubmed.ncbi.nlm.nih.gov/35056616/.

34 Prabasheela Bakthavachalu, S. Meenakshi Kannan, and M. Walid Qoronfleh, "Food Color and Autism, a Meta-Analyisis," Advances in Neurobiology 24 (2020): 481–504, https://pubmed.ncbi.nlm.nih.gov/32006369/.

35 Anna E. Kirkland, Mackenzie T. Langan, and Kathleen F. Holton, "Artificial Food Coloring Affects EEG Power and ADHD Symptoms in College Students with ADHD: A Pilot Study," Nutritional Neuroscience 25, no. 1 (2022): 159–168, https://pubmed.ncbi.nlm.nih.gov/32116139/.

36 Sari Lehto, Maria Buchweitz, Alexandra Klimm, Raphaela Straßburger, Cato Bechtold, Franz Ulberth, "Comparison of Food Colour Regulations in the EU and the US: A Review of Current Provisions," Food Additives & Contaminants: Part A: Chemistry, Analysis, Control, Exposure & Risk Assessment 34, no. 3 (2017): 335–355, https://pubmed.ncbi.nlm.nih.gov/28004607/.

37 Carlos Augusto Monteiro, Geoffrey Cannon, Mark Lawrence, Maria Laura da Costa Louzada, and Priscila Pereira Machado, Ultra-Processed Foods, Diet Quality and Health Using the NOVA Classification System (Rome: Food and Agriculture Organization of the United Nations, 2019), https://www.fao.org/3/ca5644en/ca5644en.pdf.

38 Mayo Clinic Staff. "Carbohydrates: How Carbs Fit Into a Healthy Diet." Mayo Clinic. https://www.mayoclinic.org/healthy-lifestyle/nutrition-and-healthy-eating/in-depth/carbohydrates/art-20045705

39 McKinney, Christine, RD, LDN, CDE. "Carbohydrate Goals." The Johns Hopkins Patient Guide to Diabetes. Accessed April 8, 2024. https://hopkinsdiabetesinfo.org/carbohydrate-goals/.

40 Joshi, Shashank R, Anil Bhansali, Sarita Bajaj, Subodh S Banzal, Mala Dharmalingam, Shachin Gupta, Satinath Mukhopadhyay, Parag R Shah, Rakesh Sahay, Swapan Sarkar, Pravin V Manjrekar, Rahul T Rathod, and Shilpa S Joshi. "Results from a Dietary Survey in an Indian T2DM Population: A STARCH Study." BMJ Open 4, no. 10 (October 31, 2014): e005138. https://doi.org/10.1136/bmjopen-2014-005138.

41 Wheatley, Sean D., Trudi A. Deakin, Nicola C. Arjomandkhah, Paul B. Hollinrake, and Trudi E. Reeves. "Low Carbohydrate Dietary Approaches for People With Type 2 Diabetes—A Narrative Review." Frontiers in Nutrition 8 (July 15, 2021): 687658. https://doi.org/10.3389/fnut.2021.687658.

42 Mohan, Viswanathan, Ranjit Unnikrishnan, S. Shobana, M. Malavika, R.M. Anjana, and V. Sudha. "Are Excess Carbohydrates the Main Link to Diabetes & Its Complications in Asians?" The Indian Journal of Medical Research 148, no. 5 (November 2018): 531-38. https://doi.org/10.4103/ijmr.IJMR_1698_18.

43 Alpana P. Shukla, Radu G. Iliescu, Catherine E. Thomas, Louis J. Aronne, "Food Order Has a Significant Impact on Postprandial Glucose and Insulin Levels," Diabetes Care 38, no. 7 (2015): e98–e99, https://pubmed.ncbi.nlm.nih.gov/26106234/.

44 Michelle May, Eat What You Love, Love What You Eat (Austin, TX: Greenleaf, 2009).

45 Siggins, Robert W, Patrick M McTernan, Liz Simon, Flavia M Souza-Smith, and Patricia E Molina. "Mitochondrial Dysfunction: At the Nexus between Alcohol-Associated Immunometabolic Dysregulation and Tissue Injury." International Journal of Molecular Sciences 24, no. 10 (May 23, 2023): 8650. https://doi.org/10.3390/ijms24108650.

46 Debras, Charlotte, Eloi Chazelas, Laury Sellem, Raphaëlle Porcher, Nathalie Druesne-Pecollo, Younes Esseddik, et al. "Artificial Sweeteners and Risk of Cardiovascular Diseases: Results from the Prospective NutriNet-Santé Cohort." BMJ 378 (2022): e071204. https://doi.org/10.1136/bmj-2022-071204.

47 Kim A. Williams Sr., Amanda J. Krause, Sarah Shearer, and Stephen Devries, "The 2015 Dietary Guidelines Advisory Committee Report Concerning Dietary Cholesterol," American Journal of Cardiology 116, no. 9 (2015):1479–1480, https://pubmed.ncbi.nlm.nih.gov/26341187/.

48 Jo Ann S. Carson, Alice H. Lichtenstein, Cheryl A. M. Anderson, Lawrence J. Appel, Penny M. Kris-Etherton, Katie A. Meyer, Kristina Petersen, et al., "Dietary Cholesterol and Cardiovascular Risk: A Science Advisory from the AHA," Circulation 141, no. 3 (2020): e39–e53, https://www.ahajournals.org/doi/10.1161/CIR.0000000000000743.

49 Nina Teicholz, "A Short History of Saturated Fat: The Making and Unmaking of Scientific Consensus," Current Opinion in Endocrinology, Diabetes and Obesity 30, no.1 (2023): 65–71, https://www.ncbi.nlm.nih.gov/pmc/articles/PMC9794145/.

Part 3: The Second Wheel of the Lifestyle Car: Sleep

1 Robert Lustig, The Hacking of the American Mind: The Science behind the Corporate Takeover of Our Bodies and Brains (New York: Penguin, 2018).

2 Seolbin Han, Dae-Kwang Kim, Sang-Eun Jun, and Nahyun Kim, "Association of Sleep Quality and Mitochondrial DNA Copy Number in Healthy Middle-Aged Adults," Sleep Medicine 113 (2024): 19–24, https://www.sciencedirect.com/science/article/abs/pii/S138994572300429X.

3 Karine Spiegel, Rachel Leproult, and Eve Van Cauter, "Impact of Sleep Debt on Metabolic and Endocrine Function," Lancet 354, no. 9188 (1999): 1435–1439, https://www.thelancet.com/journals/lancet/article/PIIS0140-6736(99)01376-8/fulltext?cc=y%3D.

4 Jean-Philippe Chaput and Angelo Tremblay, "Sleeping Habits Predict the Magnitude of Fat Loss in Adults Exposed to Moderate Caloric Restriction," Obesity Facts 5, no. 4 (2012): 561–566, https://www.researchgate.net/publication/230599034.

5 Adrian F. Bogh, Simon B. K. Jensen, Christian R. Juhl, Charlotte Janus, Rasmus M. Sandsdal, Julie R. Lundgren, Mikkel H. Noer, et al., "Insufficient Sleep Predicts Poor Weight Loss Maintenance after 1 Year," Sleep 46, no. 5 (2023): zsac295, https://academic.oup.com/sleep/article/46/5/zsac295/6874808.

6 Mako Nagayoshi, Naresh M. Punjabi, Elizabeth Selvin, James S. Pankow, Eyal Shahar, Hiroyasu Iso, Aaron R. Folsom, and Pamela L. Lutsey," Obstructive Sleep Apnea and Incident Type 2 Diabetes," Sleep Medicine 25 (2016): 156–161, https://pubmed.ncbi.nlm.nih.gov/27810258/

7 Isao Muraki, Hiroo Wada, and Takeshi Tanigawa, "Sleep Apnea and Type 2 Diabetes," Journal of Diabetes Investigation 9, no. 5 (2018): 991–997, https://pubmed.ncbi.nlm.nih.gov/29453905/

8 Chris Winter, The Sleep Solution: Why Your Sleep Is Broken and How to Fix It (New York: Penguin, 2017).

9 Less than six hours of sleep is the most prominent risk factor in fatal road accidents caused by falling asleep at the wheel. See: Juhani Kalsi, Timo Tervo, Adel Bachour, and Markku Partinen, "Sleep versus Non-Sleep-Related Fatal Road Accidents," Sleep Medicine 51 (2018): 148–152, https://pubmed.ncbi.nlm.nih.gov/30179735/.

10 Eric Suni and Anis Rehman, "Sleep Drive and Your Body Clock," Sleep Foundation, November 16, 2023, https://www.sleepfoundation.org/circadian-rhythm/sleep-drive-and-your-body-clock.

11 Eric Suni and Alex Dimitriu, "What Is 'Revenge Bedtime Procrastination'?" Sleep Foundation, December 8, 2023, https://www.sleepfoundation.org/sleep-hygiene/revenge-bedtime-procrastination.

12 Eckhart Tolle, A New Earth: Create a Better Life (New York: Penguin, 2009).

13 Matthew Walker, Why We Sleep (New York: Scribner, 2017).

14 Meng Zhang, Han-Yuan Wang, Xin-Hui He, Yu-Ting Jiang, Yu-Hong Zhao, Qi-Jun Wu, Hui Sun, et al., "Shift Work and Health Outcomes: An Umbrella Review of Systematic Reviews and Meta-Analyses of Epidemiological Studies," Journal of Clinical Sleep Medicine 18, no. 2 (2022): 653–662, https://jcsm.aasm.org/doi/epdf/10.5664/jcsm.9642.

15 International Agency for Research on Cancer, Night Shift Work: IARC Monographs on the Identification of Carcinogenic Hazards to Humans, vol. 124 (Lyon, France: International Agency for Research on Cancer, 2020), https://publications.iarc.fr/593.

16 Danielle Pacheco, "Treatments for Shift Work Disorder," Sleep Foundation, November 3, 2023, https://www.sleepfoundation.org/shift-work-disorder/treatment

17 Rob Newsom, "Experts Develop Sleep Guidelines Uniquely Designed for Shift Workers," Sleep Foundation, August 30, 2023, https://www.sleepfoundation.org/sleep-news/new-sleep-guidelines-tailored-for-shift-workers

18 Yool Lee, Jeffrey M. Field, Amita Sehgal, "Circadian Rhythms, Disease and Chronotherapy," Journal of Biological Rhythms 36, no. 6 (2021): 503–531, https://www.ncbi.nlm.nih.gov/pmc/articles/PMC9197224/pdf/nihms-1814239.pdf

19 Yale School of Medicine, "Sleep's Crucial Role in Preserving Memory," May 10, 2022, https://medicine.yale.edu/news-article/sleeps-crucial-role-in-preserving-memory/.

20 Daniel B. Rubin, Tommy Hosman, Jessica N. Kelemen, Anastasia Kapitonava, Francis R. Willett, Brian F. Coughlin, Eric Halgren, et al., "Learned Motor Patterns Are Replayed in Human Motor Cortex during Sleep," Journal of Neuroscience 42, no. 25 (2022): 5007–5020, https://www.jneurosci.org/content/42/25/5007.

21 Kana Okano, Jakub R. Kaczmarzyk, Neha Dave, John D. E. Gabrieli, and Jeffrey C. Grossma, "Sleep Quality, Duration and Consistency Are Associated with Better Academic Performance in College Students," npj Science of Learning 4, no. 16 (2019), https://www.nature.com/articles/s41539-019-0055-z

22 Mark Michaud, "Not All Sleep Is Equal When It Comes to Cleaning the Brain," University of Rochester Medical Center, February 27, 2019, https://www.urmc.rochester.edu/news/story/not-all-sleep-is-equal-when-it-comes-to-cleaning-the-brain.

23 Omonigho M. Bubu, Michael Brannick, James Mortimer, Ogie Umasabor-Bu-bu, Yuri V. Sebastião, Yi Wen, Skai Schwartz, et al., "Sleep, Cognitive Impairment and Alzheimer's Disease: A Systematic Review and Meta-Analysis," Sleep 40, no. 1 (2017), https://pubmed.ncbi.nlm.nih.gov/28364458/.

24 "The Basics: Defining How Much Alcohol Is Too Much," National Institute on Alcohol Abuse and Alcoholism, September 22, 2023, https://www.niaaa.nih.gov/health-professionals-communities/core-resource-on-alcohol/basics-defining-how-much-alcohol-too-much.

25 Mark T. U. Barone and Luiz Menna-Barreto, "Diabetes and Sleep: A Complex Cause-and-Effect Relationship," Diabetes Research and Clinical Practice 91, no. 2 (2011): 129–137, https://www.sciencedirect.com/science/article/pii/S0168822710003888#bib0050.

26 Karine Spiegel, Kristen Knutson, Rachel Leproult, Esra Tasali, and Eve Van Cauter, "Sleep Loss: A Novel Risk Factor for Insulin Resistance and Type 2 Diabetes," Journal of Applied Physiology 99, no. 5 (2005): 2008–2019, https://journals.physiology.org/doi/full/10.1152/japplphysiol.00660.2005?rfr_dat=cr_pub++-0pubmed&url_ver=Z39.88-2003&rfr_id=ori%3Arid%3Acrossref.org.

27 Michael Smolensky and Lynne Lamberg, The Body Clock Guide to Better Health (New York: Owl, 2001).

28 Michael Gradisar, Amy R. Wolfson, Allison G. Harvey, Lauren Hale, Russell Rosenberg, and Charles A. Czeisler, "The Sleep and Technology Use of Americans: Findings from the National Sleep Foundation's 2011 Sleep in American Poll," Journal of Clinical Sleep Medicine 9, no. 12 (2013), https://jcsm.aasm.org/doi/10.5664/jcsm.3272.

29 "Using Light for Health," Huberman Lab, January 24, 2023, https://www.hubermanlab.com/newsletter/using-light-for-health.

30 Michael K. Scullin, Madison L. Krueger, Hannah K. Ballard, Natalya Pruett, and Donald L. Bliwise, "The Effects of Bedtime Writing on Difficulty Falling Asleep," Journal of Experimental Psychology: General 147, no. 1 (2018): 139–146, https://pubmed.ncbi.nlm.nih.gov/29058942/

31 Marta Jackowska, Jennie Brown, Amy Ronaldson, and Andrew Steptoe, "The Impact of a Brief Gratitude Intervention on Subjective Well-Being, Biology and Sleep," Journal of Health Psychology 21, no. 10 (2016): 2207–2217, https://pubmed.ncbi.nlm.nih.gov/25736389/

32 M. J. Parsons, T. E. Moffitt, A. M. Gregory, S. Goldman-Mellor, P. M. Nolan, R. Poulton, and A. Caspi, "Social Jetlag, Obesity and Metabolic Disorder," International Journal of Obesity 39 (2015): 842–848, https://www.nature.com/articles/ijo2014201.

33 Karuna Datta, Manjari Tripathi, Mansi Verma, Deepika Masiwal, Hruda Nanda Mallick, "Yoga Nidra Practice Shows Improvement in Sleep in Patients with Chronic Insomnia: A Randomized Controlled Trial," National Medical Journal of India 34, no. 3 (2021): 143–150, https://pubmed.ncbi.nlm.nih.gov/34825538/.

34 Jon Kabat-Zinn, https://jonkabat-zinn.com/.

35 Dawson Church, Peta Stapleton, Anitha Vasudevan, and Tom O'Keefe, "Clinical EFT as an Evidence-Based Practice for the Treatment of Psychological and Physiological Conditions: A Systematic Review," Frontiers in Psychology 13 (2022): 951451, https://www.ncbi.nlm.nih.gov/pmc/articles/PMC9692186/pdf/fpsyg-13-951451.pdf.

Part 4: The Third Wheel of the Lifestyle Car: Stress Management

1 Andrew J. Sommerfield, Ian J. Deary, Brian M. Frier, "Acute Hyperglycemia Alters Mood State and Impairs Cognitive Performance in People with Type 2 Diabetes," Diabetes Care 27, no. 10 (2004): 2335–2340, https://pubmed.ncbi.nlm.nih.gov/15451897/

2 Zhu, Yao, Ying Li, Qiang Zhang, Yuanjian Song, Liang Wang, and Zuobin Zhu. 2022. "Interactions Between Intestinal Microbiota and Neural Mitochondria: A New Perspective on Communicating Pathway From Gut to Brain." Frontiers in Microbiology 13 (February): Article 798917. https://doi.org/10.3389/fmicb.2022.798917.

3 "Scales and Measures," Behavioral Diabetes Institute, accessed February 11, 2024, https://behavioraldiabetes.org/scales-and-measures/.

4 American Diabetes Association Professional Practice Committee, "Facilitating Positive Health Behaviors and Well-being to Improve Health Outcomes: Standards of Care in Diabetes—2024," Diabetes Care 47, supplement 1 (2024): S77–S110, https://diabetesjournals.org/care/article/47/Supplement_1/S77/153949/5-Facilitating-Positive-Health-Behaviors-and-Well?searchresult=1.

5 American Diabetes Association Professional Practice Committee, "Introduction and Methodology: Standards of Care in Diabetes—2024," Diabetes Care 47, suppl. 1, S1–S4, https://doi.org/10.2337/dc24-SINT.

6 Stephen W. Porges, "Heart Rate Variability: A Personal Journey," Applied Psychophysiology and Biofeedback 47 (2022): 259–271, https://link.springer.com/article/10.1007/s10484-022-09559-x.

7 Diabetes Prevention Program Research Group, "Reduction in the Incidence of Type 2 Diabetes with Lifestyle Intervention or Metformin," New England Journal of Medicine 346 (2002): 393–403, https://www.nejm.org/doi/full/10.1056/nejmoa012512.

8 Epel, Elissa, Rachel Lapidus, Bruce McEwen, and Kelly Brownell. "Stress May Add Bite to Appetite in Women: A Laboratory Study of Stress-Induced Cortisol and Eating Behavior." Psychoneuroendocrinology 26, no. 1 (January 2001): 37-49. https://doi.org/10.1016/s0306-4530(00)00035-4.

9 Chao, Audrey M., Ania M. Jastreboff, Marney A. White, Carlos M. Grilo, and Rajita Sinha. "Stress, Cortisol, and Other Appetite-Related Hormones: Prospective Prediction of 6-Month Changes in Food Cravings and Weight." Obesity 25, no. 4 (April 2017): 713-720. https://doi.org/10.1002/oby.21790.

10 "Diabetes Is a Fast-Growing Disease of the Poor. Here's How We Can Turn the Tide," November 14, 2017, World Economic Forum, https://www.weforum.org/agenda/2017/11/diabetes-is-a-fast-growing-disease-of-the-poor-here-s-how-we-can-turn-the-tide/

11 Mohammed K. Ali, K. M. Venkat Narayan, and Viswanathan Mohan, "Innovative Research for Equitable Diabetes Care in India," Diabetes Research and Clinical Practice 86, no. 3 (2009): 155–167, https://pubmed.ncbi.nlm.nih.gov/19796835/.

12 Felicia Hill-Briggs, Nancy E. Adler, Seth A. Berkowitz, Marshall H. Chin, Tiffany L. Gary-Webb, Ana Navas-Acien, Pamela L. Thornton, et al., "Social Determinants of Health and Diabetes: A Scientific Review," Diabetes Care 44, no. 1 (2021): 258–279, https://www.ncbi.nlm.nih.gov/pmc/articles/PMC7783927/.

13 "Personality, Anxiety, and Stress in Patients with Small Intestine Bacterial Overgrowth Syndrome. The Polish Preliminary Study." International Journal of Environmental Research and Public Health 20, no. 1 (December 21, 2022): 93. https://doi.org/10.3390/ijerph20010093.

14 Sri Ramana Maharishi, "Kaivalya Upanishad—Meaning in English, Verse 18," https://sriramanamaharishi.com/kaivalya/kaivalya-upanishad-meaning-english/.

15 Daniel Kahneman, Thinking, Fast and Slow (New York: Farrar, Straus and Giroux, 2013).

16 Susanna Søberg, Camilla H. Sandholt, Naja Z. Jespersen, Ulla Toft, Anja L. Madsen, Stephanie von Holstein-Rathlou, Trisha J. Grevengoed, Karl B. Christensen, Wender L. P. Bredie, et al., "FGF-21 Is a Sugar-Induced Hormone Associated with Sweet Intake and Preference in Humans," Cell Metabolism 25, no. 5 (2017): 1045–1053, https://pubmed.ncbi.nlm.nih.gov/28467924/.

17 Anna M. Friis, Malcolm H. Johnson, Richard G. Cutfield, and Nathan S. Consedine, "Kindness Matters: A Randomized Controlled Trial of a Mindful Self-Compassion Intervention Improves Depression, Distress and HbA1c among Patients with Diabetes," Diabetes Care 39, no. 11 (2016): 1963–1971, https://diabetesjournals.org/care/article/39/11/1963/37295/Kindness-Matters-A-Randomized-Controlled-Trial-of.

18 Aljoscha Dreisoerner, Nina M. Junker, Wolff Schlotz, Julia Heimrich, Svenja Bloemeke, Beate Ditzen, and Rolf van Dicka, "Self-Soothing Touch and Being Hugged Reduce Cortisol Responses to Stress: A Randomized Controlled Trial," Comprehensive Psychoneuroendocrinology 8 (2021): 100091, https://www.ncbi.nlm.nih.gov/pmc/articles/PMC9216399/.

19 Gagan Priya and Sanjay Kalra, "Mind-Body Interactions and Mindfulness Meditation in Diabetes," European Journal of Endocrinology 14, no. 1 (2018): 35–41, https://www.ncbi.nlm.nih.gov/pmc/articles/PMC5954593/.

20 Emily K. Lindsay, Brian Chin, Carol M. Greco, Shinzen Young, Kirk W. Brown, Aidan G. C. Wright, Joshua M. Smyth, et al., "How Mindfulness Training Promotes Positive Emotions," Journal of Personal and Social Psychology 115, no. 6 (2018): 944–973, https://www.ncbi.nlm.nih.gov/pmc/articles/PMC6296247/.

21 Ellen Vora, The Anatomy of Anxiety (New York: Harper, 2022).

22 Stephen B. Karpman, "The New Drama Triangles," August 11, 2007, https://karpmandramatriangle.com/pdf/thenewdramatriangles.pdf.

Part 5: The Fourth Wheel of the Lifestyle Car: Exercise

1 Contrepois, Kévin, Si Wu, Kegan J. Moneghetti, Hassan Chaib, Francois Haddad, and Michael P. Snyder. 2020. "Molecular Choreography of Acute Exercise." Cell 181, no. 5 (May 28): 1112-1130.e16. https://doi.org/10.1016/j.cell.2020.04.043.

2 Dawei Zhou, Chao Wang, Qing Lin and Tong Li, "The Obesity Paradox for Survivors of Critically Ill Patients," Critical Care 26 (2022):198, https://www.ncbi.nlm.nih.gov/pmc/articles/PMC9251913/pdf/13054_2022_Article_4074.pdf.

3 Karla E. Merz and Debbie C. Thurmond, "Role of Skeletal Muscle in Insulin Resistance and Glucose Uptake," Comprehensive Physiology 10, no. 3 (2020): 785–809, https://www.ncbi.nlm.nih.gov/pmc/articles/PMC8074531/.

4 Bowen, T Scott, Gerhard Schuler, and Volker Adams. "Skeletal Muscle Wasting in Cachexia and Sarcopenia: Molecular Pathophysiology and Impact of Exercise Training." Journal of Cachexia, Sarcopenia and Muscle 6, no. 3 (September 2015): 197-207. https://doi.org/10.1002/jcsm.12043.

5 Hernández-Ochoa, Erick O., Paola Llanos, and Johanna T. Lanner. "The Underlying Mechanisms of Diabetic Myopathy." Journal of Diabetes Research 2017 (2017): 7485738. https://doi.org/10.1155/2017/7485738.

6 Ibid.

7 Mauro Zamboni, Gloria Mazzali, Anna Brunelli, Tanaz Saatchi, Silvia Urbani, Anna Giani, Andrea P. Rossi, et al., "The Role of Cross-Talk between Adipose Cells and Myocytes in the Pathogenesis of Sarcopenic Obesity in the Elderly," Cells 11, no. 21 (2022): 3361, https://doi.org/10.3390/cells11213361.

8 Irshad Ahmad, Shalini Verma, Majumi M. Noohu, Mohd. Yakub Shareef, and M. Ejaz Hussain, "Sensorimotor and Gait Training Improves Proprioception, Nerve Function and Muscular Activation in Patients with Diabetic Peripheral Neuropathy: A Randomized Controlled Trial," Journal of Musculoskeletal and Neuronal Interactions 20, no. 2 (2020): 234–248, https://www.ismni.org/jmni/pdf/80/jmni_20_234.pdf.

9 Carley E. Johnson and Jody K. Takemoto, "A Review of Beneficial Low-Intensity Exercises in Diabetic Neuropathy Patients," Journal of Pharmacy & Pharmaceutical Sciences 22 (2019): 1–130, https://journals.library.ualberta.ca/jpps/index.php/JPPS/article/view/30151.

10 Munshi, Medha N., Graydon S. Meneilly, Leocadio Rodríguez Mañas, Kelly L. Close, Paul R. Conlin, Tali Cukierman-Yaffe, Angus Forbes, et al. "Diabetes in Aging: Pathways for Developing the Evidence-Base for Clinical Guidance." The Lancet Diabetes & Endocrinology 8, no. 10 (October 2020): 855-67. https://doi.org/10.1016/S2213-8587(20)30230-8.

11 Cawthon, Peggy M., and Mary Drake. "It Is Not 'Just a Fracture'." JBMR Plus 8, no. 5 (April 9, 2024): ziae022. https://doi.org/10.1093/jbmrpl/ziae022.

12 Jaime Sanz-Cánovas, Almudena López-Sampalo, Lidia Cobos-Palacios, Michele Ricci, Halbert Hernández-Negrín, Juan José Mancebo-Sevilla, Elena Álvarez-Recio, et al., "Management of Type 2 Diabetes Mellitus in Elderly Patients with Frailty and/or Sarcopenia," International Journal of Environmental Research and Public Health 19, no. 14 (2022): 8677, https://www.mdpi.com/1660-4601/19/14/8677#B37-ijerph-19-08677.

13 Grgic, Jozo, Brad J. Schoenfeld, John Orazem, and Filip Sabol. 2021. "Effects of resistance training performed to repetition failure or non-failure on muscular strength and hypertrophy: A systematic review and meta-analysis." Journal of Sport and Health Science. https://doi.org/10.1016/j.jshs.2021.01.007.

14 Renate Petschnig, Thomas Wagner, Armin Robubi, Ramon Baron, "Effect of Strength Training on Glycemic Control and Adiponectin in Diabetic Children," Medicine & Science in Sports & Exercise 52, no. 10 (2020): 2172–2178, https://pubmed.ncbi.nlm.nih.gov/32301853/.

15 Marni Armstrong, Sheri R. Colberg, and Ronald J. Sigal, "Where to Start? Physical Assessment, Readiness and Exercise Recommendations for People with Type 1 or Type 2 Diabetes," Diabetes Spectrum 36, no. 2 (2023): 105–113, https://pubmed.ncbi.nlm.nih.gov/37193205/.

16 Alicia Ann Thorp, Bronwyn A. Kingwell, Parneet Sethi, Louise Hammond, Neville Owen, and David W. Dunstan, "Alternating Bouts of Sitting and Standing Attenuate Postprandial Glucose Responses," Medicine & Science in Sports & Exercise 46(11) 2014: 2053–2061, https://pubmed.ncbi.nlm.nih.gov/24637345/.

17 Genevieve N. Healy, David W. Dunstan, Jo Salmon, Ester Cerin, Jonathan E. Shaw, Paul Z. Zimmet, and Neville Owen, "Breaks in Sedentary Time: Association with Metabolic Risk," Diabetes Care 31, no. 4 (2008): 661–666, https://pubmed.ncbi.nlm.nih.gov/18252901/.

18 Paddy C. Dempsey, Robyn N. Larsen, Parneet Sethi, Julian W. Sacre, Nora E. Straznicky, Neale D. Cohen, Ester Cerin, et al., "Benefits for Type 2 Diabetes of Interrupting Prolonged Sitting with Brief Bouts of Light Walking or Simple Resistance Activities," Diabetes Care 39, no. 6 (2016): 964–972, https://pubmed.ncbi.nlm.nih.gov/27208318/.

19 Ryan J. Pettit-Mee, Sean T. Ready, Jaume Padilla, and Jill A. Kanaley, "Leg Fidgeting during Prolonged Sitting Improves Postprandial Glycemic Control in People with Obesity," Obesity 29, no. 7 (2021): 1146–1154, https://pubmed.ncbi.nlm.nih.gov/34159757/

20 Jeff Volek and Stephen Phinney, The Art and Science of Low Carbohydrate Performance (Scotts Valley, CA: CreateSpace, 2012).

21 Kent Arnold Lorenz, Shlomo Yeshurun, Richard Aziz, Julissa Ortiz-Delatorre, James Robert Bagley, Merav Mor, and Marialice Kern, "A Handheld Metabolic Device (Lumen) to Measure Fuel Utilization in Healthy Young Adults: Device Validation Study," Interactive Journal of Medical Research 10, no. 2 (2021): e25371, https://www.ncbi.nlm.nih.gov/pmc/articles/PMC8167606/.

22 Pim Knuiman, Maria T. E. Hopman, and Marco Mensink, "Glycogen Availability and Skeletal Muscle Adaptations with Endurance and Resistance Exercise," Nutrition & Metabolism 12 (2015): 59, https://www.ncbi.nlm.nih.gov/pmc/articles/PMC4687103/.

23 Landry Bobo, "Zone 2 Training and Fat Burning," Training Peaks, accessed February 11, 2024, https://www.trainingpeaks.com/blog/zone-2-training-fat-burning/.

24 Izumi Tabata, "Tabata Training: One of the Most Energetically Effective High-Intensity Intermittent Training Methods," Journal of Physiological Sciences 69 (2019): 559–572, https://jps.biomedcentral.com/articles/10.1007/s12576-019-00676-7.

25 Alessio Bellini, Andrea Nicolò, Ilenia Bazzucchi, and Massimo Sacchetti, "The Effect of Postprandial Walking on the Glucose Response after Meals with Different Characteristics," Nutrients 14, no. 5 (2022):1080, https://pubmed.ncbi.nlm.nih.gov/35268055/.

26 Tobias Engeroff, David A. Groneberg, and Jan Wilke, "After Dinner, Rest a While, after Supper Walk a Mile?" Sports Medicine 53, no. 4 (2023): 849–869, https://pubmed.ncbi.nlm.nih.gov/36715875/

27 Kim E. Innes and Terry Kit Selfe, "Yoga for Adults with Type 2 Diabetes: A

Systematic Review of Controlled Trials," Journal of Diabetes Research (2016), https://www.hindawi.com/journals/jdr/2016/6979370/.

28 James Nestor, Breathe: The New Science of a Lost Art (New York: Riverhead Books, 2020).

29 Ted Naiman, "Type 2 Diabetes vs Bodybuilding," YouTube, 2021, https://www.youtube.com/watch?si=0aSNrc9wZ-ZE_pEL&v=z4isghAuN_0&feature=youtu.be.

30 Darren G. Candow, Scott C. Forbes, Sergej M. Ostojic, Konstantinos Prokopidis, Matt S. Stock, Kylie K. Harmon, and Paul Faulkner, "'Heads Up' for Creatine Supplementation and Its Potential Applications for Brain Health and Function," Sports Medicine 53, suppl. 1 (2023): 49–65, https://www.ncbi.nlm.nih.gov/pmc/articles/PMC10721691/.

31 Ben Bocchicchio, 15 Minutes to Fitness (New York: SelectBooks, 2017).

32 Lorcan S. Daly, Bas Van Hooren, and Philip Jakeman, "Physiological Characteristics of a 92-Year-Old Four-Time World Champion Indoor Rower," Journal of Applied Physiology 135, no. 6 (2023): 1415–1420, https://journals.physiology.org/doi/full/10.1152/japplphysiol.00698.2023.

Part 6: Taking your Lifestyle Car the Extra Mile: Fasting

1 Maayan Barnea, Tali Ganz, Miriam Menaged, Naomi Mor, Yosefa Bar-Dayan, and Oren Froy, "Reduction in Glycated Hemoglobin and Daily Insulin Dose alongside Circadian Clock Upregulation in Patients with Type 2 Diabetes Consuming a Three-Meal Diet: A Randomized Clinical Trial," Diabetes Care 42, no. 12 (2019): 2171–2180, https://diabetesjournals.org/care/article/42/12/2171/36185/Reduction-in-Glycated-Hemoglobin-and-Daily-Insulin.

2 Kathryn Doyle, "6 Years after the Biggest Loser, Metabolism Is Slower and Weight Is Back Up," Scientific American, May 11, 2016, https://www.scientificamerican.com/article/6-years-after-the-biggest-loser-metabolism-is-slower-and-weight-is-back-up/.

3 C. Zauner, B. Schneeweiss, A. Kranz, C. Madl, K. Ratheiser, L. Kramer, E. Roth, B. Schneider, and K. Lenz, "Resting Energy Expenditure in Short-Term Starvation Is Increased as a Result of an Increase in Serum Norepinephrine," American Journal of Clinical Nutrition 71, no. 6 (2000): 1511–1515, https://pubmed.ncbi.nlm.nih.gov/10837292/#:~:text=Conclusions%3A%20Resting%20energy%20expenditure%20increases,metabolic%20changes%20in%20early%20starvation.

4 Yoshinori Ohsumi, "What Is Autophagy? A Dynamic Cellular Recycling Process," YouTube, 2018, https://www.youtube.com/watch?v=6bAkvnvX0W8.

5 Mashun Onishi, Koji Yamano, Miyuki Sato, Noriyuki Matsuda, and Koji Okamoto, "Molecular Mechanisms and Physiological Functions of Mitophagy," EMBO Journal 40, no. 3 (2021): e104705, https://pubmed.ncbi.nlm.nih.gov/33438778/.

6 Daniel J. Klionsky, Giulia Petroni, Ravi K. Amaravadi, Eric H. Baehrecke, Andrea Ballabio, Patricia Boya, José Manuel Bravo-San Pedro, et al., "Autophagy in Major Human Diseases," EMBO Journal 40, no. 19 (2021): e108863, https://www.ncbi.nlm.nih.gov/pmc/articles/PMC8488577/.

7 Michael J. Wilkinson, Emily N. C. Manoogian, Adena Zadourian, Saket Navlakha, Satchidananda Panda, and Pam R. Taub, "Ten-Hour Time Restricted Eating Reduces Weight, Blood Pressure, and Atherogenic Lipids in Patients with Metabolic Syndrome," Cell Metabolism 31 (2020): 92–104, https://www.cell.com/action/showPdf?pii=S1550-4131%2819%2930611-4.

8 Edward J. Calabrese and Mark P. Mattson, "How Does Hormesis Impact Biology, Toxicology and Medicine?" npj Aging and Mechanisms of Disease 3 (2017): 13, https://www.nature.com/articles/s41514-017-0013-z.

9 Shinji Saiki, Yukiko Sasazawa, Yoko Imamichi, Sumihiro Kawajiri, Takahiro Fujimaki, Isei Tanida, Hiroki Kobayashi, et al., "Caffeine Induces Apoptosis by Enhancement of Autophagy Via PI3K/Akt/mTOR/p70S6K Inhibition," Autophagy 7, no. 2(2011): 176–187, https://www.ncbi.nlm.nih.gov/pmc/articles/PMC3039768/.

10 Marcos Martin-Rincon, Alberto Pérez-López, David Morales-Alamo, Ismael Perez-Suarez, Pedro de Pablos-Velasco, Mario Perez-Valera, and Sergio Perez-Regalado, "Exercise Prevents Muscle Loss during Fasting Due to Autophagy," Nutrients 11, no. 11 (2019): 2824, https://pubmed.ncbi.nlm.nih.gov/31752260/.

11 Sol Been Park and Soo Jin Yang, "Ketogenic Diet Preserves Muscles Mass and Strength in a Mouse Model of Type 2 Diabetes," PLoS One 19, no. 1 (2024): e0296651, https://pubmed.ncbi.nlm.nih.gov/38198459/?s=08.

12 Ameneh Madjd, Moira A. Taylor, Alireza Delavari, Reza Malekzadeh, Ian A. Macdonald, and Hamid R. Farshchi, "Effects of Consuming Later Evening Meal v. Earlier Evening Meal on Weight Loss during a Weight Loss Diet: A Randomized Clinical Trial," British Journal of Nutrition 126, no. 4 (2021): 632–640, https://pubmed.ncbi.nlm.nih.gov/33172509/.

13 Chenjuan Gu, Nga Brereton, Amy Schweitzer, Matthew Cotter, Daisy Duan, Elisabet Børsheim, Robert R. Wolfe, et al., "Metabolic Effects of Late Dinner in Healthy Volunteers—A Randomized Crossover Clinical Trial," Journal of Clinical Endocrinology and Metabolism 105, no. 8 (2020): 2789–2802, https://pubmed.ncbi.nlm.nih.gov/32525525/.

14 Robert Lustig, Metabolical: The Truth about Processed Food and How It Poisons People and the Planet (New York: Harper, 2021).

15 A. D. Booth, A. M. Magnuson, J. Fouts, Y. Wei, D. Wang, M. J. Pagliassotti, and M. T. Foster, "Subcutaneous Adipose Tissue Accumulation Protects Systemic Glucose Tolerance and Muscle Metabolism," Adipocyte 7, no. 4 (2018): 261–272, https://pubmed.ncbi.nlm.nih.gov/30230416/.

16 Patrick T. Bradshaw, "Body Composition and Cancer Survival, a Narrative Review," British Journal of Cancer 130 (2024): 176–183, https://www.nature.com/articles/s41416-023-02470-0.

17 Sandi Busch, "Does the Body Store Fat Like Carbohydrates?" Live Strong, September 9, 2019, https://www.livestrong.com/article/527281-does-the-body-store-fat-like-carbohydrates/.

18 Guillaume Henin, Audrey Loumaye, Isabelle A. Leclercq, and Nicolas Lanthier, "Myosteatosis: Diagnosis, Pathophysiology and Consequences in Metabolic Dysfunction-Associated Steatotic Liver Disease," JHEP Reports 6, no. 2 (2024): 100963, https://www.sciencedirect.com/science/article/pii/S258955592300294X-#sec3.

19 Claire Laurens and Cedric Moro, "Intramyocellular Fat Storage in Metabolic Diseases," Hormone Molecular Biology and Clinical Investigation 26, no. 1 (2015), https://www.degruyter.com/document/doi/10.1515/hmbci-2015-0045/html?lang=en.

20 Yang, Lin Ding, Xianlun Zou, Yaqi Shen, Daoyu Hu, Xuemei Hu, Zhen Li, et al., "Pathogenesis of Sarcopenia and the Relationship with Fat Mass: Descriptive Review," Obesity 28, no. 11 (2020): 2040–2048, https://www.ncbi.nlm.nih.gov/pmc/articles/PMC8977978/.

21 Yang, Lin Ding, Xianlun Zou, Yaqi Shen, Daoyu Hu, Xuemei Hu, Zhen Li, and Ihab R. Kamel, "Visceral Adiposity and High Intramuscular Fat Deposition Independently Predict Critical Illness in Patients with SARS-CoV-2," Obesity 28, no. 11 (2020): 2040–2048, https://pubmed.ncbi.nlm.nih.gov/32677752/

Part 7: Understanding investigations and prescriptions

1 Diabetes Prevention Program Research Group, "Reduction in the Incidence of Type 2 Diabetes with Lifestyle Intervention or Metformin," New England Journal of Medicine 346 (2002): 393–403, https://www.nejm.org/doi/10.1056/NEJMoa012512?url_ver=Z39.88-2003&rfr_id=ori:rid:crossref.org&rfr_dat=cr_pub%20%200.

2 Claire Laurens and Cedric Moro, "Intensive Glycemic Control and the Prevention of Vascular Events: Implications of the ACCORD, ADVANCE and VA Diabetes Trials," Hormone Molecular Biology and Clinical Investigation 26, no. 1 (2015), https://www.ncbi.nlm.nih.gov/pmc/articles/PMC2606812/.

3 Steven E. Nissen and Kathy Wolski, "Rosiglitazone Revisited: An Updated Meta-Analysis of Risk for Myocardial Infarction and Cardiovascular Mortality," Archives of Internal Medicine 170, no. 14 (2010): 1191–1201, https://jamanetwork.com/journals/jamainternalmedicine/fullarticle/225844.

4 Medtronic. "Guardian Connect Continuous Glucose Monitoring System." Medtronic Diabetes. Accessed April 9, 2024. https://www.medtronicdiabetes.com/products/guardian-connect-continuous-glucose-monitoring-system.

5 "Full Indications and Important Safety Information FreeStyle Libre 14 Day," Abbott, accessed February 11, 2024, https://www.freestyle.abbott/us-en/safety-information.html.

6 David M. Nathan, Judith Kuenen, Rikke Borg, Hui Zheng, David Schoenfeld, Robert J. Heine, and A1c-Derived Average Glucose Study Group, "Translating the HbA1c into Estimated Average Glucose Values," Diabetes Care 31, no. 8 (2008): 1473–1478, https://pubmed.ncbi.nlm.nih.gov/18540046/.

7 "HbA1c and Estimated Average Glucose," NGSP, 2010, https://ngsp.org/A1ceAG.asp.

8 Christopher D. Saudek and Jessica C. Brick, "The Clinical Use of Hemoglobin A1c," Journal of Diabetes Science and Technology 3, no. 4 (2009): 629–634, https://www.ncbi.nlm.nih.gov/pmc/articles/PMC2769940/.

9 Witold Bauer, Attila Gyenesei, and Adam Krętowski, "The Multifactorial Progression from the Islet Autoimmunity to Type 1 Diabetes in Children," International Journal of Molecular Sciences 22, no. 14 (2021): 7493, https://www.mdpi.com/1422-0067/22/14/7493.

10 Maaret Turtinen, Taina Härkönen, Anna Parkkola, Jorma Ilonen, and Mikael Knip, "Characteristics of Familial Type 1 Diabetes: Effects of the Relationship to the Affected Family Member on Phenotype and Genotype at Diagnosis," Diabetologia 62, no. 11 (2019): 2025–2039, https://pubmed.ncbi.nlm.nih.gov/31346657/.

11 Eric C. Westman, William S. Yancy Jr., Maren K. Olsen, Tara Dudley, and John R. Guyton, "Effect of a Low Carbohydrate Ketogenic Diet Program Compared to a Low Fat Diet on Fasting Lipoprotein Subclasses," International Journal of Cardiology 110, no. 2 (2006): 212–216, https://pubmed.ncbi.nlm.nih.gov/16297472/.

12 Jimmy Moore, Cholesterol Clarity: What the HDL Is Wrong with My Numbers? (Las Vegas: Victory Belt Publishing, 2013).

13 David M. Diamond, Benjamin T. Bikman, and Paul Mason, "Statin Therapy Is Not Warranted for a Person with High LDL-Cholesterol on a Low-Carbohydrate Diet," Current Opinion in Endocrinology & Diabetes and Obesity 29, no. 5 (2022): 497–511, https://journals.lww.com/co-endocrinology/Fulltext/2022/10000/Statin_therapy_is_not_warranted_for_a_person_with.14.aspx.

14 Tamara Glavinovic, George Thanassoulis, Jacqueline de Graaf, Patrick Couture, Robert A. Hegele, and Allan D. Sniderman, "Physiological Basis for the Superiority of Apolipoprotein B over Low Density Lipoprotein (LDL) Cholesterol Non-High Density Lipoprotein (nonHDL) Cholesterol as a Marker of Cardiovascular Risk," Journal of the American Heart Association 11, no. 20 (2022): e025858, https://pubmed.ncbi.nlm.nih.gov/36216435/.

15 Dave Feldman, "Cholesterol Is a Passenger, Not a Driver," YouTube, 2019, https://www.youtube.com/watch?v=0LuKwsz9Woc. I have modified Dave Feldman's analogy here.

16 Nagao, Manabu, Hideto Nakajima, Ryuji Toh, Ken-Ichi Hirata, and Tatsuro Ishida. "Cardioprotective Effects of High-Density Lipoprotein Beyond its Anti-Atherogenic Action." Journal of Atherosclerosis and Thrombosis 25, no. 10 (October 1, 2018): 985-93. https://doi.org/10.5551/jat.RV17025.

17 Weissglas-Volkov, Daphna, and Päivi Pajukanta. "Genetic Causes of High and Low Serum HDL-Cholesterol." Journal of Lipid Research 51, no. 8 (August 2010): 2032-57. https://doi.org/10.1194/jlr.R004739.

18 Castela Forte, José, Rahul Gannamani, Pytrik Folkertsma, Sridhar Kumaraswamy, Sarah Mount, Sipko van Dam, and Jan Hoogsteen. "Changes in Blood Lipid Levels After a Digitally Enabled Cardiometabolic Preventive Health Program: Pre-Post Study in an Adult Dutch General Population Cohort." JMIR Cardio 6, no. 1 (March 23, 2022): e34946. https://doi.org/10.2196/34946.

19 Gerald M. Reaven, Y.-D. Ida Chen, Jorgen Jeppesen, Pierre Maheux, and Ronald M. Krauss, "Insulin Resistance and Hyperinsulinemia," Journal of Clinical Investigation 92, no. 1 (1993), 141–146, https://www.jci.org/articles/view/116541.

20 Allan D. Sniderman, George Thanassoulis, Tamara Glavinovic, Ann Marie Navar, Michael Pencina, Alberico Catapano, and Brian A. Ference, "Apolipoprotein B Particles and Cardiovascular Disease: A Narrative Review," JAMA Cardiology 4, no. 12 (2019): 1287–1295, https://www.ncbi.nlm.nih.gov/pmc/articles/PMC7369156/.

21 Stürzebecher, Paulina E., Julius L. Katzmann, and Ulrich Laufs. "What is 'Remnant Cholesterol'?" European Heart Journal 44, no. 16 (April 21, 2023): 1446-48. https://doi.org/10.1093/eurheartj/ehac783.

22 Castañer, Olga, Xavier Pintó, Isaac Subirana, Antonio J. Amor, Emilio Ros, Álvaro Hernáez, Miguel Ángel Martínez-González, et al. "Remnant Cholesterol, Not LDL Cholesterol, Is Associated With Incident Cardiovascular Disease." Journal of the American College of Cardiology 76, no. 23 (December 8, 2020): 2712-24. https://doi.org/10.1016/j.jacc.2020.10.008.

23 J. M. Gaziano, C. H. Hennekens, C. J. O'Donnell, J. L. Breslow, and J. E. Buring, "Fasting Triglycerides, High-Density Lipoprotein, and Risk of Myocardial Infarction," Circulation 96, no. 8 (1997): 2520–2525.

24 Protasio Lemos da Luz, Desiderio Favarato, Jose Rocha Faria-Neto Junior, Pedro Lemos, and Antonio Carlos Palandri Chagas, "High Ratio of Triglycerides to HDL-Cholesterol Predicts Extensive Coronary Disease," Clinics 63, no. 4 (2008): 427–432, https://www.ncbi.nlm.nih.gov/pmc/articles/PMC2664115/.

25 R. Boizel, P. Y. Benhamou, B. Lardy, F. Laporte, T. Foulon, and S. Halimi, "Ratio of Triglycerides to HDL Cholesterol Is an Indicator of LDL Particle Size in Patients with Type 2 Diabetes and Normal HDL Cholesterol Levels," Diabetes Care 23, no. 11 (2000): 1679–1685, https://pubmed.ncbi.nlm.nih.gov/11092292/.

26 A. Cordero and Eduardo Alegria-Ezquerra, "TG/HDL Ratio as Surrogate Marker for Insulin Resistance," E-Journal of Cardiology Practice 8, no. 16 (2009), https://www.escardio.org/Journals/E-Journal-of-Cardiology-Practice/Volume-8/TG-HDL-ratio-as-surrogate-marker-for-insulin-resistance.

27 Le Wang, Hongliang Cong, Jingxia Zhang, Yuecheng Hu, Ao Wei, Yingyi Zhang, Hua Yang, et al., "Predictive Value of the TG-HDL Ratio for All-Cause Mortality and Cardiovascular Death in Diabetic Patients with Coronary Artery Disease Treated with Statins," Frontiers in Cardiovascular Medicine 8 (2021): 718604, https://www.ncbi.nlm.nih.gov/pmc/articles/PMC8333610/#B6.

28 Jørgen Jeppesen, Hans Ole Hein, Poul Suadicani, and Finn Gyntelberg, "Relation of High TG-Low HDL Cholesterol and LDL Cholesterol to the Incidence of Ischemic Heart Disease," Arteriosclerosis, Thrombosis, and Vascular Biology 17, no. 6 (1997): 1114–1120, https://www.ahajournals.org/doi/full/10.1161/01.atv.17.6.1114.

29 Constantine E. Kosmas, Shanna Rodriguez Polanco, Maria D. Bousvarou, Evangelia J. Papakonstantinou, Edilberto Peña Genao, Eliscer Guzman, and Christina E. Kostara, "The TG/HDL-C Ratio as a Risk Marker for Metabolic Syndrome and Cardiovascular Disease," Diagnostics 13, no. 5 (2023): 929, https://www.ncbi.nlm.nih.gov/pmc/articles/PMC10001260/.

30 Goldstein, Joseph L., and Michael S. Brown. "Atherosclerosis: The Low-Density Lipoprotein Receptor Hypothesis." Metabolism 26, no. 11 (November 1977): 1257-75. https://doi.org/10.1016/0026-0495(77)90119-6.

31 Sumit Oberoi and Pooja Kansra, "Economic Menace of Diabetes in India," International Journal of Diabetes in Developing Countries 40 (2020): 464–475, https://link.springer.com/article/10.1007/s13410-020-00838-z.

32 Carlos K. H. Wong, Fangfang Jiao, Eric H. M. Tang, Thaison Tong, Praveen Thokala, and Cindy L. K. Lam, "Direct Medical Costs of Diabetes in the Year of Mortality and the Year Preceding Mortality," Diabetes, Obesity, and Metabolism 20, no. 6 (2018): 1470–1478, https://dom-pubs.onlinelibrary.wiley.com/doi/abs/10.1111/dom.13253.

33 Andrea Sansone, Daniele Mollaioli, Giacomo Ciocca, Erika Limoncin, Elena Colonnello, and Emmanuele A. Jannini, "Sexual Dysfunction in Men and Women with Diabetes: A Reflection of Their Complications?" Current Diabetes Reviews 18, no. 1 (2022): e030821192147, https://pubmed.ncbi.nlm.nih.gov/33687898/.

34 Adeniyi, Ade Fatai, Jokotade Oluremilekun Adeleye, and Celia Yetunde Adeniyi. "Diabetes, Sexual Dysfunction and Therapeutic Exercise: A 20 Year Review." Current Diabetes Reviews 6, no. 4 (July 2010): 201-6. https://doi.org/10.2174/157339910791658907.

35 Geert J. Biessels and Rachel A. Whitmer, "Cognitive Dysfunction in Diabetes: How to Implement Emerging Guidelines," Diabetologia 63 (2020): 3–9, https://www.ncbi.nlm.nih.gov/pmc/articles/PMC6890615/pdf/125_2019_Article_4977.pdf.

36 "The U.S. Just Lost 26 Years of Progress on Life Expectancy," Scientific American, October 17, 2022, https://www.scientificamerican.com/article/the-u-s-just-lost-26-years-worth-of-progress-on-life-expectancy.

37 Jonathan J. Petrocelli, Alec I. McKenzie, Naomi M. M. P. de Hart, Paul T. Reidy, Ziad S. Mahmassani, Alexander R. Keeble, Katie L. Kaput, et al., "Disuse-Induced Muscle Fibrosis, Cellular Senescence, and Senescence-Associated Secretory Phenotype in Older Adults Are Alleviated During Re-ambulation with Metformin Pre-treatment," Aging Cell 22, no. 11 (2023): e13936, https://onlinelibrary.wiley.com/doi/10.1111/acel.13936.

38 Baris Afsar and Rengin Elsurer Afsar, "Sodium-Glucose Co-Transporter 2 Inhibitors and Sarcopenia: A Controversy That Must Be Solved," Clinical Nutrition 42, no. 12 (2023) 2338–2352, https://www.sciencedirect.com/science/article/abs/pii/S0261561423003229.

39 Runzhou Pan, Yan Zhang, Rongrong Wang, Yao Xu, Hong Ji, Yongcai Zhao, "Effect of SGLT-2 Inhibitors on Body Composition in Patients with Type 2 Diabetes Mellitus: A Meta-Analysis of Randomized Controlled Trials," PLoS ONE 17, no. 12 (2022): e0279889, https://www.ncbi.nlm.nih.gov/pmc/articles/PMC9803203/pdf/pone.0279889.pdf.

40 Satoshi Ida, Ryutaro Kaneko, Kanako Imataka, Kaoru Okubo, Yoshitaka Shirakura, Kentaro Azuma, Ryoko Fujiwara, Kazuya Murata, "Effects of Antidiabetic Drugs on Muscle Mass in Type 2 Diabetes," Current Diabetes Reviews 17, no. 3 (2021): 293–303, https://pubmed.ncbi.nlm.nih.gov/32628589/.

41 Satoshi Ida, Ryutaro Kaneko, Kanako Imataka, Kaoru Okubo, Yoshitaka Shirakura, Kentaro Azuma, Ryoko Fujiwara, and Kazuya Murata, "Effects of Antidiabetic Drugs on Muscle Mass in Type 2 Diabetes," Current Diabetes Reviews 17, no. 3, 2021: 293–303, https://pubmed.ncbi.nlm.nih.gov/32628589/.

42 Sandra R. Klein, Ion A. Hobai, "Semaglutide, Delayed Gastric Emptying and Intraoperative Pulmonary Aspiration: A Case Report," Canadian Journal of Anaesthesiology 70, no. 8 (2023): 1394–1396, https://pubmed.ncbi.nlm.nih.gov/36977934/.

43 Olivia Tysoe, "Sulfonylurea Secondary Failure Mechanism Identified," Nature Reviews Endocrinology 19 (2023): 189, https://www.nature.com/articles/s41574-023-00815-6.

44 Lan-Lan Jiang, Xiao-Hua Xu, Meng-Hui Luo, Hui-Ying Wang, Bo Ding, Reng-Na Yan, Yun Hu, and Jian-Hua Ma, "Association of Acarbose with Decreased Muscle Mass and Function in Patients with Type 2 Diabetes: A Retrospective and Cross-Sectional Study," Diabetes Therapy 12, no. 11 (2021): 2955–2969, https://pubmed.ncbi.nlm.nih.gov/34542866/.

45 National Institute of Diabetes and Digestive and Kidney Diseases, Alpha Glucosidase Inhibitors (Bethesda, MD: National Institute of Diabetes and Digestive and Kidney Diseases, 2012), https://www.ncbi.nlm.nih.gov/books/NBK548416.

46 Hideaki Kaneto, Atsushi Obata,Tomohiko Kimura, Masashi Shimoda, Junpei Sanada, Yoshiro Fushimi, Naoto Katakami, et al., "Notable Underlying Mechanism for Pancreatic β-Cell Dysfunction and Atherosclerosis: Pleiotropic Roles of Incretin and Insulin Signaling," International Journal of Molecular Science 21, no. 24 (2020): 944, https://www.mdpi.com/1422-0067/21/24/9444

47 Carlos E. Mendez, Christian Eiler, Rebekah J. Walker, and Leonard E. Egede, "Insulin Therapy for Insulin Resistant Patients: Harm or Benefit?" Diabetes 67, suppl. 1 (2018): 1577-P, https://diabetesjournals.org/diabetes/article/67/Supplement_1/1577-P/54779/Insulin-Therapy-for-Insulin-Resistant-Patients.

48 Ahmad Qurie, Charles V. Preuss, and Rina Musa, "Allopurinol," in StatPearls (Treasure Island, FL: StatPearls Publishing, 2024), https://www.ncbi.nlm.nih.gov/books/NBK499942/.

49 U.S. Food and Drug Administration. "FDA Adds Boxed Warning for Increased Risk of Death with Gout Medicine Uloric (Febuxostat)." FDA Drug Safety Communication, November 2017. https://www.fda.gov/drugs/drug-safety-and-availability/fda-adds-boxed-warning-increased-risk-death-gout-medicine-uloric-febuxostat.

50 Nur Izgu, Zehra Gok Metin, Canan Karadas, Leyla Ozdemir, Nuran Metinari-kan, and Demet Corapcıoglu, "Progressive Muscle Relaxation and Mindfulness Meditation on Neuropathic Pain, Fatigue and Quality of Life in Patients with Type 2 Diabetes: A Randomized Clinical Trial," Journal of Nursing Scholarship 52, no. 5 (2020): 476–487, https://pubmed.ncbi.nlm.nih.gov/32536026/.

51 Malou A. H. Nuijten, Thijs M. H. Eijsvogels, Valerie M. Monpellier, Ignace M. C. Janssen, Eric J. Hazebroek, Maria T. E. Hopman, "The Magnitude and Progress of Lean Body Mass, Fat-Free Mass and Skeletal Muscle Mass Loss Following Bariatric Surgery: A Systematic Review and Meta-Analysis," Obesity Reviews 23, no. 1 (2022): e13370, https://www.ncbi.nlm.nih.gov/pmc/articles/PMC9285034/pdf/OBR-23-0.pdf.

52 American Diabetes Association Professional Practice Committee, "Obesity and Weight Management for Prevention and Treatment of Type 2 Diabetes: Stan-dards of Care in Diabetes—2024," Diabetes Care 47, suppl. 1 (2024): S145–S157, https://doi.org/10.2337/dc24-S008.

Part 8: How to work with doctors and hospitals

1 Richard Johnson, Nature Wants Us to Be Fat (Dallas: BenBella Books, 2022); David Perlmutter, Drop Acid (New York: Little, Brown Spark, 2022).

2 Ross, R. "Atherosclerosis--an Inflammatory Disease." The New England Jour-nal of Medicine 340, no. 2 (January 14, 1999): 115-26. https://doi.org/10.1056/NEJM199901143400207.

3 Williams, Jesse W., Li-hao Huang, and Gwendalyn J. Randolph. "Cytokine Cir-cuits in Cardiovascular Disease." Immunity 50, no. 4 (April 16, 2019): 941-54. https://doi.org/10.1016/j.immuni.2019.03.007.

4 Czajka, Anna, and Afshan N. Malik. "Hyperglycemia Induced Damage to Mi-tochondrial Respiration in Renal Mesangial and Tubular Cells: Implications for Diabetic Nephropathy." Redox Biology 10 (December 2016): 100-107. https://doi.org/10.1016/j.redox.2016.09.007.

5 Davida Unwin, Jena Unwin, Dominic Crocombe, Christine Delon, Nicola Guess, and Christopher Wong, "Renal Function in Patients Following a Low Carbohydrate Diet for Type 2 Diabetes: A Review of the Literature and Analysis of Routine Clinical Data from a Primary Care Service over 7 Years," Current Opinion in Endocrinology & Diabetes and Obesity 28, no. 5 (2021): 469–479, https://journals.lww.com/co-endocrinology/fulltext/2021/10000/renal_function_in_patients_following_a_low.8.aspx.

6 Vincent Wai-Sun Wong, Mattias Ekstedt, Grace Lai-Hung Wong, and Hannes Hagström, "Changing Epidemiology, Global Trends and Implications for Outcomes of NAFLD," Journal of Hepatology 79, no. 3 (2023): P842–852, https://www.journal-of-hepatology.eu/article/S0168-8278(23)00324-0/fulltext#secsectitle0025.

7 Katherine F. Sweeny and Christine K. Lee, "NAFLD in Children," Gastroenterology & Hepatology 17, no. 12 (2021): 579–587, https://www.ncbi.nlm.nih.gov/pmc/articles/PMC9021174/.

8 Patrizia Burra, Chiara Becchetti, and Giacomo Germani, "NAFLD and Liver Transplantation: Disease Burden, Current Management and Future Challenges," JHEP Reports 2, no. 6 (2020): 100192, https://www.ncbi.nlm.nih.gov/pmc/articles/PMC7607500/.

9 Marieke de Vries, Jan Westerink, Fatima El-Morabit, H. A. H. (Karin) Kaasjager, and Harold W. de Valk, "Prevalence of NAFLD and Its Association with Surrogate Markers of Insulin Resistance in Patients with Type 1 Diabetes," Diabetes Research and Clinical Practice 186 (2022): 109827, https://www.sciencedirect.com/science/article/pii/S0168822722006398#s0085.

10 Sun, Q., Yang, P., Gu, Q. W., et al. "Increased Glycemic Variability Results in Abnormal Differentiation of T Cell Subpopulation in Type 2 Diabetes Patients." Journal of Diabetes Complications, published online March 27, 2024. https://doi.org/10.1016/j.jdiacomp.2024.108738.

11 Michelle Curll, Monica DiNardo, Michelle Noschese, and Mary T. Korytkowski, "Menu Selection, Glycemic Control and Satisfaction with Standard and Patient Controlled Consistent Carbohydrate Meal Plans in Hospitalized Patients with Diabetes," BMJ Quality and Safety 19, no. 4 (210), 355–359, https://qualitysafety.bmj.com/content/19/4/355.long

12 American Diabetes Association Professional Practice Committee, "Diabetes Care in the hospital: Standards of Care in Diabetes—2024," Diabetes Care 47, suppl. 1 (2024): S295–S306, https://doi.org/10.2337/dc24-S016.

13 American Diabetes Association Professional Practice Committee, "Diabetes Care in the hospital: Standards of Care in Diabetes—2024," Diabetes Care 47, suppl. 1 (2024): S295–S306, https://doi.org/10.2337/dc24-S016.

Part 9: Diabetes in women and children

1 Chantal Anifa Amisi, "Markers of Insulin Resistance in Polycystic Ovary Syndrome Women: An Update," World Journal of Diabetes 13, no. 3 (2022): 129–149.

2 Jacob P. Christ and Marcelle I. Cedars, "Current Guidelines for Diagnosing PCOS," Diagnostics 13, no. 6 (2023): 1113, https://www.ncbi.nlm.nih.gov/pmc/articles/PMC10047373/.

3 Helena J. Teede, Chau Thien Tay, Joop J. E. Laven, Anuja Dokras, Lisa J. Moran, Terhi T. Piltonen, Michael F. Costello, et al., "Recommendations from the 2023 International Evidence-Based Guideline for the Assessment and Management of Polycystic Ovary Syndrome," European Journal of Endocrinology 189, no. 2 (2023): G43–G64, https://doi.org/10.1093/ejendo/lvad096.

4 Shanshan Mei, Jie Ding, Kaili Wang, Zhexin Ni, and Jin Yu, "Mediterranean Diet Combined with a Low-Carbohydrate Dietary Pattern in the Treatment of Overweight PCOS Patients," Frontiers in Nutrition 9 (2022), https://www.frontiersin.org/articles/10.3389/fnut.2022.876620/full.

5 Peiseah Teo, Belinda A. Henry, Lisa J. Moran, Stephanie Cowan, and Christie Bennett, "The Role of Sleep in PCOS: What We Know and What to Consider in the Future," Expert Review of Endocrinology & Metabolism 17, no. 4 (2022): 305–318, https://pubmed.ncbi.nlm.nih.gov/35815469/.

6 Charikleia Stefanaki, Flora Bacopoulou, Sarantis Livadas, Anna Kandaraki, Athanasios Karachalios, George P. Chrousos, and Evanthia Diamanti-Kandarakis, "Impact of a Mindfulness Stress Management Program on Stress, Anxiety, Depression and Quality of Life in Women with PCOS: A Randomized Controlled Trial," Stress 18, no. 1 (2015): 57–66, https://pubmed.ncbi.nlm.nih.gov/25287137/.

7 Gislaine Satyko Kogure, Miranda-Furtado, Cristiana Libardi, Rafael Costa Silva, Anderson Sanches Melo, Rui Alberto Ferriani, Marcos Felipe Silva De Sá, et al., "Resistance Exercise Impacts Lean Muscle Mass in Women with PCOS," Medicine & Science in Sports & Exercise 48, no. 4 (2016): 589–598, https://journals.lww.com/acsm-msse/fulltext/2016/04000/resistance_exercise_impacts_lean_muscle_mass_in.2.aspx.

8 Gislaine Satyko Kogure, Iris Palma Lopes, Victor Barbosa Ribeiro, Maria Célia Mendes, Sérgio Kodato, Cristiana Libardi Miranda Furtado, and Marcos Felipe Silva de Sá, "The Effects of Aerobic Physical Exercises on Body Image among Women with PCOS," Journal of Affective Disorders 262 (2020): 350–358, https://pubmed.ncbi.nlm.nih.gov/31735408/.

9 Sehar Toosy, Ravinder Sodi, and Joseph M. Pappachan, "Lean PCOS: An Evidence Based Practical Approach," Journal of Diabetes and Metabolic Disorders 17, no. 2 (2018): 277–285, https://www.ncbi.nlm.nih.gov/pmc/articles/PMC6405408/.

10 Bihter Senem Feyzioglu, Cenk Mustafa Güven, and Zerrin Avul, "Eight-Hour Time-Restricted Feeding: A Strong Candidate Diet Protocol for First-Line Therapy in PCOS," Nutrients 15, no. 10 (2023): 2260, https://pubmed.ncbi.nlm.nih.gov/37242145/.

11 Neha Mishra, Ruchi Verma, and Payal Jadaun, "Study on the Effect of Berberine, Myoinositol and Metformin in Women with PCOS: A Prospective Randomized Study," Cureus 14, no. 1 (2022): e21781, https://www.ncbi.nlm.nih.gov/pmc/articles/PMC8890747/.

12 Mary V. Diaz-Santana, Katie M. O'Brien, Yong-Moon Mark Park, Dale P. Sandler, and Clarice R. Weinberg, "Persistence of Risk for Type 2 Diabetes after Gestational Diabetes Mellitus," Diabetes Care 45, no. 4 (2022): 864–870, https://www.ncbi.nlm.nih.gov/pmc/articles/PMC9016728/.

13 Yongfu Yu, Melissa Soohoo, Henrik Toft Sørensen, Jiong Li, and Onyebuchi A. Arah, "Gestational Diabetes and the Risks of Overall and Type-Specific Cardiovascular Diseases: A Population and Sibling-Matched Cohort Study," Diabetes Care 45, no. 1 (2022): 151–159, https://pubmed.ncbi.nlm.nih.gov/34764208/.

14 Cheryl Tatano Beck, Sue Watson, and Robert K. Gable, "Traumatic Childbirth and Its Aftermath: Is There Anything Positive?" Journal of Perinatal Education 27, no. 3 (2018): 175–184, https://www.ncbi.nlm.nih.gov/pmc/articles/PMC6193358/.

15 Erin Farah, Mary K. Barger, Carrie Klima, Beverly Rossman, and Patricia Hershberger, "Impaired Lactation: Review of Delayed Lactogenesis and Insufficient Lactation," Journal of Midwifery & Women's Health 66, no. 5 (2021): 631–640, https://pubmed.ncbi.nlm.nih.gov/34596953/.

16 Christina M. Scifres, "Short- and Long-Term Outcomes Associated with Large for Gestational Age Birth Weight," Obstetrics and Gynecology Clinics of North America 48, no. 2 (2021): 325–337, https://pubmed.ncbi.nlm.nih.gov/33972069/.

17 Olivia Curl, Uma Doshi, Nonda S. Mester, Bharti Garg, and Aaron B. Caughey, "Maternal and Neonatal Outcomes by Week in Pregnant Individuals with Gestational Diabetes," American Journal of Obstetrics and Gynecology 226, no. 1, suppl. S268 (2022), https://www.ajog.org/article/S0002-9378(21)01652-5/fulltext.

18 Jijiao Wang, Xiaochen Ji, Ting Liu, and Nan Zhao, "Maternal and Neonatal Outcomes with the Use of Long Acting, Compared to Intermediate Acting Basal Insulin (NPH) for Managing Diabetes during Pregnancy: A Systematic Review and Meta-Analysis," Diabetology & Metabolic Syndrome 14 (2022): 154, https://dmsjournal.biomedcentral.com/articles/10.1186/s13098-022-00925-7.

19 José Alberto Laredo-Aguilera, María Gallardo-Bravo, Joseba Aingerun Rabanales-Sotos, Ana Isabel Cobo-Cuenca, and Juan Manuel Carmona-Torres, "Physical Activity Programs during Pregnancy Are Effective for the Control of Gestational Diabetes Mellitus," International Journal of Environmental Research and Public Health 17, no. 17 (2020): 6151, https://www.ncbi.nlm.nih.gov/pmc/articles/PMC7503359/.

20 Jerry Guintivano, Karolina A. Aberg, Shaunna L. Clark, David R. Rubinow, Patrick F. Sullivan, Samantha Meltzer-Brody, and Edwin J. C. G. van den Oord, "Transcriptome-Wide Association Study for Postpartum Depression Implicates Altered B-Cell Activation and Insulin Resistance," Molecular Psychiatry 27 (2022): 2858–2867, https://www.ncbi.nlm.nih.gov/pmc/articles/PMC9156403/pdf/41380_2022_Article_1525.pdf.

21 Lambrinoudaki, Irene, Stavroula A. Paschou, Eleni Armeni, et al. "The Interplay Between Diabetes Mellitus and Menopause: Clinical Implications." Nature Reviews Endocrinology 18 (2022): 608-622. https://doi.org/10.1038/s41574-022-00708-0.

22 Donald K. Layman, Tracy G. Anthony, Blake B. Rasmussen, Sean H. Adams, Christopher J. Lynch, Grant D. Brinkworth, and Teresa A. Davis, "Defining Meal Requirements for Protein to Optimize Metabolic Roles of Amino Acids," American Journal of Clinical Nutrition 101, no. 6 (2015): 1330S–1338S, https://pubmed.ncbi.nlm.nih.gov/25926513/.

23 R. D. Langer, H. N. Hodis, R. A. Lobo, and M. A. Allison, "Hormone Replacement Therapy: Where Are We Now?" Climacteric 24, no. 1 (2021): 3–10, https://pubmed.ncbi.nlm.nih.gov/33403881/.

24 Charlotte Ling, Karl Bacos, and Tina Rönn, "Epigenetics of Type 2 Diabetes Mellitus and Weight Change—a Tool for Precision Medicine?" Nature Reviews Endocrinology 18 (2022): 433–448, https://www.nature.com/articles/s41574-022-00671-w.

25 Stuart Brown and Christopher Vaughan, Play: How It Shapes the Brain, Opens the Imagination and Invigorates the Soul (New York: Avery, 2010).

26 Psychwire, "The Righting Reflex in Motivational Interviewing," YouTube, https://www.youtube.com/watch?v=17qHqklweYM.

27 Diane Tavenner, Prepared: What Kids Need for a Fulfilled Life (New York: Currency, 2019).

28 Ellyn Satter, How to Get Your Kids to Eat . . . but Not Too Much (Boulder, CO: Bull, 1987).

29 "Did Coca-Cola Ever Contain Cocaine?" Just Think Twice, accessed February 11, 2024, https://www.justthinktwice.gov/article/did-coca-cola-ever-contain-cocaine.

30 Suzanne E. Cuda, Roohi Kharofa, Dominique R. Williams, Valerie O'Hara, Rushika Conroy, Sara Karjoo, Jennifer Paisley, et al., "Metabolic, Behavioral Health and Disordered Eating Comorbidities Associated with Obesity in Pediatric Patients: An Obesity Medical Association (OMA) Clinical Practice Statement 2022," Obesity Pillars 3 (2022): 100031, https://pubmed.ncbi.nlm.nih.gov/37990723/.

31 S. Berardis and E. Sokal, "Pediatric Non-Alcoholic Fatty Liver Disease: An Increasing Public Health Issue," European Journal of Pediatrics 173 (2014):131–139, https://www.ncbi.nlm.nih.gov/pmc/articles/PMC3929043/pdf/431_2013_Article_2157.pdf.

32 Anna Zenno and Evan P. Nadler, "Surgical Treatment of Type 2 Diabetes Mellitus in Youth," Advances in Experimental Medicine and Biology 1307 (2021): 321–330, https://www.ncbi.nlm.nih.gov/pmc/articles/PMC8489511/pdf/nihms-1741026.pdf.

33 Perry, Benjamin I., Jan Stochl, Rachel Upthegrove, Stan Zammit, Nick Wareham, Claudia Langenberg, Eleanor Winpenny, David Dunger, Peter B. Jones, and Golam M. Khandaker. "Longitudinal Trends in Childhood Insulin Levels and Body Mass Index and Associations With Risks of Psychosis and Depression in Young Adults." JAMA Psychiatry 78, no. 4 (April 1, 2021): 416-25. https://doi.org/10.1001/jamapsychiatry.2020.4180.

34 Holan Liang, A Sense of Belonging (London: Short Books, 2022).

35 Kelly Gfroerer, "What Are Dreikur's Four Goals of Misbehavior?" ContiuED, https://www.continued.com/early-childhood-education/ask-the-experts/what-four-goals-misbehavior-23705.

Part 10: How to handle type 1 diabetes

1 Erin Digitale, "New Research Shows How to Keep Diabetics Safer during Sleep," Scope (blog), May 8, 2014, https://scopeblog.stanford.edu/2014/05/08/new-research-keeps-diabetics-safer-during-sleep/.

2 R. P Eaton, R. C. Allen, D. S. Schade, and J. C. Standefer, "'Normal' Insulin Secretion: The Goal of Artificial Insulin Delivery Systems?" Diabetes Care 3, no. 2 (1980): 270–273, https://pubmed.ncbi.nlm.nih.gov/6993139/.

3 "Can You Have Insulin Resistance and Type 1 Diabetes?" American Diabetes Association, accessed February 11, 2024, https://diabetes.org/living-with-diabetes/type-1/can-you-have-insulin-resistance-and-type-1-diabetes.

4 Lennerz, Belinda S., Anna Barton, Richard K. Bernstein, et al. "Management of Type 1 Diabetes With a Very Low–Carbohydrate Diet." Pediatrics 141, no. 6 (2018): e20173349.

5 J. Kruger, and D. Dunning, "Unskilled and Unaware of It: How Difficulties in Recognizing One's Own Incompetence Lead to Inflated Self-Assessments," Journal of Personality and Social Psychology 77, no. 6 (1999): 1121–1134, https://psycnet.apa.org/record/1999-15054-002.

6 Riddell, Michael C., and Anne L. Peters. "Exercise in Adults with Type 1 Diabetes Mellitus." Nature Reviews Endocrinology 19 (2023): 98-111. https://doi.org/10.1038/s41574-022-00756-6.

7 Diet Doctor, "Why Run 100 Miles on a Five-Day Fast? Diet Doctor Podcast with Dr. Ian Lake," YouTube, 2021, https://www.youtube.com/watch?v=DwfB5uLk-ML4.

8 See https://www.instagram.com/jtm_fit/ and https://www.jtmfit.com/pages/jtm-fit-app.

9 Jane E. Yardley, "Reassessing the Evidence: Prandial State Dictates Glycemic Responses to Exercise in Individuals with Type 1 Diabetes to a Greater Extent Than Intensity," Diabetologia 65, no. 12 (2022): 1994–1999, https://pubmed.ncbi.nlm.nih.gov/35978179/.

10 J. Nolan, A. Rush, J. Kaye, "Glycemic Stability of a Cyclist with Type 1 Diabetes: 4011 km in Twenty Days on a Ketogenic Diet," Diabetes Medicine 36, no. 11 (2019): 1503–1507, https://pubmed.ncbi.nlm.nih.gov/31197870/.

11 Michael C. Riddell, Zoey Li, Robin L. Gal, Peter Calhoun, Peter G. Jacobs, Mark A. Clements, Corby K. Martin, et al., "Examining the Acute Glycemic Effects of Different Types of Structures Exercise in Type 1 Diabetes in a Real-World Setting: The Type 1 Diabetes and Exercise Initiative (T1DEX1)," Diabetes Care 46, no. 4 (2023): 704–713, https://pubmed.ncbi.nlm.nih.gov/36795053/.

12 Mary E. Lacy, Paola Gilsanz, Chloe Eng, Michal S. Beeri, Andrew J. Karter, and Rachel A. Whitmer, "Severe Hypoglycemia and Cognitive Function in Older Adults with Type 1 Diabetes: The Study of Longevity in Diabetes (SOLID)," Diabetes Care 43, no. 3 (2020): 541–548, https://www.ncbi.nlm.nih.gov/pmc/articles/PMC7035586/.

13 Thomas J. Songer and Rashida R. Dorsey, "High Risk Characteristics for Motor Vehicle Crashes in Persons with Diabetes by Age," Annual Proceedings of the Association for the Advancement of Automotive Medicine 50 (2006), https://www.ncbi.nlm.nih.gov/pmc/articles/PMC3217477/.

14 Munachiso Nwokolo, Stephanie A. Amiel, Owen O'Daly, Ian A. Macdonald, Fernando O. Zelaya, and Pratik Choudhary, "Restoration of Hypoglycemia Awareness Alters Brain Activity in Type 1 Diabetes," Diabetes Care 44, no. 2 (2021): 533–540, https://diabetesjournals.org/care/article/44/2/533/35492/Restoration-of-Hypoglycemia-Awareness-Alters-Brain.

15 National Institute of Diabetes and Digestive and Kidney Diseases, "How Hypoglycemia Unawareness Affects People with Diabetes," Diabetes Discoveries and Practice Blog, April 5, 2023, https://www.niddk.nih.gov/health-information/professionals/diabetes-discoveries-practice/how-hypoglycemia-unawareness-affects-people-with-diabetes.

16 Keren Zhou and Diana Isaacs, "Closed Loop Artificial Pancreas Therapy for Type 1 Diabetes," Current Cardiology Reports 24, no. 9 (2022): 1159–1167, https://pubmed.ncbi.nlm.nih.gov/35727409/.

17 Boris P. Kovatchev, Daniel J. Cox, Leon S. Farhy, Martin Straume, Linda Gonder-Frederick, and William L. Clarke, "Episodes of Severe Hypoglycemia in Type 1 Diabetes Are Preceded and Followed within 48 Hours by Measurable Disturbances in Blood Glucose," Journal of Clinical Endocrinology & Metabolism 85, no. 11 (2000): 4287–4292, https://academic.oup.com/jcem/article/85/11/4287/2856101.

18 Teresa Pearson, "Glucagon as a Treatment of Severe Hypoglycemia," The Diabetes Educator 34, no. 1 (2008): 128–134, https://journals.sagepub.com/doi/abs/10.1177/0145721707312400.

19 Wellington, Alexander. "Leonard Thompson 'Ever Remembered': The First Person to Receive Insulin." Diabetes & Vascular Disease Research 30, no. 1 (2021). https://doi.org/10.1177/0967772020974355.

20 The Nobel Prize in Physiology or Medicine was awarded in 1923 to Banting and Macleod for the discovery of insulin through research done by Paulescu, Banting, Macleod, Collip and Best between 1916 and 1922. See: Rydén, Lars, and Jan Lindsten. "The History of the Nobel Prize for the Discovery of Insulin." Diabetes Research and Clinical Practice 175 (May 2021): 108819. https://doi.org/10.1016/j.diabres.2021.108819.

21 American Diabetes Association Professional Practice Committee, "Summary of Revisions: Standards of Care in Diabetes—2024," Diabetes Care 47, suppl. 1 (2024): S5–S10.

22 Cari Berget, Laurel H. Messer, and Gregory P. Forlenza, "A Clinical Overview of Insulin Pump Therapy for the Management of Diabetes: Past, Present and Future of Intensive Therapy," Diabetes Spectrum 32, no. 3 (2019): 194–204, https://www.ncbi.nlm.nih.gov/pmc/articles/PMC6695255/.

23 Michael Erbach, Guido Freckmann, Rolf Hinzmann, Bernhard Kulzer, Ralph Ziegler, Lutz Heinemann, and Oliver Schnell, "Interferences and Limitations in Blood Glucose Self-Testing," Journal of Diabetes Science and Technology 10, no.

5 (2016): 1161–1168, https://www.ncbi.nlm.nih.gov/pmc/articles/PMC5032951/.

24 Lutz Heinemann, Katarina Braune, Alan Carter, Amin Zayani, and Laura A. Krämer, "Insulin Storage: A Critical Reappraisal," Journal of Diabetes Science and Technology 15, no. 1 (2021): 147–159, https://www.ncbi.nlm.nih.gov/pmc/articles/PMC7783014/.

25 "Diabetes Distress," Behavioral Diabetes Institute, accessed February 11, 2024, https://behavioraldiabetes.org/scales-and-measures/#1700008262720-4edd9098-4166.

26 Vicki S. Helgeson, "Diabetes Burnout among Emerging Adults with Type 1 Diabetes: A Mixed Methods Investigation," Journal of Behavioral Medicine 44, no. 3 (2021): 368–378, https://pubmed.ncbi.nlm.nih.gov/33566266/.

27 Margo E. Hanlan, Julie Griffith, Niral Patel, and Sarah S. Jaser, "Eating Disorders and Disordered Eating in Type 1 Diabetes: Prevalence, Screening and Treatment Options," Current Diabetes Reports (2013), https://www.ncbi.nlm.nih.gov/pmc/articles/PMC4002640/

28 June Alexander, My Kid Is Back: Empowering Parents to Beat Anorexia Nervosa (London: Routledge, 2010).

29 Diabetes UK. "Diabulimia." Diabetes UK. Accessed April 9, 2024. https://www.diabetes.org.uk/guide-to-diabetes/life-with-diabetes/diabulimia.

Part 11: The journey ahead

1 Juan P. Munoz, Tammy C. Bleak, and Gloria M. Calaf, "Glyphosate and the Key Characteristics of an Endocrine Disruptor: A Review," Chemosphere (2020), https://usrtk.org/wp-content/uploads/2020/11/Glyphosate-and-the-key-characteristics-of-an-endocrine-disruptor-A-review.pdf.

2 Vanessa Vigar, Stephen Myers, Christopher Oliver, Jacinta Arellano, Shelley Robinson, and Carlo Leifert, "A Systematic Review of Organic versus Conventional Food Consumption: Is There a Measurable Benefit for Human Health?" Nutrients 12, no. 1 (2020): 7, https://www.ncbi.nlm.nih.gov/pmc/articles/PMC7019963/.

3 Jerrold J. Heindel, Robert H. Lustig, Sarah Howard, and Barbara E. Corkey, "Obesogens: A Unifying Theory for the Global Rise in Obesity," International Journal of Obesity (2024), https://www.nature.com/articles/s41366-024-01460-3.epdf?sharing_token=9UhHngJpGLTdwAtKadFaeNRgN-0jAjWel9jnR3ZoTv0MUG4Gc1kXCk0AqVnRqaAc1VyJpzpSqk-__wXxUIX-liI5itHBkQZf-ItMaDP1TongLhPffKkWl4fW-orgnhsFgKOPunErI64fpfYy7d-7SialLReosCFKzqbgpNIKndntIk%3D

4 A. Agha, A. Basu, and W. Hanif, "Burnout in Diabetes and Endocrinology Specialist Registrars across England, Scotland and Wales in the Pre-COVID Era," Primary Care Diabetes 16, no. 4 (2022): 515–518, https://pubmed.ncbi.nlm.nih.gov/35667990/.

5 Robert A. Gabbay and Alana M. Barrett, "Endocrinologist Burnout: We Need to Tackle It and Bring Joy to Work," Journal of Clinical Endocrinology and Metabolism 105, no. 7 (2020): dgaa230, https://pubmed.ncbi.nlm.nih.gov/32379889/.

6 "Language Matters: Language and Diabetes," NHS England, September 7, 2023, https://www.england.nhs.uk/long-read/language-matters-language-and-diabetes/.

7 IDF Diabetes Atlas 10th edition https://www.ncbi.nlm.nih.gov/books/NBK581940/table/ch3.t4/?report=objectonly

8 World Obesity Atlas 2022 https://s3-eu-west-1.amazonaws.com/wof-files/World_Obesity_Atlas_2022.pdf

Index

Z

www.ingramcontent.com/pod-product-compliance
Lightning Source LLC
Chambersburg PA
CBHW030150310326
41914CB00103B/2028/J

9798990593015